Advance praise for *Dialogues for Discovery*

A terrific book—the fruit of both editors' years of deepening understanding, innovative clinical practice, self-reflection and growing expertise. Similar expertise illuminates chapters by CBT specialists addressing specific client groups and problems. Lively and engaging, the text skillfully embodies the curiosity, empathy, respect, and collaboration at the heart of this approach. And readers can join this journey, using chapter-by-chapter learning activities and reflection sheets. A truly significant addition to the literature on the process of effective learning in psychotherapy.

Melanie Fennell, PhD
Former Director of the Oxford Diploma and MSc in
CBT and Co-Director of the Oxford MSt in
Mindfulness-Based Cognitive Therapy

Helping people gain insights into the nature of their minds and its different brain states is common to psychotherapies, but it is no easy task. In their exciting new book international world leading cognitive therapists bring their extensive experience together to guide the reader through the use of Socratic forms of dialogue to support those therapeutic aims. The book is full of signposts of opportunities as well as roadblocks and potential traps and how to deal with them. In addition to revelation, the approach illustrated helps clients discover inner strengths and meanings. Accessible, clearly written and full of fascinating clinical insights, tips and guides, this will become a much-valued book for experienced and new therapists alike regardless of their school of therapy.

Professor Paul Gilbert, OBE
Founder of Compassion Focused Therapy

Although the use of Socratic dialogue and guided discovery have long been encouraged in psychotherapy, it is only in the last decade or so that enough data has gathered to give clear clinical guidance about their use. *Dialogues for Discovery* is an exceptional resource for therapists seeking to guide their clients towards discovery and hope. This book provides practical guidance and strategies for managing common therapy impasses and dilemmas, such as low client motivation, inflexible beliefs, and alliance ruptures. It is a clinically sophisticated guide that is grounded in empirical evidence and theoretical knowledge. The therapist-client dialogues and diverse case examples serve as powerful illustrations of common therapy traps, and clinically sound strategies offer a path forward. With its transdiagnostic approach and focus on guiding discovery, it is a valuable tool for any therapist seeking to enhance their practice and contribute to their clients' recovery and well-being.

Steven C. Hayes, PhD
Emeritus Professor of Psychology, University of Nevada, Reno
Originator of Acceptance and Commitment Therapy

Rarely are psychotherapists given a gift consisting of a combination of scholarship, clinical acumen, and practical user-friendly teaching clinical case vignettes. KUDOS to Christine Padesky and Helen Kennerley and their clinically astute colleagues for demonstrating how to use Socratic Dialogue and guided discovery procedures in psychotherapy. This book should be read, studied, and implemented by all health care providers.

Donald Meichenbaum, PhD
Research Director of the Melissa Institute for
Violence Prevention, Miami FL

Dialogues for Discovery is revolutionary. It presents a model that will resonate with therapists from all schools of therapy who want to ask more effective questions and listen/respond to client answers in ways that will help clients make active discoveries in therapy. Amply illustrated with case examples and pragmatic guidance, Padesky and Kennerley show us how placing curiosity and collaboration at the forefront of the therapeutic encounter leads to whole shifts in perspective rather than merely changing someone's mind.

Zindel Segal, PhD
Distinguished Professor of Psychology in
Mood Disorders, University of Toronto
Co-Founder, Mindfulness-Based Cognitive Therapy

Dialogues for Discovery

Dialogues for Discovery

Improving Psychotherapy's Effectiveness

Edited by

Christine A. Padesky & Helen Kennerley

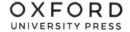

OXFORD
UNIVERSITY PRESS

OXFORD
UNIVERSITY PRESS

Great Clarendon Street, Oxford, OX2 6DP,
United Kingdom

Oxford University Press is a department of the University of Oxford.
It furthers the University's objective of excellence in research, scholarship,
and education by publishing worldwide. Oxford is a registered trade mark of
Oxford University Press in the UK and in certain other countries

Published in the United States of America by Oxford University Press
198 Madison Avenue, New York, NY 10016, United States of America

British Library Cataloguing in Publication Data
Data available

Library of Congress Control Number: 2022951656

ISBN 978–0–19–958698–1

DOI: 10.1093/med-psych/9780199586981.001.0001

Printed and bound in the UK by
Clays Ltd, Elcograf S.p.A.

Preface

Dialogues for Discovery is designed to help you discover ways to help your clients experience the hope that arises when discoveries, small or large, are made in each therapy session. This can be an exciting venture for therapists. There is no greater satisfaction than contributing to someone's recovery and increased sense of well-being, especially when you have helped them learn to help themselves.

Fortunately for therapists, the same ideas that guide client discovery also reveal clear paths for troubleshooting and managing common therapy impasses and dilemmas such as apparent low client motivation, inflexible client beliefs accompanied by repetitive therapy discussions, alliance ruptures, avoidance, and impulsive and compulsive behaviors. We address in detail these types of therapy challenges. Using therapist–client dialogues and diverse case examples to illustrate common therapy traps, we offer clinically sound strategies for moving therapy forward again.

We spent more than a decade writing *Dialogues for Discovery*. It's slow percolating evolution is its real strength. When we began, there was no empirical evidence regarding these questioning methods in psychotherapy despite their longtime use and large number of proponents. The past decade has yielded a growing body of theoretical knowledge and empirical evidence regarding the beneficial use of Socratic Dialogue and guided discovery in psychotherapy. Our contributing authors have had time to continually reflect on their practice of guiding client discovery through use of Socratic Dialogue and to hone the messages of their chapters. The resulting clinical sophistication shines through in therapist–client vignettes and the extremely helpful troubleshooting tips included throughout this book.

Originally, we considered organizing chapters around client diagnoses. In the end, we decided to focus on chapter themes, which seems a better fit with both clinical practice and recent movements toward transdiagnostic approaches to conceptualization and treatment planning. Thus, a therapist working with a client with borderline personality disorder features could find relevant and useful guidance in chapters addressing depression and suicide, inflexible beliefs, impulsive and compulsive behaviors, managing significant life adversity, and imagery. We encourage readers to read chapters that may not immediately seem to apply to your clinical practice. A good example of this is Chapter 5, "Imagery: The Language of Emotion." That chapter makes a strong case that if you are not working with imagery in nearly every therapy session, your therapy is probably less effective than it could be.

While readers can immediately peruse chapters of greatest relevance to their clinical practice, we recommend reading Chapters 1 and 2 first to get an overview of the book and how to interact with it. Chapter 1 gives an overview of the role and evolution of guided discovery methods in psychotherapy. It also defines key terms used throughout the book, addresses why and when Socratic Dialogue is recommended in psychotherapy and when it is not, illustrates a broad range of therapy methods used to guide client discovery, and summarizes current research. At the end of Chapter 1 there is a table listing some of the common therapy traps addressed in each of the following chapters. Therapists will find the 'Common Traps Addressed in Chapters' table useful for locating clinically relevant material that can help troubleshoot specific therapy impasses and roadblocks you encounter. For a complete listing of the Traps addressed in this book, see the Traps Guide in the Appendix on pp. 505–507.

Chapter 2 offers a detailed explanation of Padesky's 4-stage Model of Socratic Dialogue (informational questions, empathic listening, summaries, analytical and synthesizing questions) along with diverse clinical illustrations of each stage in action. Her four stages help therapists to stay on track and use Socratic Dialogue more effectively with clients in ways that explicitly guide client discovery. Her model is collaborative and grounded in curiosity and a genuine commitment to client discovery, wherever it might lead and whether or not the discoveries fit with the therapist's current thinking. This offers a radically client-centered approach that has been embraced by therapists of many schools of psychotherapy in the hundreds of workshops Padesky has taught internationally.

Chapters 3 through 12 can be read in any order depending upon reader interest. Expert therapists with decades of clinical experience in their area of specialty were invited to share their clinical wisdom gleaned from thousands of hours of guiding client discovery. We were fortunate that our first-choice authors for each chapter agreed to contribute to this book. Topics explored include depression and suicide (Chapter 3), anxiety (4), imagery (5), inflexible beliefs (6), impulsive and compulsive behaviors (7), life adversity (8), children and adolescents (9), group therapy (10), supervision (11), and the future of *Dialogues for Discovery* (12).

Each chapter shows how Padesky's 4-Stage Model of Socratic Dialogue and other guided discovery methods can help you avoid and manage common therapy traps often encountered when working with these themes or populations in therapy. Throughout the book, principles that help you stay on track are summarized in "Keep in Mind" boxes. At the end of each chapter, Reader Learning Activities suggest ways you can tailor what you learned to your own clinical or supervisory practice. For classroom use, these Reader Learning Activities can be assigned for student practice and learning. To further personalize and help you consolidate the skills you learn in this book, we provide Reflective Practice Worksheets in the Appendix and offer guidelines for their use in Chapter 12.

While writing and editing this book, we experienced our own excitement in the anticipation of readers unwrapping these ideas and putting them to good use in therapy sessions. We hope our enthusiasm is communicated in these pages and inspires you to creatively engage with and integrate these methods into your clinical practice, supervision, teaching, and research. We offer you *Dialogues for Discovery.* When you engage in these dialogues with your clients, see where your mutual discoveries lead!

Christine Padesky and Helen Kennerley (Editors)

Acknowledgments

The original idea for this book was developed with Dr. Joan Kirk, clinical psychologist, founder of the Oxford Cognitive Therapy Centre, and human being extraordinaire. Joan was a dear friend to us both and she mentored generations of therapists with her keen wisdom, humor, and creative contributions to psychotherapy. Sadly, Joan did not live to see the published book. We hope we have fulfilled her vision for it.

Kathleen Mooney, one of the most creative psychologists we know, graciously edited our opening chapters and played a central role in helping us sharpen the book's focus. For example, she recommended we clearly define terms such as "Socratic methods," "Socratic questioning," "Socratic Dialogue," and "guided discovery" that are often used with interchangeable and differing meanings. Her insightful suggestions throughout our writing, editing, and production stages not only improved the book, they also advance our ability to more clearly research, teach, and employ these methods in psychotherapy. Thank you, Kathleen, for your generous counsel that makes every project so much better. And thank you for designing our cover incorporating all the colors of the Progress Rainbow Flag of Colors to reflect our commitment to diversity.

Our chapter authors were extraordinary in their efforts to infuse this book with wisdom and clinical skill. They also were extremely patient with us, the editors, as some of their chapters simmered for many years waiting for the entire manuscript to be complete. They expressed understanding rather than impatience when we dealt with various life challenges that interfered with our progress. We are fortunate to count so many talented and gifted clinicians as our friends. Their warmth and caring for us throughout this process will not be forgotten.

Oxford University Press also deserves our gratitude for their patience and support. It is a rare publisher that does not pressure editors to complete a book on time "no matter what." Martin Baum and the various editors at OUP who have worked with us over the past decade have been so gracious and helpful every step of the way. Some of them watched their children grow up as this project carried on. Your commitment to us allowed this book to mature and evolve into a better work than we initially envisioned. Thank you! Our production editor, Clare Jones, deserves special thanks for carefully shepherding this project through production and working tirelessly with us to make sure it included the features we wanted.

This book is about dialogues with clients. Each clinical vignette is created from our experiences with real persons, even though details are changed to ensure confidentiality. Sometimes composites of clinical events with clients are represented. Every client seen by each of our authors deserve our sincere thanks. Throughout our long careers, our clients have taught us so much about how to carry on fruitful dialogues even in challenging circumstances. While we delight in client discoveries, we also can learn so much when client discoveries are blocked. This book is a better book for all we have collectively learned from these experiences.

Each of us also teaches and supervises psychotherapists. To our students and trainees, thank you for all the questions you have asked and the moments of confusion and struggle you have shared. You show us that there are many pathways to discovery and many ways to get lost along the way. Dialogues with you have helpfully informed our models, our strategies for teaching them, and our awareness of traps and roadblocks that require attention. We hope this book offers a fair response to the many excellent questions you have asked about Socratic Dialogue and guided discovery over the past few decades.

Special thanks to our families especially Kathleen, Udo, Eva, Noah, Susan, Bob, and Rosanne who accepted our many absences and absent-minded moments when we were wrapped up in this project. Your support and love sustain us through the best of times and the worst of times. We also benefited from the encouragement of so many friends and colleagues who assured us that this book was needed and would be welcomed.

Finally, Christine and Helen entered this project as close friends. During the course of this project we collectively navigated through the deaths of 3 parents, serious illness for each of our spouses, house moves, the pandemic, caring for younger family members, and the writing of six other books. We are delighted to report our friendship survived and thrived even during these life challenges we faced during its progress. We look forward to many more years of friendship talking about things other than "how the manuscript is coming along."

Christine Padesky and Helen Kennerley

Contents

List of Contributors

Gillian Butler, PhD, FBPsS, CPsychol
Consultant clinical psychologist (retired)

Robert D. Friedberg, PhD, ABPP
Professor and Head of Pediatric
Behavioral Health
Palo Alto University

Professor Emily A. Holmes
Distinguished Professor of Psychology
Department of Psychology
Uppsala University
Uppsala, Sweden

Helen Kennerley, DPhil
Consultant Clinical Psychologist
Oxford Cognitive Therapy Centre
Warneford Hospital, Oxford

Dr. Freda McManus
British Association of Behavioural and
Cognitive Psychotherapies

Dr. Stirling Moorey
Honorary CBT therapist (retired
consultant psychiatrist in CBT)
South London and Maudsley Trust
London, UK

Christine A. Padesky, PhD
Co-Founder & Director, Center for
Cognitive Therapy
http://www.padesky.com

James L. Shenk, PhD
Director, The Cognitive Therapy Institute,
http://www.cognitivetherapysandiego.com

Marjorie E. Weishaar, PhD
Clinical Professor Emerita
Department of Psychiatry and Human
Behavior
Alpert Medical School
Brown University

1

Dialogues for Discovery: What? Why? When?

Christine A. Padesky and Helen Kennerley

> There is no better high than discovery.
> —**E. O. Wilson,** *The Scientist Magazine,* 18:1
> (interview; 19 January 2004)

Think of the times in your life you have experienced the "high" of discovery. As children we frequently experience this thrill because we have so many opportunities for first experiences—reading words for the first time, learning to ride a bicycle, and finding a secret garden in the woods. Discoveries like these often go with a sense of awe and excitement for what the future will bring. They spark our imagination and reward us with a sense of mastery that is qualitatively different from the mastery that follows someone taking our hand and telling us step by step how to do a new task.

Discoveries we make as adults bring us similar rewards. Our secret garden becomes a beach or forest or antique shop filled with special items that we never knew existed. We learn a new language which opens up discoveries of new cultures and experiences. We make a new friend or fall in love and discover the wonders of a kindred spirt as well as new corners within our self.

As therapists, we thrive on discovery as well. Think of the sessions you have had in which you or your clients made a discovery. Even small discoveries can be transformational. Therapy can provide such fertile grounds for discovery. Imagine what it would be like to have clients making new discoveries every session and using those discoveries to either gradually or radically transform their lives. Wouldn't that be something! *Dialogues for Discovery* is designed to teach you to develop just that sort of therapy practice.

We believe discovery is the heartbeat of therapy and that therapists can learn methods to improve both the frequency and quality of discoveries their clients make. This book illustrates the richly collaborative activities of dialogue and experimentation. Every therapist can learn these processes and help their clients discover new perspectives and possibilities on the road to meaningful progress.

We titled this book and first chapter *Dialogues for Discovery* because Socratic Dialogue is a prime method for helping clients make important discoveries. As you will learn, Socratic Dialogue provides a clinically flexible strategy for navigating these rough waters of psychotherapy in ways that are client-centered, collaborative, and strengths-based. It also helps facilitate change, especially when it is embedded in all the other guided discovery methods illustrated in the case examples throughout this text.

Each of the authors brings their own clinical wisdom to their chapters, guiding readers through best practices for maintaining therapist and client curiosity, sustaining focus without forfeiting creativity, and providing methods for guiding clients towards authentic discoveries. We hope you enjoy your journey through these dialogues for discovery. In Chapter 12, the last chapter, we encourage you to make a plan that puts all your discoveries found within these pages to full effect in your own therapy practice.

Welcome All Therapists

This book is not intended for cognitive behavior therapy (CBT) therapists only, although Socratic Dialogues are most commonly associated with CBT. We have found throughout our teaching careers that practitioners of many other types of therapy also find the Socratic Dialogue approach described in this book extremely useful. Therefore, we hope all therapists who want to help their clients make more discoveries will find information, processes, and procedures here that can be readily implemented into their practices.

Dialogues for Discovery vs Changing Clients' Minds

Socratic Dialogue is one of the best skills we can develop as therapists to ensure our clients make regular and meaningful discoveries in our therapy sessions. Many of you are no doubt familiar with the concept of Socratic Dialogue. We hope you will be pleasantly surprised to learn that it is not the pale version often represented in therapy textbooks consisting of question after question designed to change a client's mind or convince them that alternative viewpoints have merit. Let's look at this in action by taking an example of a "pale version" of Socratic Dialogue and then seeing how we can improve it:

Client: I'm hopeless, really. I'll never get better.
Therapist 1: You look pained when you say that. I do recall, however, that you were feeling much improved last month. Do you remember that?
Client: Yes, but it didn't last.
Therapist 1: That's true. You've had a setback. If we look at your depression scores, how do your scores this week compare to when you started therapy?
Client: They are better than when I first came here.
Therapist 1: And what other improvements have you had since you started therapy?
Client: I'm working again. And I have had some days when my mood is better.
Therapist 1: Does that sound completely hopeless?
Client: I guess not.

Many therapists would feel satisfied after having the above dialogue with their clients, especially if it changed their client's mind about their situation being hopeless. However, we propose that the highest purpose of Socratic Dialogue in psychotherapy is to help clients make genuine and life-changing discoveries, not to momentarily change a client's mind. Notice how a second therapist begins to set the stage for new discovery in this alternative opening dialogue with the same client:

Client: I'm hopeless, really. I'll never get better.
Therapist 2: You look pained when you say that. What's going on that makes you think you'll never get better?
Client: I'm feeling much worse again. This always happens. I get my hopes up and then ... bam! I sink back into the deep pit of depression.
Therapist 2: That's tough. I can see why that is discouraging. Is this week's setback just like all the others you've experienced in the past?
Client: Pretty much. It's not full-blown yet. But I can recognize the signs that I'm slipping into that hole.
Therapist 2: That's interesting. It might really help that you can recognize signs when you are slipping into that hole. Let's talk about those signs, what you usually do when they start, and see if we can figure out anything today that might make a positive difference for you.
Client: I'm willing to give it a try.

Although the differences between these two therapist dialogues might seem subtle, they signal different intents. Therapist 1 intends to reduce her client's hopelessness by quickly gathering evidence that contradicts it. She is using Socratic questioning (without a lot of genuine dialogue) to undermine an unhelpful client belief. Therapist 2 welcomes the client's admission of hopelessness and invites her client to join in an effort to discover some paths that might lead to reasons to be more hopeful. Therapist 1 is signaling that the client is seeing things in an overly negative light which is, in fact, characteristic of depression. Therapist 2 empathizes with the client's negativity and signals that there might be reasons for hope if they join together and look for it. Both therapists are striving to end up with a more hopeful client. Therapist 1 aims to get there by eradicating the immediate basis of hopelessness. Therapist 2 suggests they actively look together for reasons to hope. By doing so, the second therapist engages the client in a collaborative investigation that can lead to unexpected and fruitful discoveries.

Readers might wonder why we don't advocate taking the more direct approach of the first therapist and simply undermine hopelessness by gathering contradictory information. When therapists use Socratic Dialogue to guide client discovery rather than to change clients' minds (Padesky, 1993), clients have an opportunity to make new discoveries that can have a more enduring impact on their moods, beliefs, behaviors, relationships, and all the other issues that bring them to therapy. Therapist 2 will guide this client to discover whether there are things that can be done in the early stages of depression relapse that will "make a positive difference." In turn, this discovery could reduce this client's hopelessness in more enduring ways than the admission sought by Therapist 1 that things may not be as hopeless as they seem in the moment.

Aaron T. Beck and his colleagues emphasized collaborative investigations in their first CBT depression treatment manual (Beck et al., 1979). In fact, actively investigating a client's existing beliefs in ways that are collaborative and guide client discovery is a core therapy process in all of Beck's cognitive therapy treatment models (Padesky, 2022). And, to varying degrees, collaboration and guided discovery have been incorporated into all CBT approaches developed by others over the following decades.

Definitions

There has been a great deal of confusion in the field in the use of terms related to guided discovery. This especially has arisen in the past when writers, including ourselves, have referred to "Socratic methods." At times this term has referred to a questioning process and at other times it has been used to

---

Box 1.1   Definitions

---

guided discovery: the *process* of designing and evolving therapy interventions to help clients discover new ideas, reach new understandings, and see new possibilities.

guided discovery methods: a broad variety of therapy interventions employed for the purposes of guided discovery. These often include Socratic questioning, Socratic Dialogue, thought records and other worksheets, behavioral experiments, imagery exercises, role play, and other types of therapy interventions (e.g., hypnosis) conducted in and outside of therapy sessions and intended to guide client discovery. Any therapy intervention (e.g., art, music) paired with Socratic Dialogue can become a part of guided discovery.

Socratic method: a teaching approach used by Socrates in which he gave no information but asked a sequence of questions in order to guide students to desired knowledge (Oxford Reference).

Socratic questioning: asking questions for the purposes of broadening a client's perspective or examining existing beliefs.

Socratic Dialogue: a four-stage collaborative process developed by Padesky (1993, 2020a) that links informational questions, empathic listening, summaries of information gathered, and analytical/synthesizing questions to guide client discovery.

---

encompass all of guided discovery. Unless citing another author who uses this term, the term Socratic method will not be used in this book. Questions used in psychotherapy will be referred to as either as Socratic questioning or Socratic Dialogue (Padesky, 1993, 2020a), depending upon which type of questioning is referenced. Therefore, at the outset, we provide the definitions in Box 1.1 as a "Rosetta stone" for those who want to link this text with other writings in the field. These are the definitions for these terms we use throughout this book.

The authors of these chapters are all therapists who are master practitioners of cognitive behavior therapy. CBT has several goals: to help clients (1) understand the interconnections among thoughts, emotions, behaviors, physical responses, and interpersonal/physical environments, (2) solve problems and relieve emotional distress, and (3) learn strategies to help themselves so they can become more resilient and function as their own therapists in the future (Kuyken et al., 2009). To accomplish these goals,

CBT emphasizes guided discovery. Although the case illustrations in this book are drawn from CBT approaches, we believe guided discovery methods can boost the effectiveness of other therapies as well. Any therapist who wants to foster client discovery can benefit from learning more about guided discovery methods.

Keep in Mind

- Many books and instructors teach therapists to use Socratic questioning as a means to gather contradictory information to undermine an unhelpful client belief.
- In this text, we advocate using Socratic Dialogue as a form of genuine exploration to help clients discover new ideas and ways of doing things that can have an enduring, constructive impact on their lives.
- Although commonly used in CBT, Socratic Dialogue and guided discovery can enhance any therapy modality practiced by readers.

Discovery Methods in Psychotherapy: What Are They?

Guided discovery is an umbrella term for a variety of therapy processes and methods that can include Socratic Dialogue, thought records, behavioral experiments, imagery exercises, core belief logs, psychodrama, in-session role plays, and a host of other structured learning exercises conducted in and outside of therapy sessions. All these methods can be used to help clients examine personal experiences in order to discover principles for adaptive and flexible living. This book explores Socratic Dialogue in detail since this process is often embedded within all the other methods and also can be used on its own as a structured approach to maximize client learning and discovery. Chapter 2 elucidates the stages and features of Socratic Dialogue that make it an ideal accelerant for discovery.

The Roots of Socratic Dialogue: A Brief History

Since it is part of the fabric of guided discovery, we begin by offering a very brief history of the roots of current day Socratic Dialogue. Instead of a comprehensive history, we reference people who have contributed in a direct genealogical lineage to of the 4-Stage Model of Socratic Dialogue described in this text (Padesky, 1993, 2019, 2020a).

Socrates

Socrates was a Greek philosopher (469–399 BC), often considered a seminal founder of Western philosophy. Although named for him, Socrates never actually spoke or wrote about the Socratic method. Instead, his student Plato wrote a series of "dialogues" in which he portrayed Socrates' teaching methods, known now as "Socratic irony" and "Socratic method." Socratic irony refers to sections of these dialogues in which Socrates described himself as ignorant and asked questions that revealed flaws in his students' thinking. Socratic method describes a teaching approach in which Socrates asked questions to elicit his students' beliefs and then pointed our logical flaws until they reached desired conclusions.

Socratic Method: Original Meaning

A teaching approach used by Socrates in which he asked questions to elicit students' beliefs and then pointed out logical flaws until they reached desired conclusions.

Socrates was not a therapist. According to Plato's descriptions of Socrates' dialogues, his questioning style was more akin to a prosecutor trying to get a witness to concede a point that Socrates already had in mind. Problems proposed by his students were broken down into small parts. For example, see how Socrates explores the meaning of courage with a student in the dialogue *Laches or Courage*[1]:

Socrates: When a person considers about applying a medicine to the eyes, would you say that he is consulting about the medicine or about the eyes?

Nicias: About the eyes.

Socrates: And when he considers whether he shall set a bridle on a horse and at what time, he is thinking of the horse and not of the bridle?

Nicias: True.

---

[1] Plato (380 BC), *Laches or Courage*, translated by Benjamin Jowett (1871), New York: C. Scribner's Sons.

Socrates: And in a word, when he considers anything for the sake of another thing, he thinks of the end and not of the means?

Nicias: Certainly.

Socrates: And when you call in an adviser, you should see whether he too is skillful in the accomplishment of the end that you have in view?

Nicias: Most true.

Although Socrates' dialogue with his student is supposedly about courage, in the section quoted, Socrates is exploring whether people generally value more the means of accomplishing something or the end result. Socrates is laying the groundwork to help his students discern that the end result of an action might be more important than the action itself in judging courage. Through inquiry, Socrates systematically uncovers his students' beliefs and untested hypotheses and, in very small steps, eliminates those that lead to contradictions with their prior and current experience. In this way, Socrates offers the first example of what we now call the scientific method of problem solving. This type of Socratic questioning is used in court rooms and law proceedings in many countries around the world.

Alfred Adler: Socratic questions in psychotherapy

Beginning in the early 1900s, Alfred Adler might have been the first psychotherapist to use Socratic questions in therapy. A contemporary who disagreed with Freud in many areas, Adler developed one of the first humanistic systems of psychotherapy. For him, use of Socratic questions was a respectful way of helping clients think for themselves and discover new and improved ways of living. As summarized by Stein (1991, 244):

> Socrates and Adler hid their insight behind questions to make their subjects think for themselves and search for a deeper truth. Neither took the role of a mentally superior authority who aggressively pointed out the mistakes of others, nor did they provide others with ready-made answers. They modeled cooperation in the role of a warm, gentle, humble co-thinker who stimulated others through skillful and sometimes playful questioning to do their own thinking and reach their own conclusions.

Aaron T. Beck: Socratic questioning in cognitive therapy

Alfred Adler is one of the therapists who influenced Aaron T. Beck, founder of cognitive therapy. While most therapists between the eras of Adler and

Beck asked clients frequent questions, purposeful questioning became the hallmark of cognitive therapy as devised by Beck in the 1970s. Beck is credited with introducing the term "Socratic questioning" in cognitive therapy although this term is not mentioned in his seminal text, *Cognitive Therapy of Depression* (Beck et al., 1979). Indeed, in a personal conversation in 2013, Beck clearly stated to the first author that he did not introduce the term Socratic questioning. "It was probably one of my students" (A. T. Beck, personal communication, October 14, 2013). Instead, he and his colleagues wrote about "questioning as a major therapeutic device" (Beck et al., 1979, 66) and cited fifteen purposes for questions in cognitive therapy. These purposes ranged from information collection to assessment; from ascertaining meanings to examining the evidence for conclusions drawn by the client (67–69). Despite not using the words "Socratic questioning," this first cognitive therapy text gives clear examples of it in sections that discuss the importance of using "questioning rather than disputation or indoctrination" (69):

> Note that every verbal expression by the therapist was in the form of a question. Also observe that the therapist was persistent in getting the patient to express *both* sides of the argument and even to challenge the validity of the reasons for engaging in a constructive activity....
>
> Questions constitute an important and powerful tool for identifying, considering, and correcting cognitions and beliefs. As with other powerful tools, they can be misused or artlessly applied. The patient may feel he is being cross-examined or that he is being attacked if questions are used to "trap" him into contradicting himself.... Questions must be carefully timed and phrased so as to help the patient recognize and consider his notions reflectively —to weigh his thoughts with objectivity.
>
> Beck et al. (1979), 71

Thus, from the beginnings of cognitive therapy, Beck emphasized the therapeutic importance of artful questioning. He even introduced the idea that it is desirable for clients to learn to use self-questioning independent of the therapist "in order to shift his mode of thinking" (195–196).

By the time his second major cognitive therapy treatment manual was published, *Anxiety Disorders and Phobias: A Cognitive Perspective*, Beck had linked his methods with current terminology, "Cognitive therapy uses primarily the Socratic method" (Beck et al., 1985, 177). Questions are of central importance in Beck and colleagues' description of Socratic methods:

> The cognitive therapist strives to use the question as a lead as often as possible. This general rule applies unless there are time restraints—in which case a therapist has to provide direct information to reach closure.

While direct suggestions and explanations may help to correct a person's anxiety-producing thoughts, they are less powerful than the Socratic method. Questions induce the patient (1) to become aware of what his thoughts are, (2) to examine them for cognitive distortions, (3) to substitute more balanced thoughts, and (4) to make plans to develop new thought patterns.

Beck et al. (1985, 177)

Again, Beck's group noted the additional advantage that patients who are asked frequent questions learn to ask themselves questions as a self-help method. "Often a patient reports that when confronted by a new anxiety-producing situation he will start by asking himself the same questions he heard from the therapist." Although subtle, the intent to help clients learn to use Socratic methods independent of the therapist is embedded in many methods developed for cognitive therapy.

Socratic Questioning: Beck's Cognitive Therapy

A system of questioning designed to: (1) bring thoughts into client awareness, (2) examine these thoughts for distortions, and (3) help the client develop more balanced thoughts in order to facilitate improved mood, greater flexibility in thinking, and better problem solving.

Over the past several decades, Socratic questioning has been routinely cited by Beck and others as central to the practice of Beck's cognitive therapy (now considered a form of cognitive behavioral therapy). Even so, Beck and his colleagues have not written extensively about Socratic questioning other than through examples. Thus, it has been left to others to specify in more detail what is meant by "Socratic questioning." The two who did so most extensively in early decades are Overholser and Padesky, who each independently presented models to guide therapist practice beginning in 1993.

James C. Overholser: The philosophy and logic of Socratic methods in psychotherapy

Overholser published three papers on Socratic questioning in the early 1990s (Overholser, 1993a, 1993b, 1994). Each one elaborated the process in terms of one of his "three main elements:" systematic questioning, inductive reasoning, and universal definitions. Overholser discussed the interplay of content and process issues, noting that the goal of Socratic questioning should be to help clients develop independent problem-solving skills. Consistent with Beck's cognitive therapy, Overholser's model described Socratic questions as a collaborative process between therapist and client.

Subsequently, Overholser published a number of papers on Socratic methods and eventually wrote a book integrating his ideas, *The Socratic Method in Psychotherapy* (2018). For Overholser, questions are an important therapy intervention in their own right. Their effectiveness requires a positive therapy alliance in which there is an agreement that both client and therapist will only say what they believe to be true and will acknowledge when they don't know something, and in which the client is willing to not agree with the therapist just to be polite. His book highlights four core strategies: "systematic questioning, inductive reasoning, universal definitions, and a sincere disavowal of knowledge, with questioning comprising the central tool" (Overholser, 2018, 32).

Overholser details a variety of ways for therapists to use *systematic questioning* to "keep the dialogue moving forward while nonetheless remaining careful to allow the client the agency to steer the answers down a chosen path" (Overholser, 2018, 38). He delineates good questions that can be used for the purposes of problem solving and/or testing beliefs with an emphasis on promoting clients' inductive reasoning skills. *Inductive reasoning* involves use of logic and hypothesis testing and is akin to Beck's vision of collaborative empiricism, client and therapist actively searching together for evidence that supports and does not support a given belief. Just as in Beck's approach, the questions asked are not random but are designed to elicit relevant information that the therapist expects to be helpful. At the same time, questions are open-ended enough to allow the therapist's expectations to be refuted.

The importance of *universal definitions* for Overholser is to clarify what clients mean and how they define the larger concepts linked to important meanings and values. What does a client who says, "No one loves me," means by love? Here, Overholser highlights the impact specific words can have on thoughts, moods, and behaviors. For example, "No one loves me," has a very different emotional impact than a more specific statement, "No one called me today to see if I've recovered from my illness."

Finally, Overholser emphasizes the importance of therapist and client embracing a *sincere disavowal of knowledge*. By this, he means each benefit by cultivating "an attitude of skepticism and uncertainty about one's factual knowledge" (2018, 93). An open mind to testing beliefs requires a willingness to consider that one's beliefs might not be accurate. Overholser emphasizes that a willingness to question one's own beliefs and assumptions is equally important for therapists as for clients: "To be effective, the therapist's disavowal of knowledge must be genuine, representing a sincere modesty and a genuine interest in the client's life, problems, and subjective experience, even when those might be different from the therapist's own views" (2018, 95).

Socratic Methods: Overholser

Overholser elucidated processes for understanding and effectively employing systematic questioning for the purposes of (1) problem solving, (2) testing beliefs, and (3) promoting clients' inductive reasoning skills. He also emphasized the importance of asking clients to define concepts linked to important meaning and values.

Christine A. Padesky: Purposes and uses of Socratic Dialogue and other guided discovery methods

At the same time Overholser was writing his initial articles on Socratic method, Padesky wrote her seminal invited address on this topic titled, "Socratic Questioning: Changing minds or guiding discovery?" (Padesky, 1993). As referenced at the beginning of this chapter, she made her case that it was better for psychotherapists to employ Socratic questioning to guide client discovery, rather than to use it in a narrow way to change clients' minds to match predetermined ideas held by the therapist or predicted by CBT theory. In this way, her approach to Socratic enquiry asks therapists to be empirical by paying close attention to client experience and comparing this with evidence-based models and *at the same time*, maintain neutrality and resist the urge to force a client's experience into a model favored by the therapist (cf. Padesky, 2020a, 2020b). Her view matches that of Beck's early guidance that CT methods are intended to be carried out in a "tactful, therapeutic, and human manner by a fallible person—the therapist" (Beck et al., 1979, 46).

Her discussion of this theme echoed many of the same ideas highlighted over the following years by Overholser such as the benefits of therapists keeping an open mind, asking questions fueled by genuine curiosity, and paying particular attention to unexpected client responses. Beck, Overholser, and Padesky each emphasize the central importance of collaboration, curiosity, and compassion during Socratic questioning.

Padesky (1993, 4) offered a new definition of Socratic questioning that incorporated the goal of guided discovery. She asserted that Socratic questioning ideally involves asking clients questions that:

a) The client has knowledge to answer;
b) Draw the client's attention to information that is relevant to the issue being discussed but which may be outside the client's current focus;
c) Generally move; from the concrete to the more abstract; and
d) Ask the client, in the end, to apply the new information to either re-evaluate a previous conclusion or construct a new idea.

Based on seven years of clinical observations of her own therapy sessions and that of trainees, Padesky also introduced a four-stage model (1993) that could be used to teach therapists of any psychotherapy school to use Socratic questioning to guide client discovery:

(1) Informational questions;
(2) Empathic listening
(3) Summary; and
(4) Analytical and synthesizing questions.

This model, as it evolved over the decades that followed, is described and elaborated in detail in Chapter 2. It was the first to equally emphasize elements of Socratic questioning unrelated to the questions themselves. For example, she pointed out that by empathically listening to various aspects of the client's experience, the therapist can notice idiosyncratic language, imagery, or details of the client's experience that are particularly relevant. She also advised therapists to notice and pay attention to important information that might be missing. For example, a man who was distressed that his life lacked love responded to his therapist's questions about this for nearly 15 minutes without mentioning his spouse. When his therapist noted this absence, he burst into tears, which redirected the dialogue to salient information that otherwise might have been missed.

Padesky noted that therapists of nearly all schools of therapy spend most of their therapy sessions engaged in the first two stages of her model. However, clients are often unaware of the potential relevance of information gathered in response to therapist questions. Therefore, she suggested that the third and fourth stages are essential to ensure true guided discovery occurs (Padesky, 2020a). Rather than pointing out the connections therapists make in their own minds, guided discovery is promoted when therapists collaborate with their clients to make a summary of the most relevant information gathered during the first two stages. When this summary is written (stage 3), the therapist can then suggest the client review the summary to make it easier to answer (stage 4) analytical ("How could you use these observations to help yourself this week?") and/or synthesizing questions ("How do these things you've told me fit with this idea that you are a bad parent?").

Throughout the 1990s, Padesky elaborated the details of her four-stage approach and began referring to it as Socratic Dialogue. Changing the word "questioning" to "dialogue" emphasized the importance of therapist listening and the interactive nature of the Socratic processes she advocated.

Socratic Dialogue linked to other guided discovery methods
In the decades following the introduction of her 4-Stage Model of Socratic Dialogue, Padesky highlighted in her workshops and teaching that Socratic Dialogue was not the only method for guiding discovery in CBT. She noted that in addition to Socratic Dialogue (a verbal method) guided discovery could take place via written methods (worksheets and other written observations) and action methods (behavioral experiments in and outside of therapy sessions, role plays, imagery exercises).

Padesky considered Socratic Dialogue a linchpin skill for therapists to master because it was often the means used to extract learning from all these other guided discovery methods. For example, when a client conducted a behavioral experiment or an imagery exercise, the therapist could use the four stages of Socratic Dialogue to extract and highlight relevant learning. The written summary of observations made along with conclusions drawn by the client in response to analytical and synthesizing questions often led to plans for post-session activities and practice.

Keep in Mind

Socratic Dialogue is a linchpin skill for therapists to master because it is often the means used to extract learning from all the other guided discovery methods.

In her invited address presented at the World Congress of Cognitive and Behavioural Therapies in Berlin in 2019, Padesky summarized more than a quarter century of her thoughts about the methods and uses of Socratic Dialogue in psychotherapy (Padesky, 2019). She highlighted a number of evolutionary shifts in her own use and teaching of Socratic Dialogue:

(1) A shift from an implicit bias for talk to an explicit bias toward action;
(2) Evolution in the methods used for each of the four stages of Socratic Dialogue;
(3) Expanding targets of Socratic Dialogue to include construction of new beliefs and behaviors; and
(4) Changes in the roles of therapist and client in Socratic Dialogue.

Each of these is briefly addressed here.

A shift from an implicit bias for talk to an explicit bias toward action

Socratic Dialogue is most potent when paired with action. Since its highest purpose is to help guide client discovery, Padesky recommends pairing it with experiential activities designed to promote learning. In particular, she recommended the regular use of interactive writing (e.g., client and therapist co-constructing models for understanding experiences or summaries of observations), behavioral experiments, imagery exercises, and role play in therapy sessions. The four stages of Socratic Dialogue can then be employed to extract, summarize, and maximize learning from these action methods. Chapters throughout this book illustrate these processes.

Pairing verbal Socratic Dialogue with active experiential therapy methods can lead to learning that is more memorable and more easily translated into steps for change. Also, action methods increase client engagement and gather here and now data about the issues being explored. For example, rather than simply talking about a depressed client's statement, "I just don't have the energy to do anything," the therapist and client can do a simple experiment in session in which they stand up and walk over to the window, look outside and talk about things they see, hear, smell, as well as other sensory responses. The therapist can prompt client observations, "See if you can identify a sight/ sound/smell/sensation that you like more than the others." By asking the client to rate their energy and mood before and after this experiment, they can gather here and now information about (a) whether the client *can* do something (e.g., walk to the window and notice sensations) even when feeling very low energy, and (b) whether doing something can change one's energy and mood (i.e., for better or worse).

Evolution in the methods used for each of the four stages
of Socratic dialogue

Action methods provide new opportunities for guided discovery in the here and now. Padesky's 4-Stage Model of Socratic Dialogue can be immediately responsive to these action methods.

Stage 1: Informational questions. Informational questions now include active observations of here and now client experiences. When behavioral experiments, role plays, imagery exercises, and interactive writing are used in session, informational questions are used to gather information about the *immediate* experiences the client is having rather than only gathering information about past events from the client's week. For example, imagine a discussion with a woman, Klarisse, who feels anger toward her adolescent son after an argument they had earlier in the week about his unwillingness to help with chores at home. Instead of simply asking informational questions about what happened several days earlier, her therapist asks her to set up the scene so the therapist can role play the adolescent and the client can re-enact what occurred. In setting the scene, her therapist asks Klarisse questions about how to role play the adolescent (e.g., questions about his demeanor, posture, language content, and tone). Her therapist asks questions about Klarisse's thoughts, feelings, physical reactions, and behavior during and after the role play.

Stage 2: Empathic listening. When we bring client experiences alive in the session through role play and other methods, we can empathically listen with our eyes and other senses as well as our ears. We can express compassion for our clients in both the tone and language used. Following the role play about her argument with her son, Klarisse's therapist made a variety of observations that illustrate this more multidimensional empathic listening that action interventions allow:

Therapist: I could hear your anger as we fought. I also noticed you were trembling.

Klarisse: Yes, I just get so angry and frustrated that he does not listen to me or treat me with respect.

Therapist: Yes. I noticed that you started out talking with him about his behavior and, as the fight progressed, you switched to talking to him about his lack of respect.

Klarisse: I think it's the lack of respect that bothers me even more than his behavior. His behavior would be different if he respected me.

Therapist: By the end, you looked like you were about to cry and asked him why he didn't respect you. I wasn't sure what he would say so I just stared at you.

Klarisse: I did start to cry last week. And that's exactly what he does. It drives me mad!

Stage 3: Summaries. Memories of experience can quickly shift and change. Writing things down soon after they occur is the best way to capture the most salient parts of a client's experience. When using active guided discovery experiences in session, it is important to make written summaries of key learning points. The best written summaries record client observations as closely as possible. "Use of a client's exact words is critically important in constructing written summaries. We want clients to look at a summary and say, 'Yes, this was my experience. These are my ideas.' In this way, they can take ownership of discoveries prompted by Socratic Dialogue" (Padesky, 2019, 8).

Stage 4: Analytical/synthesizing questions. An additional key shift over the decades in Padesky's model of Socratic Dialogue is that analytical and synthesizing questions are no longer focused only on fitting together information gathered in the summary with the client's original idea (e.g., "How do these ideas we've written in this summary fit with your belief that ... ?"). In addition, therapists can ask which ideas in a written summary are most likely to *help promote change* in the coming week. Analytical or synthesizing questions can direct a client to consider how they would like things to be in their life, how they would like to be different, what next steps they can take, and a variety of other questions that "support a CBT focus on moving forward, creating change opportunities, and identifying and reaching aspirational goals" (Padesky, 2019, 9). This expansion in focus accompanied a significant shift in Padesky's thinking about CBT's emphases as described in the next section, "Expanding targets of Socratic Dialogue to include construction of new beliefs and behaviors."

Expanding targets of Socratic Dialogue to include construction of new beliefs and behaviors

The original models of Adler, Beck, Overholser, and Padesky are largely deconstructive models. Once a person's beliefs are defined, the elements are clarified, broken down into smaller pieces, and the logical bases and connections analyzed. Mooney and Padesky (2000) proposed that an equally important process in therapy can be construction of new beliefs, assumptions, and behavioral patterns. They argue that, especially when client struggles are recurrent, a focus on helping clients construct new possibilities, beliefs, and behaviors is more engaging and motivating for clients than testing out maintaining beliefs. In addition, a focus on construction of new belief and behavior patterns can help people respond constructively when they relapse into old patterns. In Chapter 2, Padesky elucidates how the 4-Stage Model of Socratic Dialogue is modified when a therapist is pursuing this more constructive approach.

Roles of therapist and client in Socratic Dialogue

Originally, Socratic dialogue was seen as something that was primarily therapist driven. In the late 1980s, Padesky began to write down every question she asked in therapy and then send these questions home with clients to get feedback about which questions they found most helpful. This led her to develop lists of "good questions" to ask that proved particularly helpful for guided discovery. During this same time period, she began to notice that these same processes could be embedded into written worksheets and interventions that clients completed either with the therapist in session or independently between sessions.

Padesky and Greenberger wrote a client self-help book, *Mind Over Mood: Change How You Feel by Changing the Way You Think* (1995, 2016), that incorporated these "good questions" people could to ask themselves. This workbook also included a variety of worksheets that guided readers through the four stages of Socratic Dialogue by (1) asking questions relevant to particular issues, (2) providing a structured format for clients to "listen to" their own experiences prior to (3) writing down summaries of relevant information on worksheets, so that they could (4) compare their observations to beliefs they were testing (synthesizing questions) and/or make a plan to use what they learned to help themselves in the coming week (analytical questions). This format helped people learn to employ Socratic Dialogue either with or without a therapist.

Socratic Dialogue: Padesky

Padesky introduced her "4-Stage Model of Socratic Dialogue" that helps therapists facilitate client discovery processes when pursuing either deconstructive or constructive therapy goals. She encouraged the active participation of clients by pairing this four-stage model with action methods in session and worksheets between sessions that embedded Socratic Dialogue processes.

Other guided discovery methods

In this section we describe some of the guided discovery methods commonly used during therapy and reference the chapters in this book that discuss these areas in greater detail. The guided discovery methods discussed are case conceptualization, testing beliefs and images, evaluating behaviors, exploring emotions and physiological issues, and addressing environmental factors that have a bearing on client issues.

Case conceptualization

Many therapists have been taught that case conceptualization is a clinician task done outside of therapy sessions. Kuyken et al. (2009) proposed that collaborative case conceptualization done in session has greater utility for clients and enhances treatment planning as well as client motivation. Socratic dialogue is integral to conducting collaborative case conceptualization. In her article, "Collaborative Case Conceptualization: Client Knows Best," Padesky illustrates therapist–client Socratic dialogues used during the construction of two forms of collaborative case conceptualization: (1) the 5-Part Model, which is used to discover links among thoughts, emotions, behaviors, physical responses, and environments connected to therapy issues, and (2) "Box/Arrow In/Arrow Out," which is designed to help clients identify triggers and maintenance factors for specific issues (Padesky, 2020b). Her article (available from https://www.padesky.com/clinical-corner/publications) highlights specific questions and statements designed to engage clients in co-construction of these models. It also demonstrates how to make written summaries to capture key elements of the conceptualization and integrate client strengths into these models.

Testing beliefs and images

Preferred methods of testing beliefs and images depend upon the level of thought represented. Generally, three levels of thought are addressed in CBT: automatic thoughts, underlying assumptions, and core beliefs. Each of these levels of thought has its own methods designed to test them, all of which incorporate Socratic Dialogue. Thus, therapists can choose the most effective methods for testing beliefs if they first identify what level of thought is present (Padesky, 2020c).

Automatic thoughts

Automatic thoughts are those thoughts and images that pop into our minds in various situations throughout the day. These can often be tested out using

Socratic Dialogue to identify information that supports or doesn't support the thought or image. Questions that help the person view the situation in which the automatic thought arose from a variety of perspectives are often the most helpful. For example, therapists can ask how other people would view the same situation, or how the person would evaluate what occurred if they were feeling a different mood, if they were looking back on it from the vantage point of some future time, or if the same circumstances happened to someone else.

The 7-Column Thought Record (Padesky, 1983) is a written exercise that teaches clients to use Socratic Dialogue to test out their own automatic thoughts and images. Detailed guidance for best practices for how to teach clients effective use of the 7-Column Thought Record is provided by Padesky (2020c). Greenberger and Padesky's (2016) popular self-help book *Mind over Mood* can also be used to teach clients step by step how to use 7-Column Thought Records to test their automatic thoughts and images. Chapter 3 illustrates this approach.

Underlying assumptions

Underlying assumptions (UAs) are conditional beliefs that can usually be stated in an "if ... then ..." format. Because UAs tend to be forward looking (e.g., "If I go to the party, then no one will talk to me"), they are best tested with behavioral experiments (e.g., go to the party, keep a friendly look on your face, and see if anyone talks to you). Some clinical issues such as anxiety disorders, substance misuse issues, self-harm behaviors, and relationship conflict are generally triggered and maintained by UAs as shown in the following examples:

- If something bad happens, then I can't handle it (generalized anxiety disorder).
- If I have an urge to use, then I may as well do it because otherwise I'll just feel worse and worse as time goes on (substance misuse).
- If I'm in emotional pain, the only way to relieve that pain is to cut myself (self-harm).
- If someone won't compromise, then that means they don't love or care about me (relationship conflict).

Each of these types of maintaining beliefs can be tested with a series of behavioral experiments as demonstrated in chapters throughout this book. As described in the classic text by Bennett-Levy and colleagues (Bennett-Levy et al., 2004), behavioral experiments involve making predictions based on the belief one is testing and sometimes an alternative belief one is considering.

Multiple experiments are usually done in order to fairly test the assumption. Cumulative evidence is analyzed, often using Socratic Dialogue, to see whether real life experience tends to support the original assumption or an alternative one.

Core beliefs

Core beliefs are absolute beliefs (all or nothing) that can be about the self, others, the world, or the future. According to cognitive theory, these come in pairs (Beck, 1967). For example, a person might hold a core belief that people can be trusted and also a core belief that people can't be trusted. While it is possible to hold in mind two possibilities at once, "some people are trustworthy and others are untrustworthy," when under threat or experiencing an intense emotion, one or the other core belief is likely to be activated. When feeling happy and secure, the core belief that others are trustworthy will be active. When anxious or in circumstances that seem dangerous, the core belief that others can't be trusted may be activated. Once activated, core beliefs play a large role in how one interprets ambiguous life events. For example, if someone you know walks by and doesn't look at you, you might think, "she must not have seen me," when your core belief "people can be trusted" is operating. However, if your core belief "people can't be trusted" is activated on that day, then you might think, "She is giving me the cold shoulder" or "She is up to no good."

The negative core belief of a pair will be activated when moods such as depression, anxiety, anger, guilt, and shame are felt strongly. Once a person is no longer depressed or anxious or enraged, their more positive core beliefs will naturally emerge. Thus, some experts caution therapists not to focus on changing core beliefs before primary mood issues are addressed in therapy (cf. Padesky, 2020c). There is some emerging evidence that working on core beliefs early in therapy can even make some presenting issues, such as depression, worse (Hawley et al., 2017).

Sometimes people with chronic issues such as those relating to moods or personality disorders have weak or absent core beliefs. In these cases, extreme core beliefs may still dominate even when circumstances are more positive. Therapists can work with clients to help them identify and build more positive core beliefs to pair with their negative core beliefs. The clinical methods for building more positive core beliefs usually include use of a continuum and core belief logs. For more detailed information about these processes, see Padesky (1994, 2020c). Again, Socratic Dialogue is typically used to boost client learning from each of these therapy methods.

A caution about working with core beliefs too early in therapy. Some therapists identify and work with core beliefs too early in therapy. Just because beliefs are called "core" does not mean they are the most important ones to work on first. One way therapists prematurely focus on core beliefs is by using the "downward arrow" technique in which, for each stated client belief, the therapist asks, "And if that were true, what would that mean about you/to you?" This is a powerful technique and the practiced therapist can become increasingly adept at "unpacking" cognitions and identifying key, fundamental beliefs. However, this is anti-therapeutic when the therapist becomes overly focused on getting to core belief meanings without proper empathic pacing or employs this method in early therapy sessions. This practice can lead to the client seeing the therapist as insensitive. Additionally, clients can feel exposed and vulnerable and become fearful of collaboration.

Negative core beliefs often trigger significant distress. Focus on them with caution and only when necessary to achieve therapy goals. Sometimes your client will have devised ways of avoiding activating them (for example, always pleasing others so as to avoid triggering "I'm unlikeable" beliefs) and in these cases, relentless downward arrowing can take them to a conclusion for which they are not well prepared. When a therapist is unpacking meaning, it is helpful to ask: "Is it alright for me to continue with these questions or do you think this is a fruitful place to stop for now?" Many clients have spent a long time, even years, trying to avoid activating the pain that is held within their core belief systems and a therapist must not underestimate the fear and distress that delving for them might elicit.

In fact, precipitous downward arrowing to access core beliefs quickly in therapy can also result in missed opportunities to help clients learn more about the nature of their problem, associated cognitions, and ways of managing them. There is much material to be worked with en route to core beliefs as shown in the following case example.

Thirty-year-old Niamh felt depressed after her divorce and had not been able to stick with any jobs or relationships since that time. She was reluctant to collaborate in the exploration of her affect. Niamh tended to minimize her emotional responses, dismissing them or laughing about her feelings but never clearly saying that she was distressed by the process. She was not comfortable identifying core beliefs (which could be summarized as, "I am worthless and others will reject me").

The slow pace Niamh's therapist followed in unpacking her cognitions afforded many opportunities to look at cognitive processes and to engage in thought records and behavioral experiments that addressed cognitions "…that were…." were less distressing than her core beliefs. Niamh had many assumptions which were ripe for further exploration, such as, "If I'm not good enough, then there's no point in trying: I have to be the best." These assumptions provided opportunities to address thinking biases, examine the pros and cons of holding particular assumptions, construct models explaining the maintenance of unhelpful assumptions, look at evidence for and against assumptions, question unhelpful automatic thoughts, and introduce techniques such as continuum work and behavioral experiments. By doing all this work first, Niamh was more highly skilled and prepared to focus on her core beliefs later in therapy. Our Chapter 6 illustrates how to effectively work with core beliefs.

Evaluating behaviors

Behaviors are usually maintained by underlying assumptions. The impact or consequences of particular behaviors compared to others is generally tested using behavioral experiments. Role plays can also be employed in session to evaluate client skills and to conduct in session experiments. Role plays allow clients to try out and practice new behaviors or communication strategies. When clients switch perspectives during a role play we can use Socratic Dialogue to help them discover how particular behaviors might be experienced by other people in an interaction. For behaviors that can't be re-enacted easily in session (e.g., boarding an airplane and experiencing turbulence in flight), imagery can be used for purposes of exposure, practice, and rehearsal of new behaviors. See Chapter 5 for a more detailed exploration of imagery and guided discovery. Chapter 7 of this book offers a variety of examples of using guided discovery when working with impulsive and compulsive behaviors.

Exploring emotions

Some of the most well-known CBT protocols address the understanding and management of emotions such as depression and anxiety. Clients who come to therapy with these moods will be met with a wide range of well-established evidence-based practices that incorporate guided discovery. These include exercises involving behavioral activation, thought records, and behavioral experiments for depression (see Chapter 3); behavioral experiments and exposure exercises for anxiety disorders (see Chapter 4). Other emotions often explored in therapy such as anger, guilt, and shame can also be addressed using a variety of guided discovery processes such as responsibility pies, worksheets for evaluating the seriousness of actions taken or not taken, and forgiveness letters (cf. Greenberger & Padesky, 2016; Padesky, 2020c).

When clients are less aware of or less willing to discuss emotions, therapists can use guided discovery methods such as imagery and role playing to re-create emotional situations. Client and therapist observations of physical and emotional reactions can be explored during and after these experiences using Socratic dialogue. As described in Chapter 9, creative play methods can be used to guide children's awareness and processing of emotional reactions.

Physiological inquiries

Clients also frequently come to therapy for help with health worries, chronic pain, serious illness, functional symptoms, debilitating insomnia, and other physiological concerns. As is true for all presenting issues, a variety of guided discovery methods such as behavioral experiments, imagery exercises, and acceptance and mindfulness practices can be employed to identify the central features of these concerns and to explore remedies to help clients either manage or alleviate them. Socratic Dialogue can be integrated with all of these methods. Use of imagery to manage pain is illustrated in Chapter 5, and Chapter 8 details a variety of approaches for working with health adversities.

Environmental factors

Environmental factors can be the root cause and/or an exacerbating factor for many human struggles. These include personal physical environments such a noisy or crowded living situation, interpersonal environments such as one's family or workplace, or broader social environments such as one's community or country. Both past and current environmental factors can influence one's mental health and well-being. For example, a person's childhood relationship history often links to current interpersonal patterns. Sometimes challenges in one's environment can be addressed with problem solving, which often involves making observations and considering alternative responses to make. Guided discovery methods including Socratic Dialogue, role play, imagery rehearsal, and behavioral experiments are often used to explore potential responses to environmental issues.

Broad social patterns such as systemic racism, homophobia, and oppression of certain groups (e.g., based on culture, religion, race, ethnicity, gender nonconformity, economics, or physical or mental health status) are linked to depression, anxiety, relationship difficulties, trauma responses, and physical health problems (Cormack et al., 2018; Paradies et al., 2015; Van Beusekom et al., 2018). Rates of depression, suicide, and anxiety are negatively correlated with income and, in turn, poor mental health compounds poverty (Ridley et al., 2020).

Socratic Dialogue can be used to help people realize that discrimination, oppression, and interpersonal attacks are not warranted and do not mean the person is defective or less worthy than others. In addition, when people in a particular community (family, neighborhood, workplace, school, country) are causing harm to a client, therapists are advised not to simply look at thoughts about the harm. We help clients who are subject to adversity and social discrimination problem solve how to protect themselves, how to connect with allies, and how to consider whether it is beneficial to either leave that community or set a therapy goal to try to change it. Social and environmental change can be appropriate therapy goals.

In addition, therapists can use Socratic Dialogue to help people who oppress or harm others become more aware of the costs of their own prejudices in order to reduce their racism, homophobia, and other biased views of others. The following therapy excerpt illustrates this use of Socratic Dialogue dealing with a client's prejudice.

Roger: I'm getting so tired of this pandemic. We should just stop immigrants from coming here.

Therapist: The pandemic is really difficult, especially now that it has gone on and on. I'm curious what you think would happen if we stopped immigration.

Roger: That would control the pandemic. It's brought here by immigrants.

Therapist: I imagine some immigrants have been infected. Do you think immigrants are the only way the pandemic got to our country?

Roger: Well, it's the main way. Now it is spreading in many ways. And I can't do everything I used to do.

Therapist: I can hear how distressed you are. And I understand your frustration with all the different restrictions because of the pandemic. (Pause) You also sound angry. How angry do you feel, 0 to 10?

Roger: About an 8.

Therapist: You know how we have been talking about how your anger gets greater when you see other people's behavior as designed to hurt you?

Roger: Yeah.

Therapist: I wonder if thinking about immigrants in a way that sees them as directly hurting you is actually making you feel worse during the pandemic?

Roger: But it's true. They brought the pandemic and it is hurting me.

Therapist: Do you think immigrants come here to infect us with the virus?

Roger: No.

Therapist: Why do you think they come here?

Roger: To get the benefits in our country.

Therapist: Would you move to another country if there were better benefits there?

Roger: No.

Therapist: Why not?

Roger: Because I'm X [names his country identification].

Therapist: And it would be hard to leave a country you love.

Roger: That's right.

Therapist: So I wonder if some immigrants come here for reasons other than just getting benefits. What might be some other reasons?

Roger: Well, I know some had to come because of war or there were no jobs in their country.

Therapist: Do you think those immigrants wanted to bring the virus here when they were escaping war or looking for a way to work?

Roger: No, I suppose not.

Therapist: And do you think some of them were healthy when they arrived and they are just as frustrated with this pandemic as you are?

Roger: Probably.

Therapist: How does it affect your level of anger if you think about immigrants who came here for good reasons, who weren't sick when they came, and who are just as frustrated with this pandemic as you are?

Roger: I feel a bit less angry when I think about those immigrants.

Therapist: How much anger do you feel, from 0 to 10?

Roger: I guess about a 4.

Therapist: So thinking about immigrants as the entire cause for this pandemic in our country leads you to feel anger at about an 8. When you think about them as people who came here for many reasons and who did not want to bring the pandemic, and in fact who may be as upset by this pandemic as you are, then you feel about half as much anger . . . a 4.

Roger: Yeah.

Therapist: Can you think of a way this can help you?

Roger: Like in the other situations we've talked about, trying to look at the whole picture and consider the other person's point of view can help me feel better.

Therapist: Do you think this will be easier or harder to do with thinking about immigrants?

Roger: A little harder. I admit I don't like immigrants so much.

Therapist: What might be the benefits for you of learning to think about them as people with reasons for coming here that don't involve hurting you personally?

Roger: I guess I'd feel less riled up when I read the news or am stuck at home.

Therapist: How do you imagine you could manage to do that? Let's think of a common situation when immigrants are in the news. What can you imagine yourself doing that would help you feel less riled up?

Notice that Roger's therapist does not directly question Roger's biases about immigrants in this session and instead addresses the impact these beliefs have on him. When addressing anger, it is often important to first empathize with the person's distress and form an alliance by focusing on ways to reduce their distress, even when their reasons for anger are distorted (Padesky, 2020c). This approach is also consistent with principles of addressing racism in psychotherapy (Drustup, 2020).

Dialogues for Discovery: Why Use Them?

Dialogues for Discovery illustrates how to use Socratic Dialogue to guide client discovery in psychotherapy. It also shows how to avoid or get out of common traps that derail therapy progress with a wide variety of clients and issues. This section highlights empirical findings regarding the benefits of using Socratic questioning in psychotherapy and other settings. There is growing empirical evidence that it may be preferable compared to more direct use of psychoeducation or other therapy approaches.

Empirical research findings

It is generally asserted in educational fields that guided discovery methods foster enhanced student learning compared to other teaching approaches but this has rarely been tested. Use of Socratic questioning has been linked to the development of critical thinking skills in classrooms (cf. Sahamid, 2016), although these studies typically involve a small number of students. In terms of psychotherapy, until recent years there has been a paucity of research on Socratic dialogue (questioning) despite the frequent references to it in the CBT literature. This is especially surprising given the emphasis on empirical support for methods used in CBT and the general view that Socratic questioning is a core competency for CBT practice (Roth & Pilling, 2007).

One of the main rationales for using guided discovery methods in therapy is that asking questions, setting up experiential tests of ideas, and helping clients come to their own conclusions based on personal experience often leads to more effective learning than didactic presentations of ideas. Experimental studies provide some support for this rational of using guided discovery methods in psychotherapy.

In one study, participants were presented with a series of incomplete sentences that ended in a word fragment such as, "You wake up and feel r_f__ sh_." One group was asked to actively generate their own conclusion about how the word fragment resolved. In the other group they were simply given the correct answer—in this example, "refreshed." Those participants who had to actively come to their own conclusions showed the greatest change in both emotion and interpretation bias (Hoppitt et al., 2010). This finding is clinically relevant because negative interpretation bias (i.e., the tendency to interpret ambiguous information as negative or threatening) has been linked to many clinical disorders including depression and generalized anxiety disorder (Hirsch et al., 2018).

Clark and Egan (2015) offered one of the first comprehensive reviews of research directly pertinent to use of Socratic questioning in psychotherapy. In their article they refer to "Socratic method" which, as described there, is equivalent of what we are calling Socratic questioning. While they found no direct empirical evidence at that time for the benefits of Socratic method or even for a common understanding within the field of what Socratic methods looked and sounded like, Clark and Egan did summarize a variety of empirical findings consistent with its potential benefits. These ranged from evidence that Socratic questioning promotes student engagement (Yengin & Karahoca, 2012) to the success of motivational interviewing (Miller & Rollnick, 2013), which creates a similarly nondirective therapist–client relationship.

In their critique, Clark and Egan attributed the relative lack of research to the following:

(1) the vagueness of the definition of the Socratic Method and the potential differences that may exist in what the term connotes; (2) the lack of clarity regarding how the Socratic Method is applied across evidence-based CBT interventions; (3) the lack of a clearly operationalized mechanism through which a Socratic approach would operate; and (4) the lack of empirical data to assert whether the proposed benefits of the Socratic Method are present/absent.

(Clark & Egan, 2015, 876–877)

It is our hope that this text advances our field's understanding of these first two issues. Clark and Egan also note that research on Socratic questioning has been hampered by a lack of measures for evaluating its presence and quality. To this end, Padesky developed and published a *Socratic Dialogue Rating Scale and Manual* (Padesky, 2020a) to assess therapist use of her 4-Stage Model of Socratic Dialogue described in this text.

Since Clark and Egan's review article, they and others have conducted empirical studies to begin addressing the research gaps. Studies published to date provide additional encouragement for the utility of Socratic questioning in therapy. One study (Heiniger et al., 2018) used a video analog experiment to see whether people preferred use of Socratic questioning or didactic presentation of information in a therapy session for panic disorder. The lay observers of the video preferred the Socratic approach and rated the therapist in that video higher on alliance and empathy than the same therapist when seen in the didactic video. This study provides preliminary support for the idea that clients might find Socratic Dialogue appealing and that it can enhance treatment alliance.

In actual clinical practice, there is evidence that Socratic questioning provides benefits on therapy outcomes over and above their positive impact on therapy alliance. The first study of the relationship between Socratic questioning and symptom change found that therapist use of Socratic questioning predicted session-to-session symptom changes in depression even after controlling for client ratings of alliance (Braun et al., 2015). A study of cognitive processing therapy for PTSD (Resick et al., 2016) found that therapist skill in Socratic questioning was related to greater client improvement (Farmer et al., 2017).

To date, one study has investigated specifically whether Socratic questioning achieves symptom improvement by promoting cognitive change (Vittorio et al., 2022). This study analyzed data from 123 clients participating in CBT for depression. It found evidence consistent with the idea that cognitive change mediates the impact of Socratic questioning on depression symptom changes. In addition, the study showed that clients who entered treatment with lower levels of CBT skills benefited the most from use of Socratic questioning. This latter finding contradicts the intuition of some therapists who reserve use of Socratic questioning for more highly skilled clients. We suggest that Socratic Dialogue (questioning) is useful with most clients and maybe especially for those with lower CBT skill levels.

Studies have found that use of Socratic questioning is one of the most difficult skills for therapists to learn (Roscoe et al., 2022; Waltman et al., 2017).

Therapists in those studies were taught use of Socratic questioning through didactic lectures, clinical demonstrations, and supervision that did not use the 4-Stage Model of Socratic Dialogue taught in this text. Future research can evaluate whether a structured model like the one offered here makes it an easier skill for therapists to learn. We have anecdotal evidence from our own training programs that suggests it does.

Clearly we are still in the early stages of research on the use of Socratic Dialogue in psychotherapy. Broad questions relevant to this chapter are still unanswered:

- In what circumstances does Socratic Dialogue enhance or diminish client learning and progress compared to other types of therapist communications?
- Does use of a structured model such as proposed by Padesky (1993, 2019, 2020a) help therapists acquire and attain proficiency in use of Socratic dialogue?
- Does combining Socratic Dialogue with action in session make a difference?

It is possible that some clinical issues (e.g., phobias) might be as effectively addressed with action alone (i.e., exposure) and other issues (e.g., depression, generalized anxiety disorder) might be more effectively addressed with a combination of action and Socratic Dialogue. It is also possible, given the different ways in which people relate and learn, that clients will differentially respond to didactic or Socratic approaches—and we therapists need to be sensitive to what works best for whom (and when).

In order to study these types of questions, there is a need to develop a common understanding of what is meant by Socratic Dialogue. We hope this book offers a useful framework for clinicians and researchers to understand both Socratic Dialogue and how to best pair Socratic Dialogue with other guided discovery methods in clinical practice.

Socratic Dialogue: When to Use?

Socratic Dialogue is useful in communicating our interest in our client's situation as we explore with them their strengths, needs, and difficulties. Whenever we use Socratic Dialogue methods, we model the vital analytical and synthesizing skills that our clients can later use independently. There are a variety of therapy circumstances when Socratic Dialogue can almost always be used and other situations when Socratic Dialogue is not necessary or even helpful. Here we outline some of the most common examples of each.

When do we use Socratic Dialogue?

Socratic Dialogue is used strategically in order to enhance client learning and promote client discovery. Often it is used to explore beliefs associated with intense affect or target behaviors that clients want to change. There are three times in every therapy session that a therapist is likely to use Socratic Dialogue. It is used to promote discovery when:

(1) Debriefing between-session client-learning activities, aka homework (beginning of session);
(2) Exploring beliefs, behaviors, emotions, physiological reactions, life circumstances (middle of session); and
(3) Summarizing session learning; planning next treatment steps (throughout session/end of session).

This list might sound like Socratic Dialogue is used every moment of every session. In fact, each of these three instances might last 5 to 15 minutes. Therefore, often no more than half the session time will involve Socratic Dialogue.

Debriefing between-session client learning activities, aka homework

CBT clients generally do learning activities between sessions to practice skills, test out beliefs, or try out new behaviors. Socratic Dialogue is an ideal process to help therapists thoroughly debrief these activities. Use of Socratic Dialogue nearly always results in meaningful learning from between-session activities and accomplishes three goals:

a. Learning is identified and written down so clients are more likely to remember it;
b. The debriefing process creates a bridge between sessions by linking discussions and discoveries from the previous session with planning for the current session; and
c. These interactions highlight and underscore the value of client efforts and increase client motivation to continue to do these types of activities.

The following vignette illustrates use of Socratic Dialogue to debrief Jemma's experiences during the week when she wrote down and rated her moods before entering the house after work. Important aspects of this therapist's use of Socratic Dialogue are noted in parentheses on the transcript:

Therapist: I've been wondering what we would learn this week from your notes about your moods after work. Were you able to identify and rate your moods on some or all of the days? (Welcomes and expresses interest in Jemma's efforts.)

Jemma: I did it four of the days. I forgot to do it last night because I went shopping on the way home and was in a hurry to get the food into the house.

Therapist: (Smiles.) That's fine. We should be able to learn some important things from the four days of notes you made. (Emphasizes that the goal is learning.) Do you remember the reason we decided to ask you to write down and rate your moods before you entered the house? (Links to the previous session.)

Jemma: Yes. I want to stop yelling at the kids when I get home. I wasn't sure whether my behavior was all about them or partly about me.

Therapist: That's what I remember too. Can you show me your notes and tell me what you noticed? (Begins asking informational questions.)

Jemma: Here are the four days. My moods were different on each of the days and some days they were stronger than others.

Therapist: (Looking over Jemma's notes.) It looks like you identified feeling sad 40% on the first day, upset 80% on the second day, frustrated 75% on the third day, and discouraged 90% on the fourth day. Well done spotting and rating all those moods. Do you think those moods related to being at home or something else?

Jemma: Oh, not about home. I have a lot of time to think when I'm traveling home. I usually review my day at work and, as you can see, I don't like my job very much and it is a tough place to work. I usually feel pretty bad at the end of the day.

Therapist: And with these moods on board, I wonder if you can remember how you felt physically? For example, did you feel tired? Drained of energy? Or riled up?

Jemma: I would say deflated and exhausted. I feel like all the air is let out of me by the end of the day.

Therapist: Deflated and exhausted. All the air has been let out .... That paints quite a visual and physical picture. (Encouraging helpful imagery.) That's tough. (Empathic listening.)

Jemma: Yes. It takes all my energy to get home some days.

Her therapist continued asking informational questions and indicating to Jemma that she was listening empathically. Her therapist asked Jemma about the main thing that happened at work each day connected to that day's mood. They also considered whether the four moods were related to each other and how those moods influenced her when she walked into the house. After about a seven-minute discussion, her therapist asked Jemma to make a written summary.

Therapist: Thank you for helping me understand your experiences related to the notes you kept this week, Jemma. Let's make a summary of what we have learned so far. For example, what should we write about what moods you were already feeling when you arrived at home and how strong those moods were?

Jemma: (Writing as she speaks.) I'm usually feeling pretty strong moods when I get home. These moods are mostly about what happened at work that day.

Therapist: And we should probably write something in our summary about how those moods are linked to your energy level ... that idea that all your air has been let out. (Uses client's exact words and image.)

Keep in Mind

Mood ratings and other details of client observations are emphasized to the degree they help assess and evaluate client experiences and track progress. Although Jemma has been asked to rate her moods and she has done so, the therapist does not focus on these ratings here because this summary is intended to paint a broader picture of her experience.

Jemma: I feel really exhausted when I get home and pretty empty of any positive energy.

Therapist: Well said. You better write that down as well. (Pause.) And I remember you said something about how that affected your patience.

Jemma: When I feel beat up from work, I don't have any patience for anything out of place, loud noises, or chores left undone once I walk into the house.

Therapist: Put that on your summary as well. (Waits for Jemma to write it down.) Was there anything else important we talked about that you want to put in your summary?

Jemma: (Looking it over.) Just the idea that my moods before I walk in the house are all moods that could easily tip over into anger.

Therapist: Yes. That's important to put that in the summary as well. (Pauses while Jemma does so.) Take a moment to look at your summary. We learned a lot from the notes you took. Looking at all these ideas, does that help you understand or give you any new ideas related to your goal of not yelling at your kids when you get home from work? (Synthesizing/analytical question.)

Jemma: Well, it certainly doesn't help that I arrive home already feeling on the edge.

Therapist: Mmm hmmm. (Stays silent so Jemma can make her own discovery.)

Jemma: I think it's unfair to the kids that they get the brunt of my frustrations at work. If I could somehow get into a better frame of mind before I walk in the door that would help. I need to clean the slate on my moods and get a fresh start with them but I don't know how to do that.

Therapist: Would that be good for you as well? Learning how to clean the slate? (Therapist uses Jemma's exact words.)

Jemma: Yes. I don't like being so nasty at home.

Therapist: Should we make that our goal for today's session, then? Figuring out some ways to clean the slate and start fresh when you get home? (Therapist uses Jemma's exact words.)

Jemma: Yes. If you think that is possible.

As demonstrated in this dialogue between Jemma and her therapist, Socratic Dialogue can easily be used to debrief a client's between-session observations and experiments. When the therapist takes time to help her client extract valuable learning from between-session activities, the client often responds to analytical and synthesizing questions with ideas for the next step in treatment planning. Jemma's therapist could have surely jumped immediately from viewing Jemma's mood ratings to a suggestion that the session be spent helping her calm down before she entered the house. However, implementing a therapist-directed intervention puts Jemma in a more passive, receiving role in therapy. *Use of Socratic Dialogue puts Jemma in an active collaborative role with her therapist.* Jemma's active consideration of her own experiences puts her in a position where she can help develop her treatment plan. Socratic Dialogue also harnesses her motivation for change before treatment interventions begin.

Exploring beliefs, behaviors, emotions, physiological reactions, life circumstances

Following the debriefing of learning assignments, therapist and client begin pursuing the session's agenda. Some agenda items, as described later in this chapter, will not require use of Socratic Dialogue. Examples of times when Socratic Dialogue is likely to be used include those portions of the session in which therapist and client are conceptualizing therapy issues or zeroing in on testing beliefs, exploring emotional or physiological reactions, evaluating behavioral responses, or problem solving life challenges.

For example, Jemma and her therapist might practice mood management skills later in this session. Socratic Dialogue could be used to highlight key aspects of these skills that Jemma wants to practice in the coming week and to summarize the steps involved. Jemma and her therapist might use role play to practice alternative responses to her children when she is in "cool down" mode as she enters the house. If particular underlying assumptions are identified that could interfere with any alternative behaviors that Jemma is willing to practice, she and her therapist can write down those assumptions and devise behavioral experiments to test them out, writing out predictions for her existing assumptions and also for alternative ones. Imagery methods that Jemma could implement to dissipate the emotional fallout from her day before she enters her home can be practiced.

Jemma's therapist can choose among a wide variety of therapy methods to help her manage her moods and learn new strategies for navigating her parenting and work-related challenges. Whatever methods are chosen, her therapist can use guided discovery (via behavioral experiments, thought records, role play, imagery, Socratic Dialogue) to maximize Jemma's learning and then create a written summary of what she learns.

Summarizing session learning; planning next treatment steps

A third natural time to use Socratic Dialogue in therapy sessions is when summarizing what has been discussed in session. Use of Socratic Dialogue at this point helps consolidate learning and prompts clients to consider how to apply what has been discovered in the week(s) ahead. Informational questions (the first stage in Socratic Dialogue) can help determine what learning has been most meaningful to the client: "Let's recap today's session. What would you say have been the most important things we've talked about?" At this point, the therapist can prompt the client to make a written summary of key ideas or to refer to summaries already written earlier in the session. If important ideas are missing from the client's session summary, the therapist can remind the client of these—e.g., "Remember we also talked about how avoidance seems to make your anxiety worse. Let's make sure we add that to your list." Then the therapist can ask the client to look at their summary and answer various analytical/synthesizing questions such as, "How could these ideas help you this week?" or "What experiments could you do this week to try these ideas out?" or "What next step do you feel ready to take?" One of the benefits to this approach is that research shows clients are more likely to carry out future learning activities (aka homework) that link to the ideas a client wants to re-member from sessions (Jensen et al., 2020).

Once a client has chosen the next steps in their treatment plan, a wide range of guided discovery methods can further enhance the likelihood that clients will carry these out. If the next steps are interpersonal ones, role plays can be used to rehearse conversations and practice management of potential road-blocks. In addition, imaginal practice of planned activities increases the likeli-hood a person will carry out these activities (Libby et al., 2007). Therapists can debrief role play and imagery practice using Socratic Dialogue to highlight in-formation that supports client self-efficacy, the benefits of taking these steps, and to help the client problem-solve any barriers to action that are uncovered.

Similarly, toward the end of therapy, these same methods can be an inte-gral part of preparing for relapse management. If clients have routinely made written session summaries, these can be gathered together to make a final therapy summary. End of therapy summaries will span the whole of therapy rather than a single session. In addition, it is helpful to ask clients to consider what future events or experiences could be challenging for them. Therapists can help clients list the skills learned in therapy that might be most helpful in managing these future challenges in order to make a written plan of action (Greenberger & Padesky, 2016, 285–289). Imaginal rehearsal of challenges and the application of relevant skills/responses can be used to test out whether the person's plan of action is likely to be helpful (Padesky, 2020c).

When do we *not* use Socratic Dialogue?

Socratic Dialogue is not used every minute of a therapy session. Some ses-sions will involve more minutes when Socratic Dialogue is not being used than when it is. Questions, empathy, listening, and summaries are common elements in therapy. Therapists only need to systematically join these when we want to help clients focus on testing beliefs or systematically learn from experiences. Socratic Dialogue is not necessary when therapists are clarifying client communications, gathering information for assessment, or whenever giving direct information seems more therapeutic.

In a typical session, therapist and client will move in and out of Socratic Dialogue. The opening minutes might involve some quick checks on the client's life and even a bit of casual conversation to re-establish rapport and alliance. Therapist and client will set the session agenda, which generally involves some give and take and negotiation of topics. Socratic Dialogue is likely to be employed in debriefing the client's learning assignments. Then there might be some conversation about other agenda items, which may involve discussion, direct problem-solving, or general listening and empathy for client concerns. If a particular belief or behavior becomes the focus of the session, Socratic Dialogue might be employed to explore and investigate that belief or behavior. Next, therapist and client will use the ideas gathered and generated (and written down!) to plan future homework. This is likely to be done in a brainstorming fashion between client and therapist.

In many instances, the therapist's intention will influence whether a question is part of Socratic Dialogue or not. For example, the question, "How would you rate your anxiety when ... ?" could be asked purely for the purpose of gathering information during assessment. The very same question could be a Socratic Dialogue enquiry if used at the end of a behavioral experiment with the intention that the client will notice and reflect on it and/or compare it to predictions made.

There are three broad circumstances when Socratic Dialogue is not likely to be necessary:

(1) When exploration to understand a client's experience is sufficient;
(2) When the current therapy purpose involves gathering information or discussion (not discovery or testing beliefs); and
(3) When direct didactic teaching is a more effective approach.

Let's take a closer look at these situations.

When exploration to understand a client's experience is sufficient

With every client there will be portions of sessions in which the therapeutic dialogue is focused more on understanding and exploration than discovery. This occurs at the beginning of sessions when re-establishing alliance, when new issues are introduced by the client, when gathering information to help problem-solve crises or dilemmas, and during early assessment of issues as described in the next section, "When the current therapy purpose involves gathering information or discussion (not discovery or testing beliefs)."

Some clients may need more understanding and exploration in early therapy sessions before they are ready to actively participate in therapy discovery processes. For example, there are often a number of sessions in therapy with children and adolescents before issues are revealed that can be fruitfully explored using Socratic Dialogue. Chapter 9 of this book illustrates use of guided discovery methods that are engaging for younger clients.

Some issues such as acute grief are best addressed by listening empathically to the person's experience. When someone is experiencing a loss, it is therapeutic to ask questions and make reflections purely for the purpose of understanding and supporting the person's reactions. Grief is generally a process that takes time and offering compassion and evoking the client's memories of a lost person, pet, or capability are the essence of therapy for that issue, especially in the early months after a loss.

When the current therapy purpose involves gathering information or discussion (not discovery or testing beliefs)

It is difficult to know what areas of discovery will be most helpful for a client until you have gathered enough information to understand the client's concerns and goals. During an intake session and also in later sessions when new topics are introduced, there is generally a need to gather information and discuss with the client how, when, where, and why particular issues are important. Direct questions and written summaries are often the best approach when gathering information. Sometimes the information gathered and summarized is well suited for later discovery processes. Other times it is sufficient for its own sake.

A clear example of this is when carrying out risk assessments. Therapists pair empathy and concern with clear, unambiguous questions. Direct questions should be asked to gather the most pertinent information such as, "You say that you feel as though it's not worth the effort—do you ever have suicidal thoughts?"; "You have ticked the statement on this form that says you have thoughts of dying—do you have plans to put them into action?" Client responses will help the therapist assess risk and decide whether therapy can safely proceed as usual or whether its focus should switch to interventions to address and reduce suicide risk.

When direct didactic teaching is a more effective approach

Recall that good Socratic questions are simple questions that the client is able to answer. If a therapist wants to educate a client about sleep cycles in order to link this information to a conceptualization of a client's insomnia, direct education will be better than Socratic Dialogue, unless the client is a sleep researcher. Even so, if a point of education can be derived from the client's experience rather than told in an academic way, teaching from client experience is preferred. This is because clients are more likely to engage with, recall, and later use information that comes from their own experience. Thus, personalized direct client communication such as, "Have you ever noticed that when you are in a very deep sleep it is harder to wake up?" is preferred, even when Socratic Dialogue is not employed.

Sometimes it is important to give the client information directly. This is particularly the case when your clients do not have the knowledge to construct their own conclusions even with your help—in these instances you need to offer information or direct them to reading or audio/video materials. For example, it is necessary that someone with anorexia nervosa fully appreciates the consequences of self-starvation. Similarly, the potential hazards of taking medications erratically or overdosing needs to be directly conveyed to clients. Learning that intrusive thoughts are normal often offers clients swift relief. Once information has been given, you can continue in a discovery vein. For example, perhaps you have the hypothesis that your client will dismiss the literature on the dangers of self-starvation. You could enquire, "What do you make of this?" or "How might this apply to you?"

Often therapists will report to a supervisor that they were didactic in session because there wasn't enough time left in the session to use Socratic Dialogue to derive information about the client's experiences. This is certainly true at times. However, therapists who regularly favor didactic methods over Socratic ones are encouraged to recall research that suggests people have more positive attitudes toward therapists who are Socratic rather than didactic (Heiniger et al., 2018) and that self-generated material is better remembered. There is no harm in being didactic in therapy when this best serves the client. However, therapists who favor a didactic style because it is more comfortable or easier for them should be aware that this approach may not be as beneficial for clients for all the reasons described in this chapter. In Chapter 2, Padesky provides specific guidelines for and examples of Socratic Dialogue to help foster that skillset and build your confidence in using it.

Summary

This chapter offers a summary of how Socratic questioning and Socratic Dialogue have evolved from their introduction in therapy to the present day.

An evidence base for their use is offered as well as guidance as to when Socratic Dialogue is likely or unlikely to be helpful in therapy. Padesky's 4-Stage Model of Socratic Dialogue is briefly illustrated with an emphasis on the collaborative and empirical aspects of those processes as well as the importance of therapist curiosity and empathy.

Guided discovery is not solely comprised of verbal methods. We frequently ask clients to make observations and participate in imagery exercises, role plays, and behavioral experiments. When Socratic Dialogue is paired with these other guided discovery methods, it is used to extract client learning and consolidate client discoveries. We suggest you read Chapter 2 next to learn more about Padesky's 4-Stage Model of Socratic Dialogue. The remaining chapters of this book illustrate in greater detail how to use Socratic Dialogue and other guided discovery methods with various client issues and populations. After reading Chapter 2, read whichever chapters are most relevant to your clinical or supervisory practice.

Therapists want their clients to feel better and resolve life difficulties as quickly as possible. Paradoxically, this good intention can sometimes send therapists in suboptimal directions that can cost time and stress the therapeutic relationship. Each of the following chapters in this book identifies common traps that interfere with therapy progress and frustrate therapists and clients alike. You can see a partial listing of these traps in Box 1.2, Common Traps Addressed in Chapters. A full listing of traps addressed can be found on, pp. 505–507. By recognizing these traps early on, therapists have an opportunity to either avoid them or deal with them more effectively. These efforts increase the odds that clients will be able to make more discoveries and use these effectively to improve their lives.

Box 1.2 Common Traps Addressed in Chapters

Chapter 2: Pitfalls related to use of Socratic Dialogue itself. For example, clients who say, "Yes, but . . . ," find questions invalidating, look to therapists for answers; dialogues that address tangential thoughts instead of central ones; perils of ignoring the three speeds of therapy.

Chapter 3: Difficulties engaging depressed and/or suicidal clients in collaborative therapy; client pessimism and hopelessness; forgetting to set up a relapse management plan.

Chapter 4: Common traps in anxiety treatment such as client intolerance of uncertainty, client seeking advice and reassurance, avoidance, perceived needs for self-protection, difficulties letting go of control, and therapist fears about adding to client discomfort.

Chapter 5: Therapist neglect of mental imagery, uncertainty with how to help clients identify mental imagery, lack of therapist awareness of creative methods for evaluating imagery, uncertainty about what aspects of imagery are important to address or how to evaluate imagery that involves smells, kinesthetic sensations, or other nonverbal content.

Chapter 6: Difficulties forming and maintaining a sound working alliance in the face of inflexible beliefs, going over the same issues repetitively session after session, therapist hopelessness, dealing with alliance ruptures, and disengagement that often accompany inflexible beliefs.

Chapter 7: Poor understanding of the personal meanings and risks of impulsive and compulsive behaviors, inadequate assessment of risk, underestimations of the likelihood of relapse, the fluctuating nature of motivation to change, and the negative or dangerous consequences of change for clients with these types of behaviors.

Chapter 8: Clients dealing with adversity who find it hard to consider that their thoughts are relevant to their distress; all-or-nothing thinking regarding overcoming adversity; therapists who are too "rational" or feel overwhelmed by client adversity; narrowed options for problem solving due to adversity conditions or chronicity.

Chapter 9: Adaptations required in the use of Socratic Dialogue with children and adolescents due to developmental differences from adults—e.g., young people who experience questions as interrogation or who have low tolerance for ambiguity, abstraction, and frustration.

Chapter 10: Group therapy traps such as when particular group members dominate group therapy time or contribute to hostile group interactions, or when group members have large discrepancies in participation or skill acquisition. Also, therapist traps of passivity or overreliance on didactic methods.

Chapter 11: Supervisory traps such as being overly didactic, neglecting therapist or supervisor assumptions, losing sight of the bigger context outside of supervision and therapy, and neglecting the supervisory relationship.

Reader Learning Activities

Given this overview of Socratic Dialogue in psychotherapy,

- Do you think you use Socratic Dialogue in your therapy too little, too much, or just about the right amount of time?
- Identify one or two clients with whom you think it would be ideal to experiment with making a change in your use of Socratic Dialogue.
- Consider rating your use of Socratic Dialogue using the *Socratic Dialogue Rating Scale and Manual* (Padesky, 2020a), available from https://www.padesky.com/clinical-corner/clinical-tools/

If the ideas in this chapter are new to you, you might want to read Chapter 2 before using the rating scale or trying these ideas out with clients.

References

Beck, A. T. (1967). *Depression: Clinical, experimental, and theoretical aspects.* New York: Harper & Row. (Republished as *Depression: Causes and treatment*, Philadelphia: University of Pennsylvania Press, 1972).

Beck, A. T., Emery, G., & Greenberg, R. L. (1985). *Anxiety disorders and phobias: A cognitive perspective.* New York: Basic Books.

Beck, A. T., Rush, A. J., Shaw, B. F., & Emery, G. (1979). *Cognitive therapy of depression.* New York: Guilford Press.

Bennett-Levy, J., Butler, G., Fennell, M., Hackmann, A., Mueller, M., & Westbrook, D. (Eds.) (2004). *Oxford guide to behavioural experiments in cognitive therapy.* Oxford: Oxford University Press.

Braun, J. D., Strunk, D. R., Sasso, K. E., & Cooper, A. A. (2015). Therapist use of Socratic questioning predicts session-to-session symptom change in cognitive therapy for depression. *Behaviour Research and Therapy, 70*(7), 32–37. https://doi.org/10.1016/j.brat.2015.05.004

Clark, G. I., & Egan, S. J. (2015). The Socratic method in cognitive behavioural therapy: A narrative review. *Cognitive Therapy and Research, 39*(6), 863–879. https://doi.org/10.1007/s10 608-015-9707-3

Cormack, D., Stanley, J., & Harris, R. (2018). Multiple forms of discrimination and relationships with health and wellbeing: Findings from national cross-sectional surveys in Aotearoa/New Zealand. *International Journal for Equity in Health, 17*, 26. https://doi.org/10.1186/s12939-018-0735-y

Drustup, D. (2020). White therapists addressing racism in psychotherapy: An ethical and clinical model for practice. *Ethics & Behavior, 30*(3), 181–196. https://doi.org/10.1080/10508 422.2019.1588732

Farmer, C. C., Mitchell, K. S., Parker-Guilbert, K., & Galovski, T. E. (2017). Fidelity to the cognitive processing therapy protocol: Evaluation of critical elements. *Behavior Therapy, 48*(2), 195–206. https://doi.org/10.1016/j.beth.2016.02.009

Greenberger, D., & Padesky, C. A. (2016). *Mind over mood: Change how you feel by changing the way you think* (2nd ed.). New York: Guilford Press.

Hawley, L. L., Padesky, C. A., Hollon, S. D., Mancuso, E., Laposa, J. M., Brozina, K., & Segal, Z. V. (2017). Cognitive behavioral therapy for depression using Mind Over Mood: CBT skill use and differential symptom alleviation. *Behavior Therapy, 48*(1), 29–44. https://doi.org/10.1016/j.beth.2016.09.003

Heiniger, L. E., Clark, G. I., & Egan, S. J. (2018). Perceptions of Socratic and non-Socratic presentation of information in cognitive behaviour therapy. *Journal of Behavior Therapy and Experimental Psychiatry, 58*, 106–113. https://doi.org/10.1016/j.jbtep.2017.09.004

Hirsch, C. R., Krahé C., Whyte J., Loizou S., Bridge L., Norton S., & Mathews A. (2018). Interpretation training to target repetitive negative thinking in generalized anxiety disorder and depression. *Journal of Consulting and Clinical Psychology, 86* (12),1017–1030. https://doi.org/10.1037/ccp0000310

Hoppitt, L. Mathews, A., Yiend, J., & Mackintosh, B. (2010). Cognitive bias modification: The critical role of active training in modifying emotional responses. *Behavior Therapy, 41*(1), 73–81. https://doi.org/10.1016/j.beth.2009.01.002

Jensen, A., Fee, C., Miles, A. L., Beckner, V. L., Owen, D., & Persons, J. B. (2020). Congruence of patient takeaways and homework assignment content predicts homework compliance in psychotherapy. *Behavior Therapy, 51*(3), 424–433. https://doi.org/10.1016/j.beth.2019.07.005

Kuyken, W., Padesky, C. A., & Dudley, R. (2009). *Collaborative case conceptualization: Working effectively with clients in cognitive-behavioral therapy*. New York: Guilford Press.

Libby, L. K., Shaeffer, E. M., Eibach, R. P., & Slemmer, J. A. (2007). Picture yourself at the polls: Visual perspective in mental imagery affects self-perception and behavior. *Psychological Science, 18*(3), 199–203. https://doi.org/10.1111/j.1467-9280.2007.01872.x

Miller, W. R., & Rollnick, S. (2013). *Motivational interviewing: Helping people change* (3rd ed.). New York: Guilford Press.

Mooney, K. A., & Padesky, C. A. (2000). Applying client creativity to recurrent problems: Constructing possibilities and tolerating doubt. *Journal of Cognitive Psychotherapy: An International Quarterly, 14*(2), 149–161. https://doi.org/10.1891/0889-8391.14.2.149

Overholser, J. C. (1993a). Elements of the Socratic method: I. Systematic questioning. *Psychotherapy, 30*(1), 67–74. https://doi.org/10.1037/0033-3204.30.1.67

Overholser, J. C. (1993b). Elements of the Socratic method: II. Inductive reasoning. *Psychotherapy, 30*(1), 75–85. https://doi.org/10.1037/0033-3204.30.1.75

Overholser, J. C. (1994). Elements of the Socratic method: III. Universal definitions. *Psychotherapy, 31*(2), 286–293. https://doi.org/10.1037/h0090222

Overholser, J. C. (2018). *The Socratic method of psychotherapy*. New York: Columbia University Press.

Oxford Reference. (n.d.) Retrieved August 8, 2022 from https://www.oxfordreference.com

Padesky, C. A. (1983). *7-Column Thought Record*. Huntington Beach, CA: Center for Cognitive Therapy, Huntington Beach. Retrieved from https://www.mindovermood.com/workshe ets.html

Padesky, C. A. (1993, September 24). *Socratic questioning: Changing minds or guiding discovery?* Invited speech delivered at the European Congress of Behavioural and Cognitive Therapies, London. Retrieved from https://www.padesky.com/clinical-corner/publications/

Padesky, C. A. (1994). Schema change processes in cognitive therapy, *Clinical Psychology and Psychotherapy, 1*(5), 267–278. https://doi.org/10.1002/cpp.5640010502

Padesky, C.A. (2019, July 18). *Action, dialogue & discovery: Reflections on Socratic questioning 25 years later*. Invited address presented at the Ninth World Congress of Behavioural and Cognitive Therapies, Berlin, Germany. Retrieved from https://www.padesky.com/clinical-corner/publications/

Padesky, C. A. (2020a). *Socratic dialogue rating scale and manual*. https://www.padesky.com/clinical-corner/clinical-tools/

Padesky, C. A. (2020b). Collaborative case conceptualization: Client knows best. *Cognitive and Behavioral Practice, 27*, 392–404. https://doi.org/10.1016/j.cbpra.2020.06.003

Padesky, C. A. (2020c). *The clinician's guide to CBT using Mind over Mood* (2nd ed.). New York: Guilford Press.

Padesky, C. A. (2022). Collaboration and guided discovery. *Journal of Cognitive and Behavioral Practice, 29*(3), 545–548. https://doi.org/10.1016/j.cbpra.2022.02.003

Paradies, Y., Ben, J., Denson, N., Elias, A., Priest, N., et al. (2015). Racism as a determinant of health: A systematic review and meta-analysis. *PLoS ONE 10*(9): e0138511. https://doi.org/10.1371/journal.pone.0138511

Resick, P. A., Monson, C. M., & Chard, K. M. (2016). *Cognitive processing therapy for PTSD: A comprehensive manual.* New York: Guilford Press.

Ridley, M., Rao, G., Schilbach, F., & Patel, V. (2020). Poverty, depression, and anxiety: Causal evidence and mechanisms. *Science, 370*(6522). https://doi.org/10.1126/science.aay0214

Roscoe, J., Bates, E.A., and Blackley, R. (2022). "It was like the unicorn of the therapeutic world": CBT trainee experiences of acquiring skills in guided discovery. *The Cognitive Behaviour Therapist, 15*(32), e32. https://doi.org/10.1017/S1754470X22000277

Roth, A. D., & Pilling, S. (2007). *The competences required to deliver effective cognitive and behavioural therapy for people with depression and with anxiety disorders.* London: HMSO, Department of Health.

Sahamid, H. (2016). Developing critical thinking through Socratic questioning: An action research study. *International Journal of Education and Literacy Studies, 4*(3), 62–72. https://doi.org/10.7575/aiac.ijels.v.4n.3p.62

Stein, H. T. (1991) Adler and Socrates: Similarities and difference. *Individual Psychology, 47*, 241–246.

Van Beusekom, G., Bos, H. M. W., Kuyper, L., Overbeek, G., & Sandfort, T. G. M. (2018). Gender nonconformity and mental health among lesbian, gay, and bisexual adults: Homophobic stigmatization and internalized homophobia as mediators. *Journal of Health Psychology, 23*(9), 1211–1222. https://doi.org/10.1177/1359105316643378

Vittorio, L. N., Murphy, S. T., Braun, J. D., & Strunk, D. R. (2022). Using Socratic questioning to promote cognitive change and achieve depressive symptom reduction: Evidence of cognitive change as a mediator. *Behaviour Research and Therapy, 150*, 104035. https://doi.org/10.1016/j.brat.2022.104035

Waltman, S., Hall, B. C., McFarr, L. M., Beck, A. T., & Creed, T. A. (2017). In-session stuck points and pitfalls of community clinicians learning CBT: Qualitative investigation. *Cognitive and Behavioral Practice, 24*(2), 256–267. https://doi.org/10.1016/j.cbpra.2016.04.002

Yengin, I., & Karahoca, A. (2012). "What is Socratic method?" The analysis of Socratic method through "self determination theory" and "unified learning model". *Global Journal on Technology, 2*, 357–365.

2

The 4-Stage Model of Socratic Dialogue

Christine A. Padesky

> *People are generally better persuaded by the reasons which they have themselves discovered than by those which have come into the minds of others.*
>
> **—Blaise Pascal (1623–1662)**

The term Socratic questioning has been linked to Beck's cognitive therapy since the late 1970s. So, how and why did I develop my own understanding that it would help create better psychotherapy practices if we progressed from Socratic questioning to Socratic dialogue? In 1986 I was teaching an intensive cognitive behavioral therapy (CBT) training course and had just done a clinical demonstration when a therapist asked me, "But how do you know what questions to ask?" My quick reply was, "Follow your curiosity. I simply ask the questions that pop into my head." As I heard myself answer in this way I had a series of automatic thoughts: "That is a really unhelpful answer to a valid student question. I must be following some principles. What are they? My answer implies therapists need to practice for a number of years and then they will become a Socratic savant. Do I really believe this?"

It is a testimony to the power of a good question that this trainee inquiry prompted me to examine the questions I asked in therapy with much greater curiosity. For the next seven years I paid close attention and reflected on the questions I asked. When listening to trainee session recordings, I paid closer attention to therapist questions and their responses to client replies. For some of this time period, I wrote down every question I asked of my own clients in therapy. When clients said a session was particularly helpful, I asked, "What do you think was most helpful?" If clients indicated the questions I asked were useful, I made of copy for them of all the questions I had asked in that session. I sent clients home with these lists of questions and asked them to tell me which ones that they found most meaningful or helpful.

From Socratic Questioning to Socratic Dialogue

My reflections on my own interventions as a therapist and observations of therapists I was teaching in the 1980s and 1990s led me to conclude that it was more therapeutic when Socratic questioning was used to guide client discovery rather than trying to change client beliefs. I observed that the specific questions asked by the therapist were often less important than what happened after the questions were asked. For example, I heard therapists asking wonderful questions and then, when their clients replied in unexpected and clinically significant ways, they simply moved on to their next question rather than responding with empathy and curiosity to their clients' replies. Therefore, rather than using the term "Socratic questioning" which emphasizes the questions asked, I began using the phrase "Socratic dialogue."

Socratic dialogue better described the process I observed when Socratic enquiries appeared to be particularly helpful for clients. By 1993 I had developed and published a four-step model of Socratic questioning (Padesky, 1993) which I finally thought adequately answered the question, "How do you know what questions to ask?" Subsequently, this has evolved into what I now refer to as the 4-Stage Model of Socratic Dialogue. As briefly described in Chapter 1, the four stages of Socratic Dialogue are:

1. informational questions,
2. empathic listening,
3. summary of information gathered, and
4. analytical or synthesizing questions.

There is some back-and-forth movement among these stages but over the course of Socratic Dialogue, all four stages generally progress in this order as illustrated throughout this chapter.

3 Speeds of Therapy

Around this same time period, I began to talk with therapists about attending to what I called the 3 Speeds of Therapy (Padesky & Mooney, 1993). This concept helped therapists be more thoughtful about the questions they asked, the empathic replies they made, and the pacing of proceeding through Socratic dialogue and other therapy interventions. What do I mean by 3 Speeds of Therapy?

In my view, the fastest speed of therapy is the pace of thoughts racing through a therapist's mind. When doing therapy we think about what our client is saying, watch for nonverbal signals that might be relevant, weigh hypotheses of what we think is going on, and consider and weigh the possible benefits of interventions we think might prove helpful. Most therapists understand it is not therapeutic to blurt out all these thoughts to the client. Yet, when therapists pepper clients with questions it is usually because they have already a set of questions in their mind that they are eager to ask and they proceed to ask them without considering their client's response.

The second speed of therapy is what we actually say aloud to the client. This speed should be slower and reflect the best and most helpful of all the ideas going through our mind. What we say to the client should be paced to the client's level of understanding, mood, personal style, and the ideas most likely to provide immediate benefit. We consider what is likely to be most helpful for this particular client at this particular moment in time.

The third speed of therapy is what we ask clients to do between sessions. In my view, this should generally be slower than what has happened in session because it can take some practice for clients to independently apply new ideas in their life. So, for example, early in a second session we might begin to mentally make a treatment plan for a client who struggles with moderate depression. We mentally record the life pressures and thinking patterns that might be maintaining their low mood and begin to think about how to effectively set up behavioral activation experiments so they can learn what types of activities boost their mood the most (fastest speed, in our mind). Rather than saying all this to the client, we might ask a few questions about what they do during the day and talk to them about how it might be helpful to learn more about the links between what they do and how they feel (slower speed). Then, recognizing that it can be hard to remember things, especially when we feel depressed, we set up a simple chart for the client to fill out listing their activities throughout the day along with mood ratings. We practice filling out this chart in session to make sure the client can do it and then send them home to "do as much as they can" in the coming week to help us both learn what we can about links between the activities they do during the week and their mood (slowest speed).

Paying attention to the 3 Speeds of Therapy encourages us to constantly consider the impact on our clients of what we say and do. It asks us to imagine how our clients might be hearing what we say and experiencing what we do in therapy sessions. It reminds us that therapy does not go "faster" if we overload clients with learning assignments (aka homework) that are overwhelming or confusing or if we jump from intervention to intervention. Thus, it is a good companion concept to the 4-Stage Model of Socratic Dialogue which is designed to create a guided discovery process that is paced to each client's current learning needs and capacities.

Throughout this book, therapist–client dialogues illustrate the second speed of therapy and sometimes describe the at-home learning activities planned in that session (third speed). Many of these dialogues are accompanied by an "In the Therapist's Mind" box to describe what is going on in the first and fastest speed of therapy so you can learn what is guiding that therapist's intervention choices.

---

3 Speeds of Therapy

1. Fastest speed: thoughts racing through the therapist's mind
2. Slower speed: what we actually say aloud to the client
3. Slowest speed: what we ask clients to do between sessions

4-Stage Model of Socratic Dialogue

This chapter highlights how to effectively employ Socratic Dialogue in order to investigate beliefs, behavioral responses, and other therapy targets. It also introduces ways to use Socratic Dialogue to maximize client learning from other methods of guided discovery such as behavioral experiments, role play, and imagery exercises (Padesky, 2019, 2020a). Finally, use of Socratic Dialogue to help construct new beliefs, emotional reactions, and behavioral patterns is discussed in terms of its applications in Strengths-Based CBT (Padesky & Mooney, 2012).

There are two benefits I propose for learning this 4-Stage Model of Socratic Dialogue. The first is that, in my experience from more than 40 years conducting clinical training, this model helps therapists acquire the skills of Socratic Dialogue more quickly. Secondly, these four stages offer clear paths to overcoming common therapy traps therapists often encounter when using Socratic Dialogue. The first four of these five traps listed in Box 2.1 will be addressed throughout our discussion of the four stages. The fifth trap is discussed later in this chapter in the section titled "When Socratic Dialogue is Not Helpful."

The following sections offer detailed explorations of the processes and rationales for each stage of Socratic dialogue. You will learn how to use Socratic dialogue to guide client discovery rather than fall into the trap of

---

Box 2.1 Socratic Dialogue: Common Traps

Trap 1
Therapists ask so many questions clients feel bombarded and think their therapists don't understand or accept their point of view.

Trap 2
The therapist asks a variety of good questions and gathers helpful information but neither therapist nor client knows how to apply this information to the client's issues.

Trap 3
A client looks to the therapist for answers. The therapist works harder and harder over time while therapy progresses quite slowly.

Trap 4
A client asks the therapist for suggestions. Whenever the therapist offers helpful ideas, the client responds, "Yes, but . . . ."

Trap 5
The therapist uses Socratic Dialogue appropriately but it is not helpful because it does not address the central and maintaining beliefs or behaviors related to a client's issues.

---

asking questions to try to change your client's mind which often weakens therapeutic trust and alliance. As part of this process, I encourage therapists to take a stance of neutrality toward client beliefs and not prejudge them as "rational" or "irrational," as "adaptive" or "maladaptive." Instead, therapists are well served by genuine curiosity, compassion for a client's existing points of view, and an investigative spirit.

Stage 1: Informational questions

The purpose of asking a client informational questions is to gather a range of relevant information that the client can use to evaluate particular beliefs, behaviors, or decisions. Over the years, I've identified seven guidelines that inform my own choice of questions to ask, as shown in Box 2.2.

Box 2.2 Guidelines for Informational Questions

---

1. Ask questions the client can answer.
2. Get specific.
3. Begin by asking for information consistent with client beliefs.
4. Express neutral curiosity.
5. Ask questions that broaden your client's perspective.
6. Draw from your own relevant knowledge bases:
   (a) Relevant curiosity,
   (b) Knowledge of common human experiences,
   (c) Client history and culture, and
   (d) Shared history of client and therapist.
7. Allow silence.

Let's consider each of these guidelines in turn.

Ask questions the client can answer

Informational questions are designed to help someone access information they already know even if it is outside awareness. For example, Brianna has always been a reclusive woman and wants to improve her social skills. It would *not* be most helpful to ask her, "What are common topics of discussion at a party?" If Brianna has not been to parties recently, she would not know how to answer this question. Such a question can reinforce her view (and perhaps the reality) that she is socially unskilled. Instead, it would be better to ask, "What have you done, read, or heard about recently that interests you?"

The concept of drawing the client's attention to information relevant to the discussion at hand but outside the client's current awareness sounds difficult in the abstract but in reality it is straightforward. One common type of informational question is to ask someone to search their memories for life experiences dissimilar to those currently in mind. For example, you could ask Brianna, "Is there anyone at any of the shops you visit that you chat with, even for a minute?" Follow-up questions could explore her experiences with these conversations.

Socratic Dialogue is often used to explore beliefs that are highly associated with intense affect. Whenever affect is high, people cognitively retrieve information consistent with that affect and forget information contradictory to the activated emotions (Dalgleish & Watts, 1990). In addition, once new memories are accessed (e.g., associated with a different mood or content) people are more able and likely to remember events consistent with that new primed content (Mace & Petersen, 2020). Therefore, you could ask a depressed person, "How might you see this situation differently if you were happy and everything was going well for you?"

Get specific

As illustrated with the question to Brianna about chats she might have in shops she visits, informational questions are most useful when they probe for specific experiences in the client's life. In fact, a generic informational question is, "Can you give me a specific example of what you mean?" Therapists gather information about who, what, where, when, and how. It is helpful to ask clients: "How did you feel?", "What did you do?", "What thoughts went through your mind?" The latter question is better than asking, "What did you think?", because asking what went through someone's mind invites images and memories as well as word thoughts. Once the particulars of a specific situation are explored, therapists often probe for meanings ("What does this mean to you?", "What are the best/worst/most troubling parts of this for you?") and historical context ("What did you do in the past?", "How have you handled this so far?").

Begin by asking for information consistent with client beliefs

The pacing and order in which questions are asked is important. Generally, it is a good idea to begin with questions that help the client elaborate the reasons they have come to a particular conclusion. Marcus feels depressed and tells his therapist, "I'm a complete failure." If the therapist's *first* response is "Is there anything in your life that has gone even partially well?", Marcus is likely to perceive his therapist as either invalidating or invested in changing his mind. The meaning of the therapist's question changes if she first asks Marcus, "What life experiences are you thinking about when you say you are a complete failure?" Marcus easily recalls instances of failure throughout his life but does not spontaneously recall successes.

It is important that she listens to his recollections for a few minutes and even writes them down in a summary. Then, when she asks Marcus, "Is there anything in your life that has gone even partially well?", her question is now more likely to be perceived as curious and helpful. Marcus is more likely to think about the question and give a considered reply if he has already had an opportunity to discuss the idea most on his mind, his failures. Although Marcus may initially deny any successes, more specific questions which prompt a mental search will usually lead him to recall some successes (e.g., "Did you graduate from school?", "Do you think you are a good father?"). These recollections may surprise Marcus; memories of his successes will be far removed from his current awareness until prompted by specific inquiries.

Express neutral curiosity

In addition to the pace and order in which questions are asked, a therapist's tone of voice, facial expression, and other nonverbal communications signal to the client whether the therapist is really curious or trying to change their mind. Imagine after he has described some failures that trouble him, his therapist asks Marcus in a cheerful tone, "Is there anything in your life that has gone even partially well?" Although the question is well-timed, the tone is an abrupt shift. It would be much better for her to maintain a thoughtful look on her face, make direct eye contact, and ask this question in a quietly curious tone of voice. Words can also underscore therapist neutrality. For example, his therapist could preface the question in this way, "Just to be fair, before we go on, is there anything in your life that has gone even partially well?"

Expressing neutrality in curiosity means the therapist does not write down distressing information with reluctance and write down encouraging information with gusto. It is better to demonstrate an equal level of interest in all the information the client offers. In fact, distressing details of the client's life that support their beliefs are really crucial details for us to understand. We really need to know whether Marcus' "failures" relate to behaviors like, "I yell at the children, my boss says I'm always late to work" or personal disappointments such as, "I never finished school and therefore never became a doctor like I dreamed."

Ask questions that broaden your client's perspective

One goal of Socratic Dialogue is to broaden the client's perspective. There are a variety of informational questions that help do this (cf. Greenberger & Padesky, 2016, 75) such as:

- "What would you tell a friend if they thought this?"
- "What would someone who cared about you (name a specific other person) point out if they were part of this discussion?"
- "When you are not feeling the way you are right now, do you think any differently about these things?"
- "If you were looking back on this moment five years from now, how do you think you might see things differently?"

Each of these questions asks clients to step outside their current personal experience, either by shifting to another person's mind-set (the first two questions) or by shifting their mood (third question) or the timeframe (fourth question). When people shift perspective in these ways, they commonly are able to recall new information and think more flexibly.

Draw from your own relevant knowledge bases

There are an infinite number of informational questions that can be asked in therapy. The therapist at the beginning of this chapter asked, "How do you know which questions to ask?" Embedded in this question is a recognition that some informational questions are likely to be more useful than others. For example, a highly successful engineer, Ben, states, "Anything less than perfection is worthless." Asking Ben informational questions such as, "What would you tell a friend if she thought like this?" may not be useful because Ben is likely to reply, "I'd tell her she was absolutely right!" How does a therapist decide what informational questions to ask? Here are four knowledge bases I've learned to draw on:

    a. Relevant curiosity,
    b. Knowledge of common human experiences,
    c. Client history and culture, and
    d. Shared history in therapy.

Relevant curiosity

Relevant curiosity refers to the questions that occur to me that flow naturally from listening to the client talk about the matter at hand. When Ben says, "Anything less than perfection is worthless," I am immediately curious to ask Ben to define his terms so I can understand what he means by his statement. These questions include: "What do you mean by perfection?", "Can you give me an example of what you mean?", and "Do you think this is true for everyone or just you?" If true for everyone, I'd be curious to ask, "So if I help you 99% then you'd rate my effort worthless?" Or if he only applies this rule to himself, I'd be curious to know, "So how do you evaluate other people's performance that is less than perfect?"

    Therapists tend to be curious by nature so many curious questions will pop into your mind during therapy (fastest speed of therapy). Be careful to only ask those questions that are *relevant* to the issue at hand (second and slower speed). For example, Ben might mention a large city engineering project he is working on that I have been following in the news. It is not appropriate for me to ask questions about that project to satisfy my personal curiosity about it if these questions are unrelated to Ben's concerns. This example might seem obvious but I have observed many therapists asking questions about things that interest them but which have little relevance to addressing the client's immediate needs.

Knowledge of common human experiences

After these initial questions of relevant curiosity are asked and answered, I begin to wonder what questions might broaden Ben's perspective. The first arena for exploration is often guided by my knowledge of normative human experience. With Ben, I ask myself, what are common human experiences that are not perfect and yet most people value? The answer to this question will bring us to new territory that may not fit with Ben's current belief.

In my life I have observed most people cherish imperfect gifts from children, enjoy the process of skill improvement even if perfection is not attained, and prize falling in love above other human endeavors. Reflecting on these human experiences can lead me to ask a series of questions in as many of these areas as necessary until our discussion begins to intrigue Ben and I can see that he is showing greater curiosity or even some doubt in the universality of his statement, "Anything less than perfection is worthless." Observe how informational questions build one upon the other.

Therapist: Have you ever received a gift from a child?

Ben: Sure, my nephew gives me presents at the holidays.

Therapist: What's his name? (How old is he? ... a series of questions to personalize the inquiry)

Ben: (Answers all questions, becoming relaxed as he proudly describes his 6-year-old nephew.)

Therapist: What's a gift he gave you that pleased you the most?

Ben: He gave me a coffee cup. He made it in a pottery workshop at the community center.

Therapist: Was it a well-made cup?

Ben: (Laughing.) Well, for a six-year-old. It was a bit lop-sided but he painted it red and blue, my favorite colors. So I like it.

Therapist: So it was not perfect but it sounds like you value it a lot.

Ben: Yeah. Well, like I said, it's nearly perfect for a six-year-old. It wouldn't have any value in a pottery shop.

Therapist: Yes, I understand. At the same time, I'm a bit fuzzy on how it can be as valuable to you as it is, given it definitely is not perfect?

Ben: Well ... sometimes I guess the value is in the meaning of something.

Therapist: Tell me more what you mean by that.

Most minutes of dialogue do not lead to significant shifts in client beliefs and therefore it is useful for a therapist to be flexible and think of several paths of enquiry to follow in turn. For example, Ben may participate in this conversation for a while and then assert, "Once you are no longer a child, anything less than perfection is worthless." This could signal a dead end in this line of discussion although his therapist could ask, "At what age does perfection begin to be required?" "Is the age the same for someone with great intellect and talent as it is for someone who lacks intellectual and other types of talent?" It is important these questions are asked with genuine curiosity and not with a goal of changing Ben's mind or "catching him" in a logical error. Instead, the goal of these questions is to help him develop a more flexible belief system, although Ben is the arbiter of what beliefs he holds.

In addition to drawing on personal experience and knowledge of other people's experiences as source material for questions, therapists can consider books, movies, and social archetypes in the search for questions that tap different aspects of human experience. For example, the therapist might ask Ben if he is familiar with the movie *Cast Away* (Zemeckis, 2000). This movie depicts a time-pressured, perfectionistic supervisor who is marooned on a desert island and cannot rely on any of his normal strategies for success in life. All that he values is stripped away. If the client has seen this movie, there can be a discussion of whether and how the client identified with the man in the movie. Links can be drawn to his current dilemmas regarding perfection and value. If the client has not seen the movie and the therapist thinks it would be a thematic match for the client's struggles, the therapist can ask the client to see the movie before the next session so they can discuss it.

Client history and culture

Therapists can also search their knowledge of client history and culture to discover good paths for enquiry. Using the client's history as a source of questions is wise because most people consider their own experience as more relevant than the experiences of other people. This is especially true of people who view themselves as different or somehow standing outside social "norms." People from marginalized groups are often justifiably sensitive to being compared to others who come from more privileged groups in the community. Thus, searching within the client's personal history for experiences that supports more flexible beliefs can have a more powerful impact than telling your own personal stories or that of other people you have known.

Beliefs and behaviors targeted in therapy are almost always embedded in cultures that are part of the client's life. Therefore, it is important to be familiar with those cultures whether they are ethnic, racial, generational, gender-based, religious, or grounded in any of the many intersecting dimensions of culture (cf. Iwamasa & Hays, 2018). Some cultures highly value achievement and the perfectionistic strivings of individuals. Others are more likely to value community membership and group rapport. Therapy with Ben will look quite different depending upon his cultural background and current values. In fact, Ben grew up in a family and religious community that did value achievement over almost everything else. His parents endorsed the same perfectionistic beliefs that he expressed.

Nonetheless, Ben's therapist remembers incidents from Ben's personal history that he reported in prior sessions that run contrary to his belief, "If something is not perfect, it has no value:"

Therapist: I just remembered a conversation we had last month when you told me about your new boss at work.

Ben: Which one?

Therapist: You were telling me how your boss seemed to come in and begin criticizing everyone. You didn't think she was a very good manager.

Ben: No, I still don't.

Therapist: You told me about a project you were starting and you thought she was really unreasonable to be criticizing the flaws because it was a work in progress.

Ben: That's right. I remember.

Therapist: Our conversation today makes me wonder if your supervisor has the belief, "If something is not perfect, it has no value." Maybe that is why she attacked it when she found flaws in your project.

Ben: I don't think so. I think she is just a nasty person.

Therapist: Even so, if she said to you, "Your project has no value because it isn't perfect," what would you say back to her?

Ben: I'd tell her it needs more time. No project can be perfect out the gate. One of the ways we are figuring out how to set it up is by trying things and using the failures and weaknesses to guide our design.

Therapist: Hmmm. That's interesting. Is that something you usually do on projects like this?

Ben: Yes. There's no way to ultimately know how something will work in the real world until you try it out.

Therapist: So the trial-and-error process really helps you get the project working in the best way possible even though there may be flaws along the way.

Ben: That's right. She just doesn't understand how our work needs to operate.

Therapist: If we set your supervisor aside for a moment, do you think there is any possibility that you are like your project at work?

Ben: I don't know what you mean.

Therapist: What I mean is, is it possible that sometimes you can't be expected to be perfect out the gate. That maybe your failures and mistakes could guide you rather than be signs your efforts lack value?

Ben: (Pause.) I don't know. (Looking thoughtful.) I'd have to think about that.

In the Therapist's Mind

Ben's therapist scanned her memory for a time when Ben's perfectionistic rule was applied to him by someone else with the hope this would contribute to a shift in his perception of this issue. When she recalled his irritation with his new boss's criticism of his flawed work in progress, this seemed like an ideal situation to mine for new ideas. Notice she did not quickly react to Ben's remarks about "trying new things and ... using the failures to ... guide our design" even though she recognized this idea could be used to shift his belief. If she had done so, it might have seemed like she was trying to change his mind rather than maintain a stance of neutral curiosity to guide Ben's discovery process. Once Ben seems to strongly state his view about the helpfulness of trial and error, she tentatively asks whether this could be connected to his perfectionistic beliefs, "do you think there is any possibility ...." When Ben says he would have to think about it, she allows silence rather than pressing him to form a conclusion at that time. It is more important to her for Ben to deeply consider this idea than to get him to prematurely say, "Oh, that's right."

Shared history of client and therapist

Similarly, guided discovery that uses your own shared history with your client can be emotionally and cognitively very meaningful. Using shared interpersonal experiences as a basis for Socratic Dialogue often increases the emotional intensity of the discussion. This is particularly desirable with clients who tend to avoid emotion or those who approach therapy discussions with abstract intellectualism. The following example captures the spirit of what occurs when the therapy relationship is used as a source of information in a Socratic dialogue:

Therapist: Can you think of a time when I have been less than perfect as a therapist for you?

Ben: Well, I suppose.

Therapist: What's one time that comes to mind? (Gets specific.)

Ben: (Slowly.) Well, there was that time I came to your office and you weren't there yet. I had to wait 10 minutes and almost left before you showed up.

Therapist: OK. Let's take that as an example. Do you remember that session?

Ben: I sure do. I got really angry with you.

Therapist: I remember. What else do you remember about that session?

Ben: I was going to quit therapy. I said you were a real flake as a therapist.

Therapist: What else?

Ben: You listened to me, even while I yelled at you. Then you apologized.

Therapist: What happened then?

Ben: Once I stopped yelling, we started to talk about therapy and how it was going. I told you some of the things I didn't like about you. I think that was also the first time I told you I wanted to kill myself.

Therapist: Yes, I think it was.

Ben: It's funny. That session turned the corner for me.

Therapist: How so?

Ben: I began to trust you then.

Therapist: So even though I was imperfect by arriving at my office so late, something good came of the session; something that hadn't happened in other sessions when I was there on time.

Ben: Yes. I think when I got angry and you agreed with my anger and didn't put me down it surprised me. Usually people fight me when I point out their mistakes. So that got me thinking you were maybe different … different from the other therapists I have seen.

Therapist: That was a turning point in our relationship. Do you think we can learn anything from it that can help us with this idea that you see yourself as worthless when you are not perfect?

Ben: (Laughing.) Maybe if you yelled at me when I wasn't perfect we'd get somewhere.

Therapist: (Laughing.) That would be one approach! (Silent until Ben speaks.)

Ben: I guess I appreciated that you seemed to care about doing a good job even though you had messed up. Maybe there's something in that. (Silent for a few seconds.) When I make a mistake I focus on the mistake. Maybe if I paid attention to how much I am trying to do a good job I would feel differently. I mean I don't want to mess up. If I could trust you after you did what you did, maybe I could learn to trust myself a little more, even when I make a mistake.

Therapist: Those are interesting ideas. Let's write them down so we remember them and can consider them some more in the weeks ahead.

Notice this therapist asks a variety of informational questions related to the shared interpersonal experience Ben remembered. All the questions are ones Ben can easily answer. As he answers, Ben actively remembers the event and recalls details more vividly. It recreates an emotional closeness between Ben and his therapist in this session. Ben's joke and laughter indicates a shift in perspective. He finds humor in the concept of the therapist yelling at him when he makes a mistake, even though this is what he commonly does to himself with grim seriousness.

Allow silence

Also notice in the previous dialogue how Ben's therapist uses periods of silence to allow Ben space to create new learning from their shared therapy experience. Ben's final remarks reflect a deep thoughtfulness and serious consideration of a different approach to making mistakes that may not have occurred to him if his therapist continued talking. Silence is an important part of asking informational questions. As we will see in the section "Stage 2: Empathic listening," it is also a crucial part of the second stage of Socratic Dialogue, empathic listening.

Keep in Mind: Informational Questions

- Informational questions are intended to gather a range of relevant information outside the clients' current awareness that can help them evaluate beliefs, behaviors, and decisions.

- When affect is intense, information congruent with that affect is more easily retrieved. Therefore, sometimes it is helpful to ask how they might see the same situation if they had a difference mood.

- Ask for specific examples—Who? What? When? Where? How?—before probing for meanings: "What went through your mind?"

- The order in which questions are asked is important. Begin asking about memories and experiences that support client beliefs and write these down before asking for information that does not support their beliefs. Then when you ask whether there have been experiences that don't support their beliefs, this is more likely to be received as genuine interest.

- Informational questions are designed to broaden the client's perspective. When questions prompt the client to view something from someone else's perspective or a different time frame, they may recall new or different information and begin to think more flexibly.

- The most useful informational questions reflect neutral and relevant curiosity, knowledge of common human experiences, the client's personal history and culture, and your shared history in therapy with the client.

- Allow silence so your client has time to reflect on and consider new ideas.

Stage 2: Empathic listening

Most therapists are curious and usually ask questions with ease. Unfortunately, sometimes we have so many questions in our mind we forget to listen empathically to our client's reply before we ask the next question. And yet, empathic listening is crucial to the guided discovery process. Otherwise, clients are likely to feel bombarded by the questions we ask and can even begin to think we don't understand or accept their point of view. Such a questioning style will often derail the therapeutic alliance as illustrated in the following example:

Trap 1

Therapists ask so many questions, clients feel bombarded and think their therapists don't understand or accept their point of view.

Jindal: I really just can't do anything right anymore.
Therapist: What leads you to think that?
Jindal: I keep messing up on everything. I make so many mistakes. I'm disappointing everyone in my life.
Therapist: How long as this been going on?
Jindal: Most of the past year.
Therapist: Is there anything you have not messed up in the past year?
Jindal: I'm sure. But I mess up most things.

Therapist:	Let's look at today. Did you get to my office on time?
Jindal:	Yes.
Therapist:	Did you make any mistakes in traveling here?
Jindal:	No, not really.
Therapist:	Do you think you are disappointing me?
Jindal:	I'm not sure.

In this dialogue the therapist is so focused on questioning Jindal's belief that he can't do anything right that the bigger issues are missed. Consider how the interview might be different if, rather than trying to directly change the client's mind about whether he can do anything right, the therapist stays curious, listens with empathy, and guides the client to consider various different bits of information that might contribute eventually to the client reaching his own new conclusion:

Jindal:	I really just can't do anything right anymore.
Therapist:	What leads you to think that?
Jindal:	I keep messing up on everything. I make so many mistakes. I'm disappointing everyone in my life.
Therapist:	How long as this been going on?
Jindal:	Most of the past year.
Therapist:	That must be tough. That's a long time to feel like you aren't doing anything right.
Jindal:	Yes, it really is discouraging.
Therapist:	I hear that. Can you tell me about something that happened recently that stands out in your mind?
Jindal:	Sure. Yesterday I was supposed to be home early to help prepare for my daughter's birthday party. My boss gave me a big stack of work to do in the middle of the afternoon and I didn't finish it for hours. I got home late rather than early.
Therapist:	Oh no! How was that for you?
Jindal:	I felt terrible. The whole way home I was imaging my daughter's disappointment and my wife's anger.
Therapist:	What happened when you got home?
Jindal:	My wife was actually pretty understanding. I texted her in the afternoon to let her know what happened. And my daughter was so excited about the party she didn't say anything.
Therapist:	How did you feel when they reacted like that?
Jindal:	Terrible. They shouldn't have to always accept me messing everything up.

Therapist: So it sounds like even though they didn't express disappointment, you felt very disappointed and upset with yourself that you didn't keep your promise to get home early.

Jindal: Yes, exactly!

Even though this therapist is asking a lot of questions, they are paced and responsive to what Jindal is saying. Also, the questions are not designed to change Jindal's mind but to understand his perspective. By listening with empathy, the therapist stays responsive to what Jindal is saying and also begins to uncover details that will prove helpful in broadening Jindal's perspective on his problem later in this session. For example, in this instance Jindal's "messing up" came about because he faced a dilemma in that he was likely to "mess up" either at work or at home. It also is not clear that others are as disappointed in him as he is in himself. His therapist is gathering lots of useful information about his issue and, at the same time, she is expressing empathy and concern for his reactions.

As you can see in this example, listening with empathy maintains a therapeutic alliance. This is the first of six positive outcomes listed in Box 2.3, Positive Outcomes of Empathic Listening. The following sections explore each of these in turn.

Maintains the therapeutic alliance

Empathic listening maintains the therapeutic alliance which can become strained if clients perceive we don't care about what they think and feel. How we listen can convey empathy and caring to the client, crucial building blocks of a positive therapy alliance (Del Re et al., 2021; Nienhuis et al., 2018). Empathic listening is at the heart of the second stage of Socratic Dialogue. Therapists convey empathy via verbal and nonverbal listening cues. Verbal

---

Box 2.3 Positive Outcomes of Empathic Listening

1. Maintains the therapeutic alliance.
2. Helps therapist choose fruitful paths of enquiry.
3. Develops language resonant with client.
4. Alerts therapist to hidden or missing content.
5. Uses silence to encourage clients to consider, process and react.
6. Provides clues to understanding client culture.

signals of empathic listening include periodic markers of attention such as "Uh huh," "I see," or "Really?" as well as reflective comments such as, "It sounds like that was a difficult time for you," "I can see how important this is to you," "I bet you felt relieved when that was over." Nonverbal signals are equally important and should be congruent with verbal statements made. Attentiveness via eye contact, relaxed posture, or even leaning forward with an interested facial expression can convey openness, concern, and caring. Hand gestures and facial expressions (furrowed brow, smile) also contribute to client perceptions of therapist empathy and connectedness.

Vocal tone is another element that can be interpreted as empathic or not. Quiet, calm tones are likely to convey thoughtful listening. Loud, energetic comments can convey enthusiastic engagement with the client's communication or dismissal of it, depending on the context. Vocal tone and pacing are best when matched closely to client's tone (e.g., quiet reflections in response to quiet client communications, staccato-paced reflections to rapid client communications). The exception to this rule is when the therapist is trying to therapeutically shift the client's tone. In this case, the therapist's tone and pacing should be only slightly afield of the client's in order to maintain and enhance rapport.

For example, a therapist may signal empathic listening in a slightly upbeat tone in response to a client reporting despondent feelings:

Client: Things seem pretty hopeless right now. (Sigh and shrug.)

Therapist: Let's see if we can figure out some things that will help you feel more hopeful before you leave today. (Concerned eye contact, gentle smile and head nod.)

This therapist response injects some hope at the same time she signals that the depth of the client's despair has been heard. This is a more empathic reply to this highly depressed client than an enthusiastic, "I'm sure we can figure out some solutions to these problems!", which is overly cheery and can be perceived as denying the seriousness of this client's desperation.

Helps therapist choose fruitful paths of enquiry

In addition to conveying empathy to the client, listening helps focus the therapist's attention on information that can guide the choice of fruitful paths for Socratic enquiries. Skilled therapists listen to more than the straightforward content of what the client is saying. Clients reveal the meanings that events have, emotional reactions, behavioral habits, social connections, and many other types of information as they speak. Fortunately, there are usually ample opportunities to "hear" the client's message even if we miss the first one or two clues. And there are often multiple messages beneath the surface.

Recall the previous example with Jindal. He described how his boss gave him extra work mid-afternoon and this led him to arrive home late the day of his daughter's birthday party. His wife was not upset with him and his daughter did not express disappointment as he expected. This brief example tells us a lot about Jindal and his life. First, he seems highly responsible. He stayed at work even though he wanted to go home. We are not sure why he didn't communicate to his boss that he wanted to leave early for his daughter's party. Does Jindal lack assertion skills? Is his job one that requires all work done in a certain time frame? Is his boss unlikely to respond positively to a personal request?

Listening carefully also indicates that Jindal seems to have a good relationship with his wife. He was considerate in texting her in advance to say he needed to work later than planned, she was not upset with him when he arrived home, and his daughter was excited for her party, which suggests she might feel secure and happy in their family.

All these details taken together suggest that Jindal's distress about "messing up on everything. I make so many mistakes. I'm disappointing everyone in my life" might relate more to his internal values and standards than to external feedback he is getting from others in his life. This hypothesis will need to be checked out with Jindal, of course. If it is right, it may be more fruitful to begin exploring his definitions of "messing up" and his personal assumptions about what it means to "make mistakes" and "disappoint people" than to initiate enquiries about others' reactions to him.

Develops language resonant with client

As we listen, we can carefully notice the language, metaphors, and images our clients use. Pay close attention to each client's choice of language, metaphors, and images and incorporate these into your empathic comments and therapy lexicon going forward. In this way, we develop a language that is resonant with our clients' hearts and minds. The form of a client's language offers clues to their internal identity and world.

Jose had a narcissistic personality style and described himself as "a maverick" in his business dealings. His therapist explored the images associated with Jose's self-identity as a maverick and learned Jose had developed a fantasy of himself as a lonesome cowboy riding solo with a shotgun into situations and then "leaving town" when he had completed his business. This fantasy captured both the ruthlessness and loneliness that marked his life. Jose and his therapist explored this metaphor extensively early in therapy. These discussions helped Jose consider new options for his life and relationships more easily than direct discussions of his real-life strategies.

Use of exact client wording and images in both verbal and written summaries in session enhances rapport and also facilitates client collaboration. Kim said, "I'm a limp rag when it comes to confrontation." Her therapist noted this image and later, when debriefing an argument Kim had with her husband, asked, "Did you become a limp rag when he raised his voice?" Use of client language, especially language packed with emotional and kinesthetic associations, helps engage clients more fully because it evokes both their experiential and rational minds (Epstein, 2014; Teasdale, 1996, 1997). Personalized language such as "limp rag" evokes deeper meaning structures than asking a standard non-personalized question such as, "Did you back down when he raised his voice?"

In the same way, therapists are encouraged to match a client's general language in educational level, linguistic complexity, casualness, or formality. A close match in language allows the therapy conversation to flow more easily because the client does not need to mentally translate therapist comments into familiar language before replying. For example, a client who says, "I toss and turn all night even when I'm sleepy," is likely to struggle if the therapist asks, "Did you experience intermittent, nocturnal awakening again this week?"

Such an extreme example highlights the importance of congruence between the language of therapists and clients. Few therapists would miss the mark so widely. Yet careful listening can help a therapist say, "Did you feel good this week?" instead of the more grammatically correct, "Did you feel well this week?" which might create a small barrier in communication with some clients. Similarly, calling an older adult client "Mrs. Guidugli" rather than "Klara" may keep the therapy alliance on track, especially if the client in the first session introduced herself as Mrs. Guidugli and called you "Dr." throughout the session.

Matching our language to our clients' language also helps guard against introducing therapist influence on client imagery and memories. Loftus and Palmer (1974) conducted a now classic experiment in which they showed participants a film of a car crash. After watching the film, participants were asked to estimate the speed of the moving vehicles in the crash. If the question was asked, "What speed were the cars going when they 'smashed'?" participants gave much higher speed estimates than when they were asked, "What speed were the cars going when they 'contacted'?" Different words evoke different images. In this way, the language we use as therapists can actually change our clients' memories of events. For this reason, I recommend therapists play the role of "humble parrot" and try to use clients' exact words during empathic reflections (Padesky, 2019). Chapter 5 explores the impact of imagery in greater depth.

Alerts therapist to hidden or missing content

Noticing what we don't hear when we listen closely to our clients can alert us to hidden or missing content that might be important to understanding and helping them. We need to pay as much attention to what clients do not say as to what they do say. Tashi came to see me because he felt there was no meaning in his life. During the initial 15 minutes of our first appointment, I asked him to tell me about his life. He described his work pressures and physical fatigue in great detail. Never once did he mention his wife or 3 young children. This seemed significant to me. For many people, relationships are the center of life's meaning. When I asked about his family he described them in a somewhat detached way, as if they were people he visited on occasion. The things Tashi did not say in this initial conversation provided many clues about why his life lacked meaning.

Sometimes clients neglect to say things in more subtle ways. Serenity always was quick to describe her feelings in particular situations and yet was silent on this subject during discussion of lunch with a friend. Upon therapist enquiry, she revealed she felt angry with her friend yet did not think this was an appropriate emotion to feel so she was embarrassed to mention it. Another client, Yimmi engaged in frequent self-cutting behavior. When Yimmi wore a long sleeve shirt to a summer therapy session her therapist noted the shirt and Yimmi's careful descriptions of an unusually bland week which somehow seemed avoidant and decided to directly ask about self-harm.

As these examples show, when a therapist notes that something expected is missing from a client's report of events or reactions, there are several possibilities. It is possible what the therapist perceives as missing was not actually present in the client's experience. The missing elements may have been present but out of the client's awareness. The client may be actively avoiding the missing pieces. Sometimes clients are aware of their experiences and intentionally leave details out of accounts given to their therapists because they are uneasy about revealing them. Paying attention to what we don't hear can help uncover hidden clues which, in turn, lead to a better shared understanding of a client's desires and issues.

Uses silence to encourage clients to consider, process and react

Once, when we were editing a filmed therapy session, a sound engineer told me he could shorten the film considerably by simply removing the silences.

What a mistake that would have been! Silence is a critical component of empathic listening. It allows space for the client to hear, consider, react, and process what is being discussed. It is perfectly okay to make an empathic comment and then sit in silence. When we do so, clients often will follow up with a more in-depth observation or emotional response.

Chidinma: When I arrived back at university, I finally could breathe again.
Therapist: (Quietly, taking a deep breath.) You could breathe again. (Silence.)
Chidinma: Yes. (After about 20 seconds of silence) You know, it's funny. I guess the university is where I feel most at home. It's my happy place. I now know I belong here. That's what I always wanted to feel. I never thought I'd have this feeling.

Provides clues to understanding client culture

Empathic listening can be especially helpful as a means to understand and validate client culture. When we hear and incorporate client language, metaphors, and images into therapy we increase the depth of our engagement with our client. Use of client language can also validate a client's culture and values as demonstrated in the following dialogue with Isabella and Mia, a lesbian couple struggling with decisions about having a child:

Isabella: I would like to have a baby with Mia. But I know if we have a child, our child will be bullied. I'm not sure I want to put another child through that.
Mia: But we can start to change things. If we are loving parents, we can help our child cope with the mean things other people say.
Isabella: Two nice moms are not enough to soothe the pain from Internet trolls and schoolyard bullies. I don't want my child to always have a bloody nose.
Therapist: This is a real dilemma. You both want a child and know you could be loving mothers. Mia thinks your love will be protective and yet Isabella worries that all your love won't be able to be enough to stop trolls and bullies from bloodying your child's life. How do these feelings about having a child relate to your own experiences?
Isabella: I was bullied throughout school because I was different. Kids called me lesbo and said hateful things to me. And social media was not even a thing kids did when I was a child. I cringe to think what I would have had to endure if that had been around.

Mia:	I know Isabella went through hell. I didn't have to face that so much because I dated guys until just a few years ago. But I see the world changing so fast, I don't think it will be as bad for our child as Isabella thinks.
Therapist:	So each of you grew up in different realities. It makes sense that your personal history affects your view of the future you see for your child. I hear both of you wanting the best for your child.

(Isabella and Mia nod their heads.)

Therapist:	For you, Isabella, that means protecting a child from trolls and bullies, even if that means giving up the chance to have a child. And, Mia, you think the world will be a better place in the years ahead. Am I understanding you both?
Isabella & Mia:	Yes.
Therapist:	None of us really knows what a child's life will be like. But we could take the worst-case scenario from this discussion and talk about how you would respond as a couple if trolls and bullies attacked your child. It seems important to consider whether your collective mom power could handle bullies in the real world and on social media.

In this session, their therapist asks Isabella and Mia to describe life experiences that fit with their concerns and ideas about having a child. In doing so, the therapist uncovers that this lesbian couple come from very different cultural backgrounds. Isabella self-identified as lesbian throughout her childhood and adolescence and was bullied for her identity. Mia grew up with a heterosexual identity and did not experience bullying of any kind. Their therapist labels their common goal, "wanting the best for their child," and, at the same time, validates that different cultural backgrounds can lead to very different ideas about achieving this goal. By asking them to consider how they would respond as a couple to trolls and bullies who attacked their child, the therapist validates both cultural viewpoints using client language.

Culture is multifaceted and these different parts of our experience intersect. The previous example only considers one aspect of Isabella's and Mia's cultural backgrounds. Race, gender, generation, economic status, religion, ethnicity, cultural identity, physical and neurological abilities or differences, and many other dimensions of culture and identity can be relevant to understanding clients, our own reactions and biases, and our therapy relationship. Listening to client language, expressing curiosity about our clients' cultural experiences and identities, and maintaining an active awareness of our own cultural identities and biases are all part of culturally responsive therapy practices (Iwamasa & Hays, 2018).

Keep in Mind: Empathic Listening

- Empathic listening is one of the crucial building blocks to a positive therapy alliance.
- Therapists convey empathy when there is congruence between their verbal, nonverbal, tonal, and language choices and when these accurately reflect what the client is saying about their experiences.
- Careful listening helps therapists understand the meanings events hold for a client, emotional reactions, behavioral habits, and social connections, and it helps identify fruitful paths for Socratic enquiries.
- Pay attention to client language, metaphors, and images as windows into the client's internal world.
- Adopt client language, metaphors, and images and reference these to support client engagement in sessions.
- Therapists are encouraged to be a "humble parrot" and reflect clients' exact words in reflective statements.
- Notice what the client does not say, especially when expected information is missing. Enquiries about missing elements can reveal important clues for understanding client desires and issues.
- Silence allows space for the client to hear, consider, react, and process what is being discussed. Silence after an expression of empathy often leads to deeper processing of experiences.
- Listening to client language, expressing curiosity about our clients' cultural experiences and identities, and maintaining an active awareness of our own cultural identities and biases are all part of culturally responsive therapy practices.

Stage 3: Summary of information gathered

Almost all types of therapy teach therapists guidelines for asking questions and listening empathically to clients' replies. If only these two stages of Socratic Dialogue are followed, there is a risk of falling into the situation in which neither the therapist nor client know how to effectively apply the information gathered to the client's issues.

Trap 2

The therapist asks a variety of good questions and gathers helpful information but neither therapist nor client knows how to apply this information to the client's issues.

Summaries are the linchpin of Socratic Dialogue and provide a platform for new discoveries. They give tangible feedback to the client that the therapist is listening and allow therapist and client to mutually know what has been said and heard. This is so important because clients are not usually tracking their answers to questions. A summary helps clients see the collective potential relevance of what they have already said about the issues being discussed. When therapists misunderstand or miss making note of an important comment, clients can make crucial modifications to the summary. In this context, written summaries are better than verbal summaries especially if the client is expected to make connections or see patterns in the information discussed.

To begin co-constructing a written summary, a therapist might say after a period of discussion, "Let's make a list of some of the key parts of your experience and what you've told me so far. This might help us decide how this information can be helpful." A written summary creates a bridge between the gathering of helpful information and the fourth stage of Socratic Dialogue, asking the client analytical/synthesizing questions. Without a written summary, clients can be at a loss to describe what they have learned or what to do next. Also, a copy of the written summary can be placed in both therapist and client therapy notes for future review.

Make frequent oral and written summaries

Frequent summaries are necessary to facilitate client learning. When listening to recordings of my own therapy sessions I have counted as many as six summary statements within five minutes. Some of these summaries are brief lists of points just made by the client. In addition to these brief oral summaries, other summaries span several topics to allow my client and me to see links between issues discussed. It is important to write summaries down because clients often are either so caught up in or detached from emotion when speaking that they are not really aware of all the possible relationships among bits of information conveyed. When the summary has been written down by the therapist, the client is invited to review, comment, correct, and amend it. Clients often pay a leading, or at least collaborative, role in writing the summary.

Written summaries often lead to more detailed and in-depth commentary by the client. This is perhaps because written summaries frequently evoke greater emotion than oral summaries. One woman spoke calmly about her experiences in a house fire. Her therapist wrote a summary of her description using the woman's own words to capture key moments. When the woman read the written summary, she was visibly shaken. She remarked tearily, "I didn't realize until I saw those words just how frightening this has been for me. My god, I'm homeless!"

As already discussed, one of the principles of good listening is to pay attention to and use the client's language. This listening practice makes it easier to provide summaries that use clients' exact language. Using their language is validating and also encourages more to be said, as illustrated in the following example:

Therapist: When you say you are not sure you can trust me, what things come to mind that make you question my trustworthiness?

Megan: I've had bad experiences with therapists before.

Therapist: Yes, you've described some of those bad experiences to me. Is there anything in our relationship so far that also makes you think I will be another bad experience?

Megan: (After a pause.) You sometimes seem a bit distant to me.

Therapist: Is this an intuitive feeling you get or do I do things or act in certain ways that seem distant?

Megan: You sometimes stare at me. I think you think I'm a bit strange. And you look at your watch every now and then so it seems like you want to get rid of me as quickly as possible.

Therapist: I can see how those things might seem "distant." Anything else?

Megan: You smile like my last therapist. It creeps me out.

Therapist: Because your last therapist made a sexual pass at you? Does my smile make you worry I'll make a sexual pass at you?

Megan: Yes, sometimes. I've had bad experiences.

Therapist: Yes, you have. And it sounds like you think you are likely to have bad experiences with me too.

Megan: Uh, huh.

Therapist: Partly because of your past experiences with other therapists and specifically because I sometimes stare at you and look at my watch. And also when I smile that reminds you of the last therapist who was sexual with you and that creeps you out.

Megan: Yes.

Therapist: Let's make a list here on this piece of paper. Is that okay with you if we write this down?

Megan: Okay.

Therapist: It sounds like there are two main ways you think I might betray your trust. One way is by being distant. We'll make a "too distant" list here: I stare at you and I look at my watch. How about if we make a second column that describes what that behavior means to you?

Megan: Okay.

Therapist: You think my stare means I think you are a bit strange. We'll write that across from "you stare at me."

Megan: (Leaning in to look at the summary.) Yes.

Therapist: The next way I seem too distant is that I sometimes look at my watch. I'll write that in the "too distant" column. You think I want to get rid of you. We'll write that across from "look at your watch" in the "what it means" to you column. Is that right?

Megan: Yes.

Therapist: The second way you think I'll betray your trust is by being too close. Let's also make a "too close" list and with a second column about what those things mean to you. My smile reminds you of the therapist who sexually abused you. We'll write that here under "too close." What should we write here under what that means to you?

Megan: It makes me think you might abuse me too.

Therapist: Do you want to write that or do you want me to write it?

Megan: You write it. (Therapist does as shown in Figure 2.1.)

Therapist: Do these lists capture what makes you not trust me?

Megan: Yes. There's also the fact that you wouldn't see me two Saturdays ago when I felt sort of suicidal.

Therapist: Where should we write that?

Megan: Under "too distant."

Therapist: Here, why don't you take this pen and write it there. (Hands pen to client.) Write what that means to you. (Pauses while she writes, "You don't really care about me.") What else?

[If therapy is via teletherapy, both would be writing same summary and therapist would say, "I'll write that on my summary and you write it on yours".]

Megan: Once you called me "Meg" instead of "Megan." That is what my sister calls me.

Therapist: Where should that go?

Too Distant	What it means to me
You stare at me.	You think I'm a bit strange
You look at your watch.	You want to get rid of me.
You wouldn't see me two Saturdays ago when I felt suicidal.	You don't really care about me.

Too Close	What it means to me
Your smile reminds me of the therapist who sexually abused me.	You might abuse me too.
You once called me Meg like my sister does.	You are acting closer to me than you should.

Figure 2.1 Summary of Megan's observations of her therapist being too distant or too close.

Megan: Under "too close." (Writes that observation in the "too close" list and what it means to her across from it, as shown in Figure 2.1.)

Therapist: Anything else?

Megan: Don't you think that's enough?

Therapist: That's a lot of danger signals. Let's look at all the things that lead you to be unsure you can trust me. (Reads all the items.) What do you notice when you look at these things (pointing to summary in Figure 2.1)?

Megan: Well, I didn't realize I won't trust you if you get either too close or too distant.

Therapist: Sounds like there is a "just right" place for trusting me and that you worry things will get too close or too distant and sometimes my behavior seems to tilt one way or the other.

Megan: That's right.

Therapist: I don't want our therapy to be too close or too distant to be trustworthy either. Do you think it would help to talk some more about these items on the list we've made? It might help us to come to an understanding about how and why I behave the ways I do as your therapist. And how we might work out the things that bother you in a way that supports your trust rather than betraying it.

Megan: OK. I'm actually a little surprised you are willing to talk about this.

This vignette demonstrates how summaries help build clarity in a dialogue with a client. Use of client language validates a client's concerns and shows that the therapist is not defensive in the face of criticism. Notice how this therapist first completed the list of client concerns and wrote down all their meanings. Only then did she propose they talk more to understand how and why the therapist was behaving in certain ways. This created an atmosphere that encouraged Megan to bring additional concerns into the open. You can imagine this session would have been less productive if the therapist had immediately provided alternative explanations for "staring" or "looking at my watch." This could have provided additional evidence to Megan that her therapist didn't care about her feelings and couldn't be trusted.

Writing the summary down adds to its power. As shown in Figure 2.1, a written summary can be more organized than a verbal discussion. Two major concerns are identified in the written summary with specifics examples of each listed: fears the therapist is too close and fears the therapist is too distant. When the client sees the written summary, she remembers additional concerns in each area. The therapist makes this a more personal and also more collaborative process by handing the pen to the client so she can begin adding items to the list. This nonverbal gesture conveys trust in the client and therapist openness to learn more from the client's perspective. From a practical standpoint, as the client writes, the therapist has time to reflect and consider avenues for processing the information gathered.

A written summary ensures that information is not lost. It provides a structure for organizing client information that sometimes actually increases its value (e.g., "I didn't realize I won't trust you if you get either too close or too distant"). In this way, sometimes the organizational structure of a summary can highlight important dimensions of a client's concerns. It also helps therapist and client remember critical points of information that may require further discussion. Finally, the summary provides an important platform for guided discovery. It presents the client with everything he or she needs to know to answer the analytical or synthesizing questions, which complete the Socratic Dialogue process.

Notice in this example of Megan's therapy session that even before the final stage of Socratic Dialogue when analytical and synthesizing questions are asked, *a written summary has already begun a rich discovery process*. Megan is already learning new things about her trust of this therapist. She observes that trust is threatened either when her therapist seems too distant or too close. Megan spontaneously comments, "I'm actually a little surprised you are willing to talk about this," which indicates another important discovery about this therapist compared with her previous ones. Megan's perspectives on trusting her therapist are beginning to shift in response to her therapist's curious (neutral curiosity) and respectful interactions throughout the first three stages of Socratic Dialogue. This lays the groundwork for discovering new possibilities for building, repairing, and maintaining trust.

Keep in Mind: Summary of Information Gathered

- Summaries are the linchpin of Socratic Dialogue.
- Summaries demonstrate to the client that the therapist has been deeply listening.
- Summaries provide a bridge between clients' answers to informational questions and analytical/synthesizing questions.
- Written summaries are best. They are co-constructed with the client and use the client's exact words, images, and metaphors.
- Written summaries are often more organized than verbal discussions; sometimes the organizational structure can highlight important dimensions of the client's concerns.
- Written summaries provide a platform for discovery because they allow client and therapist to recall and reflect on all the relevant information gathered.

Stage 4: Analytical and synthesizing questions

Once a summary is made, the therapist asks the client to examine the information gathered and see how it applies to whatever is being evaluated. This final stage of Socratic Dialogue is designed to ensure clients have a chance to make a new discovery and call it their own. Therapists set the stage for clients to make their own discoveries by asking analytical and/or synthesizing questions that link the summary of information collected to the original belief or idea that is being evaluated through the Socratic Dialogue process.

The best synthesizing and analytical questions can be quite simple ones. For example, a good synthesizing question is "How does this information we've written here in the summary fit with your idea that [fill in the original thought which is being evaluated]?" The therapist could also ask in a puzzled voice, "I'm trying to see how this information fits with your idea [client's original statement that began the guided discovery process]. Can you help me out?" Good analytical questions include (while pointing at the summary of information collected), "When you look at this list, what do you notice?", "What do you make of this?", and "Given these experiences, what do you think will help?"

When written summaries are combined with analytical or synthesizing questions, therapists can quite easily manage the situation in which the client looks to the therapist for answers instead of staying engaged in a process of discovery.

Trap 3

A client looks to the therapist for answers. The therapist works harder and harder over time while therapy progresses quite slowly.

If the therapist is working harder than the client or the client is sitting back and watching the therapist work, these are signs that client engagement is suboptimal. Three common reasons clients disengage are (1) they don't know how to help themselves, (2) they don't believe they have the knowledge to help themselves, or (3) they feel hopeless. When clients don't know how to help themselves or don't believe they have the knowledge to help themselves, a written summary of information discussed in that session provides a great platform to help them answer the question "Can you think of a way these ideas might help you this week?" If the client is uncertain how to answer, the therapist can become even more specific: "Let's take the first observation we wrote down. How could you use this idea to help yourself this week?"

Asking clients to look at summaries and consider ways to apply these ideas to their issues increases engagement. In addition, clients who derive their own plans for action, experiments, or alternative ways of thinking about things are more likely to follow through on their implementation. Thus, analytical and synthesizing questions give clients a chance to experience ownership of new learning and creative problem solving. This process also often reduces client hopelessness. Chapter 3 describes additional ideas for using Socratic Dialogue with clients who view situations as hopeless, especially when their hopelessness is linked to depression and suicidal ideation.

Analytical and synthesizing questions also provide the solution to the fourth trap discussed in this chapter, clients who say "Yes, but..." to therapist suggestions.

Trap 4

A client asks the therapist for suggestions. Whenever the therapist offers helpful ideas, the client responds, "Yes, but...."

A common error therapists make is to follow the first three stages of Socratic Dialogue and then enthusiastically point out a new idea to the client. They ask informational questions (Stage 1), listen empathically (Stage 2), summarize the information gathered (Stage 3), but do not ask analytical and synthesizing questions (Stage 4). In other words, the therapist stops using Socratic Dialogue. Commonly, therapists do this by either highlighting a logical conclusion for the client or giving advice based on the information collected:

- *So it looks like, based on this summary of what you've told me today, you can succeed at this new job if you just give it a few more weeks.*
- *It looks like from what you said you should get out of bed thirty minutes earlier to make sure you arrive at work on time.*

Fortunately, when therapists make these errors, our clients supervise us by saying, "Yes, but . . . ." Whenever your client says this, pay attention to what you just said. Almost every time you will have either just given them some advice or drawn a conclusion for them.

When therapists draw conclusions for their client or offer advice, clients are free to return to their old belief systems and behavioral habits. In contrast, when therapists maintain a guided discovery stance (i.e., asking analytical and synthesizing questions), clients are asked to come up with their own new conclusions or ideas for what they could do. They are asked to fit together the information they gave you (summarized in their own exact words) with their goals, understanding of their distress, and plans for improvement. The active process of working with their own ideas helps clients either generate new ideas or discover incompatibilities between a familiar idea and their experience. Clients rarely say, "Yes, but . . ." to these types of self-generated discoveries. Instead, clients often exhibit genuine curiosity or surprise, reactions which can increase energy, motivation, and hope.

Keep in Mind: Analytical and Synthesizing Questions

- Analytical and synthesizing questions allow the client to make their own discoveries.
- Asking clients to look at summaries and consider ways to *apply* these ideas to their issues increases engagement and can reduce hopelessness.
- The best analytical and synthesizing questions are quite simple ones such as "How does this fit with that?" and "How can you use these ideas to help yourself this week?"

- Analytical and synthesizing questions prompt clients to apply the information gathered in session with their goals, understanding of their distress, and plans for improvement.

- Clients say, "Yes, but ... ," when therapists make suggestions, give advice, or draw conclusions from the summary for them. They are not likely to respond this way to their own ideas. Therefore, asking analytical and synthesizing questions nearly always eliminates clients' "Yes, but ..." responses.

Clinical illustration—debriefing a between-session learning assignment

As described previously, Socratic Dialogue is often used to debrief learning assignments (aka homework) done between sessions. These assignments can include observations, behavioral experiments, imagery exercises, written worksheets, and a whole variety of other action or observational tasks. In the following vignette, the therapist is using Socratic Dialogue to help Martin capture relevant information from his between session activities. Martin is a 73-year-old man being treated for depression. The following dialogue illustrates how Socratic Dialogue is used to debrief Martin's experiences with behavioral activation.

To highlight the Socratic Dialogue process, each therapist comment in the following vignette is marked according to which of the four stages is being expressed. Additional parenthetical comments point out other significant aspects of client and therapist remarks. Note that there is some flow back and forth among the stages and yet there is a general forward movement through the four stages:

Therapist: Hello, Martin. How are you feeling this week? *(Stage 1 Informational question)*

Martin: Still pretty down.

Therapist: I'm sorry to hear that. *(Stage 2 Empathic listening)* Let's see what we can figure out this week to help you.

Martin: Okay.

Therapist: *(Continues asking informational questions with empathic listening)* Did you manage to try out some of those experiments we discussed last time?

Martin: Yes. I got out of bed right away like we discussed on Tuesday and Thursday.

Therapist: And did you stay in bed on Wednesday and take some notes about how you felt each of those days? *(Informational question)*

Martin: I have my notes here. (Taps his mobile phone.)

Therapist: Good for you. Was that easy or difficult for you to do? To take the notes? *(Informational questions)*

Martin: Not too difficult. I'm not sure if I did it right, though.

Therapist: Let's see what you noticed. Can you show me? *(Informational question)*

Martin: On Tuesday I got up and made some coffee right away. I was feeling depressed about 9 out of 10 when I woke up. By the time I sat down to drink my coffee, my mood was about an 8.

Therapist: That's useful information. I'm glad you remembered to rate your mood. Just like you predicted, you felt really depressed when you woke up. Then what happened? *(Empathic listening; informational question)*

Martin: I read the news and then got dressed and went for a walk like we agreed.

Therapist: And what was your mood like while walking? *(Informational question)*

Martin: At first it dropped to about a 7 but by the time I got home it went up to a 9.

Therapist: That's interesting. What do you think was going on there? *(Informational question)*

Martin: I was happy I stuck to our plan and felt good about that when I started. But then my hip started to hurt and I began to think I was just too old for this therapy to work for me.

Therapist: So you started to feel discouraged. A sore hip is no fun. Would it be OK with you if we debrief all three mornings first and see if we can learn something to help know what to do with that thought? *(Empathic listening; informational question)*

Martin: Sure. (Martin and his therapist continue debriefing all three morning's experiments.)

Martin is seriously depressed. Empathy deepens emotional responses. Therefore, rather than making deep empathic remarks such as "Oh, I'm so sorry you were feeling so depressed when you woke up," Martin's therapist chooses to make encouraging factual remarks, "I'm glad you remembered to rate your mood" or makes lightly empathic comments paired with an action statement, "A sore hip is no fun. Would it be OK with you if we debrief all three mornings first and see if we can learn something to help … ?" By using light empathy paired with action/learning statements, his therapist is trying to ignite some hope in Martin. At the same time, his therapist is watching Martin to make sure this approach is having the intended effect. Martin continues participating in the conversation and appears engaged so this level of empathy seems to be appropriate for this session.

Therapist: (*Stage 3: Written summary of information gathered*) I appreciate all your useful observations, Martin. I've been taking some notes and want to show them to you to make sure I've captured everything important (shows Martin the written summary in Figure 2.2*).*

Therapist: Does what I wrote match your notes? (*Informational question*)

Martin: Yes. I see that's a different way of writing it out. I didn't think to do it that way.

Therapist: Oh, your notes are just fine the way you did them. As you talked, I was just trying to think of some way to compare the days. That's not what you were meant to do. (*Clarification*)

Martin: I see.

Therapist: Would you change or add anything to this list? (*Written summary*)

Martin: I'm not sure I'd put my hip hurting as the worst point on Tuesday.

Therapist: Okay. What should we write instead? (*Written summary*)

Martin: I can handle my hip hurting. It was more the idea that this therapy won't help me.

Therapist: I'm glad you pointed that out. That's good to know. Yes, let's change the worst point on Tuesday to that thought you had. Here's the pen, why don't you make the change? (Pauses while Martin crosses out "hip hurts" and writes "I'm too old to do this therapy.") (*Written summary*)

	Tue/Thurs - Got Out of Bed	Wed - Stayed in Bed
Wake up Mood	9, 8	9
Mood 1 hour later	9, 6	10
Best mood	7, 6	9
Best point	Starting to walk (Tue) Talking to Frank (Thurs)	(none)
Worst point	Hip hurts (Tue) Waking up (Thurs)	Thinking I'm worthless

Figure 2.2 Summary of Martin's behavioral experiments.

In the Therapist's Mind

Martin's therapist is feeling a bit embarrassed and foolish for choosing the aching hip rather than the depressed thought to write down as the worst point on Tuesday. On the other hand, his therapist recognizes that this was a lucky mistake. Martin has an opportunity to see himself as competent in correcting his therapist's error. By letting Martin make the change on the summary, Martin becomes more engaged and an active participant in the summary. His therapist notes that Martin's mood seems a bit brighter even while he writes down his depressed thought about "being too old" for this therapy.

Therapist: Thanks for making that correction, Martin. Does this summary look right to you now? (*Written summary*)

Martin: I think so.

Therapist: Good. Let's look at it for a minute and see what we can learn from it. (Quietly after few moments) What do you notice? (*Stage 4: Synthesizing question*)

Martin: I had some good points on the days I got up and not when I stayed in bed.

Therapist: What can we learn from that? (*Stage 4: Analytical question*)

Martin: I guess it's like the lottery. You don't have a chance to win unless you buy a ticket.

Therapist: (Smiling) I like that. Let's write that down below the summary. (Martin writes.)
   I think I know what you mean, but how might that idea help you when you are feeling depressed? (*Analytical question*)

Martin: When I feel really depressed I don't want to do anything. But I see there is a chance I might feel better if I do something.

Therapist: Yes. I can see that too. Will you remember that idea when you read about the lottery ticket or do you want to write that idea down also? (*Written summary*)

Martin: I guess I could write, "Doing nothing gets you nothing. Doing something might help." (Therapist nods and Martin writes this down.)

Therapist: I notice that your mood was best the morning you met Frank while you were out walking. Is there anything you can learn from that to help yourself this week? (*Analytical question*)

Martin: I tend to stay inside and by myself when my mood is bad. But I think I feel better when I have someone to talk with.

Therapist: How can you use that idea to help yourself this week? (*Analytical question*)

Martin: Maybe it would help to see or talk to my friends on the phone. (Long pause.) And maybe it is better to get outside the house every day—even if I just go to the shops and see people there.

As this example illustrates, the 4-Stage Model of Socratic Dialogue is ideally suited as a template for helping clients learn from homework assignments and other experiences in and outside of session:

(1) Informational questions are used to gather relevant observations.
(2) Empathic listening can be modulated to fit client needs and provide optimal support for client efforts.
(3) Written summaries of client observations help draw client attention to helpful and challenging aspects of their experiences. These summaries guide the client's attention to useful ideas and metaphors ("lottery ticket") that might provide a springboard for new learning.
(4) Analytical and synthesizing questions are the therapist's tools to prompt clients to derive new helpful ideas from their experiences.

In turn, the new ideas prompted by the analytical and synthesizing questions can be written down to begin making a "learning summary" for the session. Learning summaries can be used to plan future experiments and homework assignments. In this way, Socratic Dialogue fosters clients' ability to learn from experience and creates a written record so that each therapy session builds on prior learning.

Keep in Mind

- In practice, there is some back and forth flow among the four stages of Socratic Dialogue with a general forward movement through them.
- New ideas prompted by the analytical and synthesizing questions can be written down to begin making a "learning summary" for the session.
- Socratic Dialogue fosters clients' ability to learn from experience and creates a written record so that each therapy session can build on prior learning.

Socratic Dialogue is embedded in the 7-Column Thought Record

I developed the 7-Column Thought Record to help people use Socratic Dialogue processes with themselves to evaluate the central beliefs that maintain their distressed moods (Padesky, 1983). This thought record helps clients develop skills to test out and evaluate their thoughts, as described in the popular self-help workbook *Mind over Mood* (Greenberger & Padesky, 2016). Thought record chapters in that workbook guide readers to ask themselves a series of informational questions (Socratic Dialogue Stage 1). First, people are asked simple questions about the situation in which they had a strong mood (Where were you? Who were you with? What were you doing? When was it?). Second, they are asked to identify and rate the strength of their moods. Third, a series of questions helps them to identify the automatic thoughts and images they had in this situation that are connected to their moods. Then they are asked to determine which thoughts are "hot thoughts," or thoughts most closely tied to the mood they want to investigate. A final set of informational questions helps 7-ColumnThought Record users look for information that supports and does not support their hot thoughts.

Writing all this information on the 7-Column Thought Record acts as both an opportunity for the person to empathically listen (Socratic Dialogue Stage 2) to themselves and also to make a written summary (Socratic Dialogue Stage 3) of what is going on during an intense mood. Analytical and synthesizing questions (Socratic Dialogue Stage 4) are introduced when the person fills out the sixth column of the Thought Record, which is called "Alternative or Balanced Thought." To fill out this column, people are asked to review all the written evidence from columns four and five of the Thought Record and write either a balanced summary of this evidence and/or an alternative view to their original distressing hot thought. If the evidence supports their hot thought, then the person is asked to make an action plan to solve the problem encapsulated by this 7-Column Thought Record or to develop greater acceptance or ways of coping with the situation linked to their distress (Padesky, 2020b).

Embedding Socratic Dialogue in other guided discovery methods

Socratic Dialogues can be embedded within many therapy interventions. Clients who do behavioral experiments or who use a continuum to rate their experiences can be asked a variety of informational questions about their rat-ings and observations. Then, they can be prompted to view these ratings with self-compassion (empathic listening), write down observations that seem helpful (summary), and ask themselves, "How can I use these ideas to help myself this week?" which is an excellent analytical/synthesizing question. For a more detailed discussion and exploration of how to link Socratic Dialogue with client worksheets, see Padesky (2020b).

Constructive use of Socratic Dialogue

In classic CBT, Socratic Dialogue is used to test out existing beliefs and to ex-tract learning from client experiences (deconstructive use). As part of their Strengths-Based CBT approach (SB-CBT), Mooney and Padesky demonstrate that Socratic Dialogue can also be used to help clients construct new beliefs or aspirations and evaluate their utility (Mooney & Padesky, 2000; Padesky & Mooney, 2012). When used to construct new beliefs or aspirations, mod-ifications in therapist behavior are made at each of the four stages (Padesky, 2019) as highlighted in the following sections.

Informational questions

Common informational questions when trying to help someone develop new beliefs or aspirations are "How would you like it to be?" or "How would you like to be/see yourself?" When asking questions meant to evoke new and desired possibilities, nonverbal aspects of Socratic Dialogue are as important as verbal ones. Clients tune into therapist nonverbal behaviors for guidance. If this question is asked by a therapist holding a neutral face or a furrowed brow, the person is likely to give a cautious response. If the therapist instead asks an aspirational question with sparkling eyes and an encouraging smile, leaning forward to demonstrate a keen interest in the answer, then the client is more likely to express a heartfelt wish.

Nonverbal body language is considered a key aspect of constructive use of Socratic Dialogue. Padesky emphasizes what she calls the "therapeutic smile" (Padesky, 2005):

> Imagine me asking with a calm, neutral face and tone, "How would you like things to be in your life?" Next imagine me asking with an inviting smile and softer vocal tone of deep interest, "How would you like things to be in your life?"
>
> (Padesky, 2019, 11)

A therapist's smile changes the entire context of this meaningful question. When asked by someone with a serious or neutral expression, it can be perceived as a challenge and even evoke anxiety or hostility in the client. Anxiety and hostility are linked to amygdalae activation of a fear or anger network, which puts the person in survival mode rather than a space of creative imagining. A genuine human smile activates the reward learning network and stimulates the amygdalae to generate a positive emotion instead of the fear/anger network (Mühlberger et al., 2010). The human smile also activates the orbitofrontal cortex (OFC) which, among other functions, is active in encoding and remembering reward experiences (Tsukiura & Cabeza, 2008).

A genuine human smile involves the eyes as well as the mouth. Vocal tones also change with a smile. Fortunately, when people are unable to see the therapist's face (e.g., if a client's eyes are closed, therapy is done by telephone, or the therapist is wearing a mask), people perceive auditory cues of a smile. Research demonstrates that people respond in the same ways to a smile that is heard and not seen (Arias et al., 2018).

Empathic listening

Once clients offer responses to constructive questions, therapists are encouraged to listen as a supportive ally rather than a neutral observer. In Strengths-Based CBT, therapists respond in ways that actively support client ideas rather than making neutral reflections of client responses. For example, a therapist might say with a big smile, "You'd like to be more connected to people. I can see how that would be so good for you!" When clients give more cautious answers, the SB-CBT therapist encourages clients to imagine the best possible changes as illustrated in the following dialogue:

Therapist: How would you like to be in your relationships?

Devante: I guess I'd like to be a little more ... friendly.

Therapist: Friendly (Smiling). I can see how that might be good for you! (Pause.) You know, when you say "friendly," I wonder if an image comes to mind of how you would look or come across. (Inclines head, looking curious with a slight smile.)

Devante: Uh. I dunno. I guess I'd walk up to people and seem interested.

Therapist: Interested. OK. (Smiling.) What else?

Devante: Well, I guess I'd maybe joke with them a bit.

Therapist: Okay. So you'd be friendly, seem interested, joke with them a bit. (Pause.) Since we're imagining the best ways you'd like to be,

	I figure we may as well dream big. (Smiling.) Is that the best you can imagine or is there even more?
Devante:	(Long silence.) I'm not sure more change is even possible.
Therapist:	Let's not get hung up on what's possible right now. We're just dreaming together about the best it could be (Smiling). If absolutely anything was possible, how would you like it to be?
Devante:	(Pause, then speaking quietly with heartfelt emotion.) I'd like to walk up to people with confidence. Like I really believed in myself. I'd like to think they were interested in me and happy to see me. It would be a real connection.
Therapist:	Wow. (Nodding head.) That would be really something, wouldn't it? (Said quietly with heartfelt emotion followed by a pause.) I'd sure like to help you get to that point of real connection. (Smiling with direct eye contact.)

Although Devante's initial answers were positive, he spoke them in a somewhat flat tone. His therapist was looking for Devante to have some enthusiasm or even a sparkle in his eye. By smiling at each response and encouraging him to say a bit more, she hoped Devante would begin to imagine even bigger changes. When Devante expressed skepticism that more change would be possible, his therapist added the language of "dreaming" of "anything possible." She also allowed silence, noting that Devante seemed to be thinking about her questions. In his final remarks of this session, Devante showed some deep emotion connected to his words. She tried to match his quiet emotionality and endorsed his dream both verbally and nonverbally.

Whereas deconstructive questions such as "What happened?" can usually be answered quite quickly, constructive questions such as "How would you like to be?" often require time for reflection. Therefore, silence is an important therapy intervention during constructive use of Socratic Dialogue. When questions require someone to generate new ideas or imagine different ways of being in the world, the most meaningful answers often require time for deep consideration. Thus, therapists who provide relaxed silence with occasional encouragement, "Take some time and see what comes to mind," are more likely to help their clients construct new ideas. I often recommend "friendly silence" in which the therapist holds a relaxed and open posture with a slight smile or expression of curiosity. It can be helpful to encourage clients to consider a question between sessions and see what ideas occur to them over an even longer period of time.

Like Devante, clients often express skepticism or self-criticism even while they are being asked constructive questions. When the current therapy goals are constructive, therapists are encouraged to listen for these negative comments and respond to them with redirecting constructive questions or comments. For example, if someone says, "I'm such an idiot," the therapist might respond, "When you see yourself that way, it can't feel good. If anything were possible, how would you like to think about yourself instead?"

Written summaries

When using Socratic Dialogue for constructive purposes, the written summary will capture *only* the constructive ideas offered by the client. Since aspirational dreams are often linked with imagery and metaphors, it is especially important that written summaries capture these as well. For example, later in the session excerpted above, Devante equated the connection he wanted to feel with others to the "Band of Brothers" feeling he had with fellow soldiers during combat. It was important to include that phrase "Band of Brothers" in the written summary. That one brief phrase connected to deeply emotional memories and experiences that closely captured many aspects of connection important to Devante. Other words only captured this essence in vague, intellectual ways that did not resonate with his deepest wishes.

Analytical and synthesizing questions

When using Socratic Dialogue to help clients construct something new, analytical and synthesizing questions often take a forward-looking perspective. For example:

- How much would you like this to happen?
- What would it be like for you to achieve this dream?
- If it/you were like this, what would you be able to do? Think? Feel?
- What qualities do you already possess that could help you achieve this?
- What would be a step you could take to try out this new way?

In addition to verbal responses to these types of enquiries, it can also be very helpful to ask clients to use their imagination to envision the answers. For example, you might say to your client, "Take a few minutes and imagine walking into a room of people. You are just the way you'd like to be and they are just the way you'd like others to be. Imagine the situation unfolding in the best ways possible." As elaborated in Chapter 5, use of imagination can capture emotions, physical sensations, memories, and metaphors often missed when enquiries and responses are purely verbal. As described for informational questions, analytical and synthesizing questions are enhanced when the therapist smiles when asking these questions, allows sufficient silence for a meaningful answer to emerge, and offers encouragement to the client throughout.

Keep in Mind: Constructive Use of Socratic Dialogue

When Socratic Dialogue is used to help clients construct new beliefs or aspirations, therapists are advised to modify their implementation of each stage:

- Therapist nonverbal behavior can be a determining factor in whether clients fully engage in constructive therapy processes.
- Aspirational questions are best when paired with a smile expressed in the eyes as well as the mouth to demonstrate keen interest in the answer.
- Pairing aspirational questions with a neutral therapist facial expression can evoke client anxiety instead of constructive imagining.
- People perceive and respond to auditory cues of a smile so therapist smiling is important even when clients cannot see the therapist.
- Therapists are encouraged to actively express support of client ideas as an ally rather than make neutral reflections of client aspirational statements.
- Silence is an important therapy intervention in order to give time for deep consideration of constructive questions such as "How would you like to be?" Allow for relaxed and "friendly" silences.
- Written summaries should include images and metaphors connected to aspirational dreams.
- Analytical and synthesizing questions often take a forward-looking perspective, such as "What could you do to try out this new way?"
- Use of imagery to imagine a better future can capture emotions, physical sensations, memories, and metaphors often missed when enquiries and responses are purely verbal.

Whether used in classic ways or for constructive purposes, Socratic Dialogue relies on the therapist's ability to conversationally blend questions that elicit relevant client experiences with empathic comments. Careful listening leads to more fruitful questions and useful summaries. Written summaries focus both client and therapist on the relationship between information gathered and the ideas being either tested or constructed. Analytical and synthesizing questions help guide the client to develop new ideas and enjoy the experience of discovery.

When to use Socratic Dialogue

As described in Chapter 1, Socratic Dialogue is likely to be used in every session but not in every moment of psychotherapy. In addition, it is often used when developing a collaborative case conceptualization and linking that conceptualization to treatment planning (Padesky, 2020c).

When to Use Socratic Dialogue

1. Debriefing between-session client learning activities, aka homework (beginning of session);
2. Exploring beliefs, behaviors, emotions, physiological reactions, life circumstances (middle of session);
3. Summarizing session learning; planning next treatment steps (throughout/end of session); and
4. Developing a collaborative case conceptualization and linking it to treatment planning.

When Socratic Dialogue is not helpful

Even the most elegant Socratic Dialogue is unlikely to be helpful when it is applied to evaluating beliefs or behaviors that don't play a central role in triggering or maintaining clients' issues. When Socratic Dialogue leads nowhere even when you follow the principles detailed in this chapter, consider whether you are targeting the most relevant aspects of your client's experience.

Trap 5

The therapist uses Socratic Dialogue appropriately but it is not helpful because it does not address the central and maintaining beliefs or behaviors related to a client's issues.

Collaborative case conceptualization is a good first step for identifying the most important triggers and maintenance cycles linked to client concerns (Kuyken et al., 2009). In fact, Socratic Dialogue is often embedded within collaborative case conceptualization. In a method I call "Box, Arrow In, Arrow Out", clients are asked to identify emotional, cognitive, behavioral, interpersonal, and situational triggers for a particular issue along with their responses to it once it is has been triggered (Padesky, 2020c). This method of case conceptualization guides clients to discover which of their cognitive, behavioral, interpersonal, or emotional responses are helpful and which actually maintain the issues they want to address. During the processes of collaborative case conceptualization, clients and therapists often become aware of triggers or responses that need to be addressed.

It is also helpful for therapists to have a good working knowledge of what types of beliefs and behaviors are usually central to common client concerns such as depression, anxiety, relationship problems, eating disorders, or other treatment targets. For example, with OCD it is much less likely to be helpful to use Socratic dialogue to evaluate an automatic thought such as, "I need to say a prayer to protect her when I think about my mother getting into an accident," than it is to test the more central underlying assumption, "If I have a disturbing thought, then that means something bad will happen." The remaining chapters of this book take a deeper dive into particular diagnoses, types of clients, and therapy processes to highlight how Socratic Dialogue can best be applied to central issues for each.

Summary

Socratic Dialogue can be a powerful tool for guiding client discovery and learning. In this chapter, you learned the 4-Stages of Socratic Dialogue process that emphasizes:

(1) informational questions,
(2) empathic listening,
(3) written summaries, and
(4) analytical/synthesizing questions.

Detailed guidance for how to effectively navigate these stages was illustrated in case examples throughout this chapter. This 4-Stage Model of Socratic Dialogue can help achieve a positive therapy alliance, maintain optimal client engagement in therapy, foster deep learning, and create a platform for consistent and memorable client discovery. It can support both deconstructive and constructive therapy processes as long as therapists adapt their verbal and nonverbal processes to the needs of each.

Therapists are encouraged to also attend to the 3 Speeds of Therapy and consider which ideas racing through their mind (1st—fastest speed) will be most beneficial to express to the client (2nd—slower speed) at any given moment in therapy. The ideas that the client will be applying or practicing between session (3rd—slowest speed) will often be at least partly generated by the client in response to analytical questions asked during Socratic Dialogue. Thus, the 3 Speeds of Therapy and Socratic dialogue can work together to keep the client's point of view always in the forefront of a therapist's mind.

While Socratic dialogue is not used all the time in therapy, it is a preferred method to actively engage clients to use their knowledge and experience to evaluate the beliefs, behaviors, emotions, physical responses, and environmental contexts central to their concerns. This process maximizes client learning, discovery and recall by providing frequent written summaries of client observations and insights. These written summaries provide a growing knowledge base to help each successive therapy session build on prior learning.

Reader Learning Activities

Now that the 4-Stage Model of Socratic Dialogue has been described,

- Notice and identify these four stages in vignettes throughout this book.
- Practice the elements of Socratic Dialogue as described in this chapter in your therapy sessions. It is often helpful to begin your practice by using Socratic Dialogue to debrief something the client tried or practiced between therapy sessions.
- Consider rating your use of Socratic Dialogue using the *Socratic Dialogue Rating Scale and Manual* (Padesky, 2020a), available from https://www.padesky.com/clinical-corner/clinical-tools/.
- Remember a CBT therapist does not always use Socratic Dialogue. Often therapists ask questions, listen, or make summaries just to clarify understanding of client communications. It is only necessary to use this 4-Stage Model of Socratic Dialogue in a systematic way when the goal of a dialogue is to actively test out beliefs or to foster client discovery.

References

Arias, P., Belin, P., & Aucouturier, J-J. (2018). Auditory smiles trigger unconscious facial imitation. *Current Biology, 28*(14), R782–783. https://doi.org/10.1016/j.cub.2018.05.084

Dalgleish T., & Watts, F. N. (1990). Biases of attention and memory in disorders of anxiety and depression. *Clinical Psychology Review, 10*(5), 589–604. https://doi.org/10.1016/0272-7358(90)90098-U

Del Re, A. C., Flückiger, C., Horvath, A. O., & Wampold, B. E. (2021). Examining therapist effects in the alliance–outcome relationship: A multilevel meta-analysis. *Journal of Consulting and Clinical Psychology, 89*(5), 371–378. https://doi.org/10.1037/ccp0000637

Epstein, S. (2014). *Cognitive-experiential theory: An integrative theory of personality.* Oxford: Oxford University Press.

Greenberger, D., & Padesky, C. A. (2016). *Mind over mood: Change how you feel by changing the way you think* (2nd ed.). New York: Guilford Press.

Iwamasa, G. Y., & Hays, P. A. (2018). *Culturally Responsive Cognitive Behavior Therapy: Practice and Supervision* (2nd ed.). Washington, DC: American Psychological Association.

Kuyken, W., Padesky, C. A., & Dudley, R. (2009). *Collaborative case conceptualization: Working effectively with clients in cognitive-behavioral therapy.* New York: Guilford Press.

Loftus, E. F., & Palmer, J. C. (1974). Reconstruction of automobile destruction: An example of the interaction between language and memory. *Journal of Verbal Learning and Verbal Behavior, 13*(5), 585–589. https://doi.org/10.1016/S0022-5371(74)80011-3

Mace, J. H., & Petersen, E. P. (2020). Priming autobiographical memories: How recalling the past may affect everyday forms of autobiographical remembering. *Consciousness and Cognition, 85,* 103018. https://doi.org/10.1016/j.concog.2020.103018

Mooney, K. A., & Padesky, C. A. (2000). Applying client creativity to recurrent problems: Constructing possibilities and tolerating doubt. *Journal of Cognitive Psychotherapy: An International Quarterly, 14*(2), 149–161. https://doi.org/10.1891/0889-8391.14.2.149

Mühlberger, A., Wieser, M. J., Gerdes, A. B. M., Frey, M. C. M., Weyers, P., & Pauli, P. (2010). Stop looking angry and smile, please: Start and stop of the very same facial expression differentially activate threat- and reward-related brain networks. *Social and Cognitive Affective Neuroscience, 6*(3), 321–329. https://doi.org/10.1093/scan/nsq039

Nienhuis, J. B., Owen, J., Valentine, J. C., Winkeljohn Black, S., Halford, T. C., Parazak, S. E., Budge, S., & Hilsenroth, M. (2018). Therapeutic alliance, empathy, and genuineness in individual adult psychotherapy: A meta-analytic review, *Psychotherapy Research, 28*(4), 593–605. https://doi.org/10.1080/10503307.2016.1204023

Padesky, C. A. (1983). *7-Column Thought Record.* Huntington Beach, CA: Center for Cognitive Therapy, Huntington Beach. Retrieved from https://www.mindovermood.com/worksheets.html

Padesky, C. A. (1993, September 24). *Socratic questioning: Changing minds or guiding discovery?* Invited speech delivered at the European Congress of Behavioural and Cognitive Therapies, London. Retrieved fromhttps://www.padesky.com/clinical-corner/publications/

Padesky, C. A. (2005, May). *Constructing a NEW self: Cognitive therapy for personality disorders.* 12-hour workshop presented London, UK.

Padesky, C. A. (2019, July 18). *Action, dialogue & discovery: Reflections on Socratic Questioning 25 years later.* Invited address presented at the Ninth World Congress of Behavioural and Cognitive Therapies, Berlin, Germany. Retrieved from https://www.padesky.com/clinical-corner/publications/

Padesky, C. A. (2020a). *Socratic dialogue rating scale and manual.* Retrieved from https://www.padesky.com/clinical-corner/clinical-tools/

Padesky, C. A. (2020b). *The clinician's guide to CBT using mind over mood* (2nd ed.). New York: Guilford Press.

Padesky, C. A., (2020c). Collaborative case conceptualization: Client knows best. *Cognitive and Behavioral Practice, 27*, 392–404. https://doi.org/10.1016/j.cbpra.2020.06.003

Padesky, C. A., & Mooney, K. A. (1993, February). *Winter workshop cognitive therapy: essential skills and supervised application to complex cases.* 24-hour workshop presented in Palm Desert, CA.

Padesky, C. A., & Mooney, K. A. (2012). Strengths-based cognitive-behavioural therapy: A four-step model to build resilience. *Clinical Psychology and Psychotherapy, 19*(4), 283–90. https://doi.org/10.1002/cpp.1795

Teasdale, J. D. (1996). Clinically relevant theory: Integrating clinical insight with cognitive science. In P. M. Salkovskis (Ed.), *Frontiers of Cognitive Therapy* (pp. 26–47). New York: Guilford Press.

Teasdale, J. D. (1997). The transformation of meaning: The Interacting Cognitive Subsystems approach. In M. J. Power & C. R. Brewin (Eds.), *The transformation of meaning in psychological therapies: Integrating theory and practice* (pp. 141–156). New York: Wiley.

Tsukiura, T., & Cabeza, R. (2008). Orbitofrontal and hippocampal contributions to memory for face-name associations: The rewarding power of a smile. *Neuropsychologia, 46*(9). 2310–2319. https://doi.org/10.1016/j.neuropsychologia.2008.03.013

Zemeckis, R. (Director). (2000). *Cast away.* [Film].Twentieth Century Fox.

3

Guided Discovery for Depression and Suicide

Marjorie E. Weishaar

> *If you try to give me solutions, I will dismiss you and if you agree with me that things are hopeless, I will kill myself.*
>
> **—Jamal, a depressed and suicidal client**

The dilemma posed by this client's statement captures some of the difficulties encountered in working with depressed and suicidal people. The reasoning is rigid, dangerously dichotomous, and not readily open to hypothesis testing. Collaboration is sometimes refused. Problem-solving, a mainstay in therapy with depressed clients, is compromised by client hopelessness and pessimism. This, in turn, can lead therapists to wanting to give advice and reassurance. How can one be Socratic and curious when the life-or-death stakes seem so high?

This chapter illustrates how guided discovery can reduce client hopelessness and help clients learn to unravel their own negative thinking. Case examples illustrate methods for navigating common traps in therapy for depressed and suicidal clients including times when therapists do more and more of the work rather than collaborating for the following reasons:

- Clients are shut down or passive in therapy.
- Clients display low energy with little motivation, or, in contrast, are agitated or ruminative.
- Clients have meager evidence to counter their negative thoughts and therapists feel stuck along with them.
- Therapists are unsure how to overcome persistent client hopelessness.

Depression Overview

Marianne is a single mother who works cleaning houses with two other women she employs. Due to an economic downturn, business has been slow. Marianne has had to stop employing the other women and now works alone. Lately, she has felt sad and guilty about firing the other women, anxious about the economy, and unable to see her way to a better future. She is able to get her children off to school in the morning, but then finds herself watching television all day and thinking about her life's regrets. Despite feeling extremely lonely, she does not want to see friends or even go to church, previously a source of spiritual strength for her as well as a connection to a caring community.

Marianne illustrates many symptoms of depression, a mood disorder characterized by profound sadness. Regret, guilt, a sense of failure, powerlessness, helplessness, hopelessness, irritability, and anxiety are often part of the picture. Social withdrawal, lethargy, and loss of interest in things previously enjoyed result from negative thoughts and expectations. Reduced engagement in life activities, in turn, fuels more negative feelings. Depressed thinking is slowed and inflexible, concentration and recall are poor, and errors in logic, or cognitive distortions, skew thoughts in a negative direction (Beck, 1967, 1976; Beck et al., 1979).

Just as there can be biological contributions to depression such as genetics, physical illnesses, brain injuries and drug reactions, there are cognitive ones as well. The negative beliefs and assumptions people have about themselves, other people, and the future can predispose them to depression. When these beliefs and assumptions get triggered by life events, people experience a shift in their thinking so that they pay attention only to information that seems to support their negative beliefs. Marianne, for example, had worked extremely hard for all she had accomplished in life. Her parents had given her little emotional or practical support growing up. Her positive beliefs about being self-reliant were also accompanied by beliefs that no one would help her and that she was responsible for other people. Thus, she felt helpless and especially distressed when she needed to stop employing the women who worked for her.

The shift in thinking that occurs in depression even includes negatively biased memories. As Marianne lay on the couch, she ruminated on other times in her life when she struggled financially. She dismissed her repeated triumphs over economic instability. Raising healthy children and being a good parent didn't even cross her mind when she judged her life. Her difficulty sleeping and loss of appetite contributed to her fatigue, and she had no interest in seeing other people. Her social withdrawal from friends and church became a problem itself, for lack of contact with other people prevented Marianne from obtaining new information and other perspectives on her situation. She was left alone with her negative, unchallenged thoughts, including negative judgments about how miserable she felt and how little she was doing. At her lowest, Marianne wondered whether suicide was the only way out of her unbearable pain, and imagined that her children could be raised just as well by her sister.

When depressed people become suicidal, the cognitive features of depression are even more pronounced to the point they become suicide risk factors. Marianne shows some of them. They include poor problem-solving, rumination (a never-ending litany of worry and remorse), cognitive rigidity (including perfectionism and all-or-nothing thinking), dysfunctional assumptions, overgeneralized memory (the inability to remember specific events, especially positive ones), and hopelessness (Wenzel et al., 2009). These risk factors become even more dangerous when paired with impulsivity.

This chapter illustrates how a therapist can engage depressed and suicidal clients and motivate them to stay in therapy despite these various challenges. At the same time, it considers how to manage the traps that present obstacles to engaging these clients in collaborative treatment. Next, it addresses the content of the depressed person's inner world and how guided discovery is used to help shift unproductive thoughts and actions. Finally, but crucially, the chapter addresses how to use guided discovery to keep a client safe when hopelessness and thoughts of suicide are present. Strategies for recognizing and managing the therapist trap of vicarious hopelessness are also described. To set the stage for these discussions, a brief overview of cognitive behavior therapy (CBT) for depression follows.

CBT for Depression

CBT for depression weaves cognitive and behavioral methods as needed throughout the course of therapy. Typically, behavioral interventions are begun first, particularly with more severely depressed clients who are inactive, lethargic, relatively isolated, and unable to concentrate for long periods of time (Beck et al., 1979; Young et al., 2008). Behavioral activation, a plan of gradually increasing the client's engagement in pleasurable and satisfying activities, is used to stimulate the client's interest in therapy (Wright et al., 2009), decrease avoidance of tasks or other people, decrease rumination (Dimidjian et al., 2008), and expose the client to experiences and information that contradict negative beliefs about themselves or their situation. The latter offers a powerful opportunity for guided discovery.

For example, as an experiment recommended by her therapist, one day Marianne took a short walk instead of watching a television program. This experience helped her begin to see links between her behavior and mood. Marianne noticed that even this mild exercise outdoors helped her feel a bit better. In this way, behavioral activation can serve as a form of affect regulation (Jobes, 2016). Other behavioral strategies include self-reliance training or assuming more responsibility for daily tasks and self-care, role playing in the therapy session to practice new behaviors, physical activity, and social contact (Young et al., 2008).

Behavioral experiments, tasks designed to examine a client's beliefs through in vivo exposure to new information or the use of new skills (Beck et al., 1979), are extremely important in CBT for depression. Behavioral experiments are not conducted simply to practice a new behavior (e.g., assertiveness, planning one's day), but to see whether a new way of thinking, revealed through new behaviors, is possible and helpful (e.g., "I can ask for what I want from him without arguing about it," "I was able to get shopping done because I planned for it."). In this way, they are an important method for guided discovery in a therapist's repertoire.

As described in Chapter 1, when behavioral experiments are designed to test specific beliefs they can enhance therapy's effectiveness because demonstration and personal experiences are usually more effective and memorable than verbal persuasion. Behavioral experiments influence cognitive change by testing old beliefs and, at the same time, providing information to support new beliefs. Behavioral experiments are usually debriefed using Socratic Dialogue, which can sharpen the focus on the examined belief and help make accurate interpretations and attributions of the results of the experiments.

Marianne met with a CBT therapist at her sister's urging. Her improved mood when she took a brief walk demonstrated to her that it might be a good idea to get out of the house and interact more with her neighborhood. Her therapist helped her identify some other behaviors, which Marianne agreed to try to see how they affected her mood. She chose to go to church one Sunday and stay for the coffee hour after the service. As Marianne discovered and began to pursue the activities that helped her mood, she and her therapist began to explore her negative thoughts and assumptions that seemed to contribute to her depression. Her thought "Unless I provide for my children, I am nothing" was important to examine. Marianne prided herself on being dependable and rising above poverty.

A therapist who was not familiar with Socratic Dialogue might try to convince Marianne that she was worthwhile even though she wasn't currently providing for her children economically. This would be tough to do, given her beliefs. Two other avenues seemed more helpful, taking into account Marianne's belief system described in the section "Depression Overview." The first was taking the long view and problem-solving what Marianne could do to help her family over time. She could ask for help to get her business back on a solid footing. This required testing her belief that she should not ask for help from anyone. Her therapist developed hypotheses which could be explored using Socratic Dialogue: if she were willing to have her sister look after her children, was she willing to ask for other kinds of help from her? What about asking others for work?

A second avenue was to look at all the ways Marianne could be and was dependable, even during this challenging time in her life. When could she better demonstrate her dependability than during tough times? How could she demonstrate her dependability now?

Examining a client's beliefs and assumptions is more likely to be helpful when the therapist maintains an appreciation of which thoughts and assumptions are helpful to test and which ones are important to maintain because they bolster the client. For Marianne, it was helpful for her to continue to see herself as a dependable breadwinner and not shift the focus away from that identity to something like how worthwhile she was as a person for other reasons. It was more productive to test her belief that dependable, self-reliant people must not seek help. In testing this belief, she was able to see that dependable people are able to use many resources, including other people. This was a new idea and gave her some hope she could resolve her difficulties.

In the depths of her depression, Marianne struggled to concentrate and stay focused on daily tasks such as making lunches for her children and getting them off to school. The structure of her CBT sessions, which included agenda setting, goal setting, behavioral assignments, frequent summaries, and continuous feedback between herself and her therapist, helped Marianne stay focused and organized. She was able to use these same skills outside of therapy to structure her day and complete tasks step-by-step.

The many skills learned in therapy—identifying triggers to low mood, testing negative thoughts and beliefs, and responding more adaptively to difficult situations—are reinforced throughout therapy. By regularly practicing these skills outside of session and using Socratic Dialogue to debrief these experiences in session, a goal of CBT is to make these skills an explicit part of the client's repertoire when therapy ends. In this way, the skills learned over the course of CBT also help clients prepare for and manage relapse. This is very important since depression is a recurring illness for many.

One challenging aspect of working with depressed clients is that, when you first see them, their faulty logic is air-tight. Depression oversimplifies. Therapy can be a frustrating endeavor if the therapist approaches depression without opening up the situation by being curious, asking a lot of questions and getting details. Just at the time when a client desperately wants an answer, the therapist must ask questions to get a clearer picture of the situation, how the client is thinking about it, what the client may have tried to resolve problems, what resources the client has, and how best to help the client discover these resources.

This is not an easy task, especially when a client's depression symptoms pose challenges for a therapist and the therapist's responses to these challenges trap them in unhelpful dead ends. For example, therapists run the risk of giving advice or becoming argumentative in response to clients' rigid thinking. Similarly, a therapist's ability to listen and empathize can be compromised if they feel too much urgency to alter a client's suicidal thinking. Further, a therapist may become overly talkative to counteract client silence or become hopeless in the face of a client's overwhelming pessimism. The following clinical examples demonstrate how Padesky's (1993) 4-Stage Model of Socratic Dialogue—informational questions, empathic listening, written summaries, and analytical and synthesizing questions—can help therapists and their clients get out of these traps.

Engaging Depressed Clients in Collaborative Treatment

One challenge for therapists working with depressed and suicidal clients is engaging them in collaborative treatment. Negative, rigid, and hopeless thoughts often lead clients to conclude there is no use in trying new things or testing out beliefs. Guided discovery methods provide helpful tools for achieving this goal as illustrated in numerous case examples throughout this chapter. Common signs that therapy is not currently collaborative include the following:

- A client frequently asks for advice and the therapist gives it.
- A therapist becomes frustrated when a client agrees with everything the therapist suggests, but does not follow through outside therapy sessions.

- A therapist becomes complacent and does less and less with a client who is inactive outside of therapy.
- The client is disengaged and the therapist gives advice or becomes overly directive or optimistic to add energy to their interactions.

Clients cannot be expected to understand how to collaborate in their own treatment unless the therapist educates them about this and shows how this can work and be helpful. Clients come to therapy with a model of treatment just as the therapist does. Identifying client and therapist thoughts and assumptions and evaluating their helpfulness can be key. Engagement is a continuous process throughout the course of therapy. The following questions, prompts, and suggestions can be used to begin to share treatment expectations and assumptions:

- How did you choose this type of therapy? What do you hope will happen as a result of being here?
- Have you been in therapy before? What was it like? What was helpful? What was not helpful? Did you learn skills to help your mood? Did you have things to work on between sessions?
- What have you heard about this type of therapy? What are your reactions to what you have heard?
- How would you feel about a give-and-take style of collaboration? Together we would come up with goals to work on and make a plan to accomplish those goals.
- Each time we meet, we will both contribute to an agenda or plan for our meeting in order to stay on track.
- We will measure your level of depression regularly so we can both track whether the approaches we are trying are helping.

Sometimes giving the client information about therapist expectations (e.g., "Together we'll come up with a plan that we both feel comfortable with and are committed to.") can lead to exploratory questions about their expectations. If a client has a belief that might interfere with collaboration such as, "I don't think I'm capable of doing very much in therapy," or "I can't do anything right, including therapy," the therapist and client can design a behavioral experiment to do in session and then debrief the experiment using Socratic Dialogue.

To increase collaboration, it is a good practice to always ask the client to identify items they want to add to the session's agenda. Frequent summaries during the session help the client and therapist stay on track and remember important information. In addition, the therapist can ask the client for feedback on a regular basis, including how the work done in session fits in with their goals or a belief that's being examined.

Common Traps in Engaging Depressed Clients in Therapy

Trap 1
Client is pessimistic from the outset and wants proof that therapy will work; the therapist feels challenged.

Trap 2
The client is too agitated to focus well; the therapist takes over.

When clients are highly skeptical or agitated, it can be more difficult to promote collaboration in initial sessions. The following two sections illustrate how guided discovery can help both types of clients in the initial phases of therapy.

Engaging the skeptical client in collaborative treatment

Stephen is a fifty-year-old engineer. He appears subdued in his first session and is unsure he is capable of doing the work of therapy. He reports having had periods of depression since adolescence, but the current episode is much worse than the others. He has a new boss at the engineering firm where he works who brought in his own hand-picked team of managers. Stephen was replaced as a manager and demoted despite doing very good work for many years. During his previous bouts of depression he says he just "forced myself to keep going" and eventually the depression subsided. The therapist has reviewed his history as well as the symptoms reported on Stephen's Beck Depression Inventory (BDI; Beck et al., 1961). His BDI total score was 25 which indicates a high moderate level of depression. In the following dialogue, his therapist explored Stephen's expectations and suggested a behavioral experiment to test these out.

Stephen: I've been depressed, off and on, for most of my life really. When I was young, I didn't know it was depression. I just thought there was something wrong with me. I'm on all sorts of medication. In the past, I would just pull myself out of depression by forcing myself to go to work and just get on with it, but this time is different. I just can't get over it. My psychiatrist says I need CBT.

Therapist:	How do you feel about that?
Stephen:	(Sighs.) I suppose I must.
Therapist:	You sound resigned.
Stephen:	I just don't know if it will do any good. Driving here today, I just thought, "What's the use?" Talking about my depression will only make it worse.
Therapist:	You're worried that just talking about depression will make you even more depressed.
Stephen:	(Nods and looks down.)
Therapist:	In the past, have you tried any type of psychotherapy in addition to taking medication?
Stephen:	Not really. My psychiatrist is trying his best with medication, but nothing seems to help for very long. He talks to me, but my mood doesn't get much better.
Therapist:	I can tell you've been trying to help yourself for a while. Did your psychiatrist tell you anything about CBT?
Stephen:	I heard I'll have to do homework.
Therapist:	Yes, it's true that we'll figure out things you can do between sessions to keep our work going. What do you think about that?
Stephen:	That sounds different from my understanding of therapy. I'm not sure I have the energy for that. I just thought I would talk and then you'd tell me what to do.
Therapist:	How would you feel about more of a give-and-take style, a partnership?
Stephen:	What do you mean?
Therapist:	Together we'd come up with a list of goals for therapy and decide what to work on. We'll work together to solve problems and see if there are new ways of viewing things.
Stephen:	It sounds like a lot of work. I'm not convinced it would help.
Therapist:	Would you be willing to try both styles right now to see what you think?
Stephen:	What do you mean?
Therapist:	How about telling me about your depression for about 3 minutes and I'll just listen. Then we'll see how that feels.

Stephen talks about how it feels to be depressed, why he thinks he's depressed, how he sees himself as a "brat" for complaining about life, and how he thinks his self-focus must be "narcissistic." As he talks more about being depressed, he looks downtrodden and weary.

Therapist:	Stephen, I'm going to stop you now and ask how you feel. Do you feel more depressed, less depressed, or about the same as a few minutes ago?
Stephen:	More depressed. Dwelling on depression makes it worse, but I can't help myself.

In the Therapist's Mind

Stephen appears quite skeptical about therapy. I decided to invite Stephen to talk for a few minutes since this is something Stephen thought therapy might be like: "I thought I'd talk and you'd tell me what to do." Next I described the CBT model of depression in a didactic fashion without referencing Stephen's specific thoughts, feelings, or behaviors. After this was tried for two minutes, Stephen reported feeling "spacey, numb, and absent." He said, "I wasn't really listening. After a while, I just tuned out and had more thoughts about my depression." Now I think the timing is right to portray a more active, collaborative approach and see how Stephen reacts to it.

Therapist	(Begins asking informational questions.) Let's try another way. You said you are a "brat" when you don't have the energy to do things, when you don't feel like working. To you, what is a brat?
Stephen:	A brat is a person who is spoiled, who is lazy and complains, and is bothered by the least little thing.
Therapist:	And what are you thinking about when you call yourself a brat?
Stephen:	Nothing is terribly wrong with my life. I should just suck it up and forge ahead. Instead, I feel bad that I got demoted at work.
Therapist:	You've worked hard for your company. Getting demoted feels like a loss. (*Empathic listening*)
Stephen:	Yes, it's hard for me to get my bearings, to feel I am valued at work. I feel bored there. And I feel angry.
Therapist:	All understandable. Because of what happened at work, you feel sad and angry. You are not sure of your value at work and you feel bored. (Stephen nods.) If your good friend came to you with this situation, what would you say to him? (Still asking *informational questions* but shifting his perspective so Stephen can step outside his current experience.)

Stephen:	I would feel bad for him and I would sympathize with his situation. Job changes can happen to anyone.
Therapist:	Would he be annoying for complaining?
Stephen:	No. I could probably tell he was shaken up.
Therapist:	Do you think you could give yourself the same degree of under-standing? (Trying an *analytical question*.)
Stephen:	I'm not sure. I'd have to think about it. I've never done that.
Therapist:	You told me earlier that you try to respond to your negative thoughts by being very rational, but not necessarily sympathetic, with yourself. Is that right? (*Informational question* about previous coping.)
Stephen:	Right. That's why I don't think I'll be very good at CBT. I try to be very rational on my own and it doesn't make me feel any better. I say, "No one else would be upset. Get yourself together."
Therapist:	Does that sound familiar to you? Did anyone talk that way to you?
Stephen:	Well, my parents were not warm or nurturing. Basically, they wanted me to be quiet and not bother them. They really believed in maintaining a stiff upper lip, as they say. I never saw them upset. When I was upset, I didn't show them. Because I knew they'd just tell me to "suck it up".
Therapist:	Was there anyone else, a relative or teacher perhaps, who was more compassionate? (*Informational question* about a different experience that is out of his current awareness.)
Stephen:	Yes, I would say I had many supportive teachers throughout my life.
Therapist:	Tell me about one of them.
Stephen:	(He pauses and reflects for a few seconds.) I remember one teacher when I was about seven years old, Mrs. Wetzel. Gee, I haven't thought of her in years. She was caring and supportive.
Therapist:	How so?
Stephen:	Well, as I've said, I was very talkative. (He smiles to himself.) I would ramble on about my latest interest and she would listen to me. She didn't shush me or tell me to go away. I realize now that I probably said very silly things, but she listened and was patient.
Therapist:	Were there any uncomfortable times with Mrs. Wetzel like if she had to discipline you? (How did they solve problems or how did he cope with uncomfortable feelings?)
Stephen:	I can't remember any. She would guide me to do things correctly, but not criticize me. For example, I struggled learning to read and she helped me by finding books I might really enjoy. She spent a

lot of time helping me become a better reader. (He pauses.) I think I might have even been depressed that early in my life and she saw that.

Therapist: How did she respond?

Stephen: She'd have me sit next to her when she read a story to the class. I would just sit there, but it made me feel cared for and close to her. I know this all sounds so simple, but it made me feel better.

Therapist: (Silent for a moment, letting him remember the good feelings.) When you think of how you felt learning from Mrs. Wetzel, is there anything that you can take from that experience and use in your life now? (*Analytical or synthesizing question*)

Stephen: Well, I'm not very patient with myself. I give up on a lot of things that might help me when I'm depressed and anxious—relaxation, for example—because I am impatient with myself. I expect myself to just get over this depression. Maybe when I'm trying a task I could think of her giving me all the time I need.

Therapist: (Nods and speaks gently.) You could choose a task and try to give yourself more time than usual. (Pauses.) By the way, are you feeling more depressed, less depressed, or about the same as a few minutes ago?

Stephen: I'm a bit less depressed. It's interesting what you just said about giving myself some understanding. I have to think about that some more.

In the Therapist's Mind

So far, only questions and empathic statements have been used to help Stephen identify feelings and to learn that he did not receive much comfort from his parents growing up. He reveals he did have some emotional needs met by teachers like Mrs. Wetzel. A summary at this point would consolidate that information and help him remember it in the weeks ahead. The notion of trying to be compassionate with himself is still mind-boggling to Stephen, so a written summary seems especially important. He could read that summary before the next session.

Therapist: Let's just write down a summary of where we are so far. Do you want to write it or do you want me to write it?

Stephen: I want you to write it.

Therapist: Okay, I'll write and you help me remember what we discussed. (Writing.) You suffered a demotion at work because your new boss brought in his own managers. You feel depressed, bored, and angry, but find it hard to have much understanding for your feelings, right?

Stephen: (Nods.) Right. My parents gave me no comfort when I was upset. They just couldn't deal with my sad emotions and would walk away from me.

Therapist: (Writing what he said.) And, so, what did you make of that?

Stephen: That I should not feel sad or it would drive people away. (Takes a deep breath.) But then Mrs. Wetzel let me be near her when I was upset. She took an interest in me, like some other teachers.

Therapist: Anything else?

Stephen: No, I think that's all I remember.

Therapist: It seems there was also the idea that maybe you need to give yourself more time and be more patient with yourself—like Mrs. Wetzel was.

Stephen: Oh, that's right. I already forgot that.

Therapist: Shall I write that down? (Writing, after Stephen nods.) That's good. How do you feel now compared to five minutes ago when we started this type of conversation. Better? Worse? Or about the same?

Stephen: I think a little bit better.

Therapist: Okay. I know we are just getting started, but let's compare the time you talked to me about feeling depressed with these last minutes in which we talked together about some experiences you've had that might help us figure out how to work with your depression. You seemed to feel a bit better when we talked together. Is there anything you notice about these two types of experiences? Is there a way this information can be helpful to us? (*Synthesizing questions*)

Stephen: I'm not sure. They're very different from each other. I really need to think about this.

Therapist: Okay. Well how about if you take what we wrote together and read it during the week before we meet again? Perhaps you'll remember information you'd like to add.

Stephen: Alright. I think I can do that.

Therapist: Is it okay if we shift gears? (Stephen nods.) Right now, I'd like to talk some more about both our expectations for therapy. Do you have any questions about what you've read about CBT or what I've said today?

Stephen: I don't want it to be too difficult. I don't feel very capable. Can we decide homework assignments together?

Therapist: It's a deal. You and I will decide together what we're going to work on and what you'll do between sessions. And I will keep checking with you to make sure you feel that we're making decisions together.

Stephen: That's good.

Therapist: I remember you started our session with some questions about how CBT could be helpful. Do you think you could give our work a fair trial and agree to work with me for six sessions even if you have more thoughts like, "Why bother?"

Stephen: I could try.

Therapist: In the meantime, we can work on figuring out some clear goals.

Stephen: Like what exactly?

Therapist   Well, how would you like things to be different?

In the Therapist's Mind

I shouldn't have asked it this way. This is too ambitious a question at this early stage. It is too difficult to be creative and constructive during the early stage of CBT when depression creates cognitive deficits. Plus, Stephen's sense of duty might make it hard to think about what he wants for himself. A more concrete question might work better.

Stephen: Right now, I can't imagine how I want things to be.

Therapist: Can you think of two or three things that, if we could bring them about, would make you feel better?

Stephen: I would like to find ways to deal with anxiety. I would like to feel less depressed. And I would like to find out what makes me feel happy. I don't think I've ever really learned to be happy.

Therapist: Those are good goals. (Writing them down on the summary sheet Stephen will take home.) Maybe for each of them we can identify some signposts that we are making progress. For example, what is one thing you'd be doing more of or less of in your life if you were less depressed?

Stephen and his therapist develop two or three signposts of change for depression and anxiety and agree to figure out signposts for happiness later when he is feeling a bit better.

Therapist: How do you feel if you imagine it's possible to reach these goals?

Stephen: Cautious, afraid to hope for so much change, but willing to try.

Therapist: When we started today you expressed doubts that you would be able to have the energy to do CBT. How do you feel about your ability to do CBT so far? You've identified some goals and have had a give-and-take discussion with me.

Stephen: I guess I can do this so far and I feel like I could tell you if I'm struggling.

In the Therapist's Mind

Stephen's goals can be made even more specific in future sessions. Right now, it's important enough that he can identify any goals. His caution and skepticism are useful, self-protective traits (e.g., caution may prevent him from jumping to conclusions; skepticism may help him be open to alternative views or willing to test an assumption). Further, he told me that he had been "persistent" on a project earlier in his life. All these characteristics can be harnessed for the good in future behavioral experiments and in testing out negative thoughts.

Engaging an agitated client

Some clients are so ruminative that therapists respond by trying too hard to find evidence that the client's beliefs are not true. The client's intensity is matched by the therapist's determination to challenge negative thoughts such as "I have done something terrible and deserve to be punished." A therapist may win the point, but lose the client's collaboration.

In contrast to depressed clients with slowed thinking, little energy, and reduced interest, agitated, depressed clients can have active ruminations that prevent them from focusing on the task at hand. They are so pre-occupied that they need redirection. Shea (1998) uses the term "caging" to describe how, in agitated depression, one's mind becomes trapped within a small network of themes. Such depressive ruminations "cage" or lock the person into their worries about the past, present, or future, thus preventing them from attending to and incorporating new information. Clients with agitated depression may return repeatedly to the same topic or ask the same questions again and again. It is particularly worrisome if their topic for rumination is suicide.

Sid had a severe, agitated depression. On his initial BDI (Beck et al., 1961) he endorsed the item "I have thoughts of killing myself, but I would not carry them out." He expressed suicidal thoughts in every session, and then minimized the therapist's concern about his safety by repeating that he would not kill himself. However, Sid did not seem engaged in listing his reasons for living, aspects of his life that remain stable and good, or things to do when he was trapped in ruminations. The thoughts that he deserved to die were persistent and continuous when he was not in therapy sessions. In session, Sid focused on trying to convince the therapist that he had done something really terrible and should be punished. He repeatedly said he could not tolerate the feelings of guilt and regret that plagued him. Sid's caging ruminations made it difficult to clarify the problem, much less begin to solve it. Even by session four, Sid remained stuck in ruminations.

Sid:	I did a terrible, terrible thing. I was unbelievably stupid. It's torture. Someone should put me out of my misery. I wish I could kill myself, but I have a lot of reasons to live. (He doesn't sound convincing about having a lot of reasons to live.)
Therapist:	Yes. Sid, could we return, for a minute, to your reasons for living? We began that list in our first meeting and you were going to add to it.
Sid:	Sure, sure. It's just that I ruined everyone's lives. Someone should just kill me. You have to admit that what I did is incredibly stupid.
Therapist:	I know you're in a lot of distress and that you feel trapped.
Sid:	Have you ever seen anyone as depressed as me? Have you ever worked with anyone who made a colossal mistake like me? Did they get better? Am I the most depressed person you've ever met? How does this therapy work? How can it possibly work?

In the Therapist's Mind

In order to know how to respond, I need to conceptualize what is going on. Is this the reassurance seeking of anxiety that should not be reinforced? Is he questioning my competence? Does he wish to feel special even in his depression? Is he feeling hopeless? Perhaps I can begin by asking Sid whether he is aware of his rumination. From there I can ask about how it functions for him (e.g., does he feel he has control over it, what are the consequences of thinking this way, how can he get out of his ruminative loop?). Focusing on the content of his worries and remorse might result in a debate with Sid about how bad we each believe his transgressions to be. The act of rumination is a problem in itself, so I will focus on that process.

Therapist: Sid, are you aware of how frequently you ask me these questions?
Sid: Yes, in every session, but it's really important to me to know I can get over this.
Therapist: I believe you have a very good chance of feeling better if we work together. So far, do you think I understand how you feel about what you did?
Sid: Yes.
Therapist: And do you think I understand how urgently you want help?
Sid: Yes.
Therapist: Do you think we can move on to figuring out some solutions?
Sid: Yes, alright.

When caging occurs, once the therapist has an idea of the client's intended message, it is okay, and often necessary, to interrupt and redirect. Make sure the client feels understood before moving to another topic. Interruption may not feel very Socratic, but you need to know whether there's a problem to be solved or whether mindfulness or affect regulation strategies would be helpful to calm the agitation.

After several sessions, Sid remained disconnected from therapy and his BDI score and suicide ideation were increasing. He was not engaged in treatment because, although his therapist was responsibly trying to reduce his suicide risk with a safety plan (Wenzel et al., 2009; Wright et al., 2009), a list of his reasons for living, a list of all the reasons for his decision at the time, and his identified advantages and disadvantages of forgiving himself, Sid's depressed mood was not improving. He tried repeatedly to convince his therapist of the severity of his transgression.

In the Therapist's Mind

Continuing to debate the seriousness of Sid's mistake is not helpful, however logical it may be, because Sid feels guilt and pain at a deeply emotional level. The punitive side of Sid, the side that triggers guilt for his misdeed, generally takes over between sessions because it is more emotionally charged than the side that will offer forgiveness. Rather than questioning his guilt, I think it might be more therapeutic to shift to the idea of earning self-forgiveness through reparations.

Sid: I made such a terrible mistake. How can I ever forgive myself?

Therapist: That's an important question. Do you think we could work on that?

Sid: I have thought about that constantly for months. There's no way I can forgive myself. How is that possible?

Therapist: Could we look at ways to resolve things instead of killing yourself?

Sid: I just can't let myself off the hook. Someone should just shoot me.

Therapist: Given that you feel such remorse, especially concerning your family, is there a way of making things right or at least better?

Sid: I did something really stupid.

Therapist: Would suicide fix that, would it make it right for your family?

Sid: No, it would wreck my kids' lives. I couldn't do that to them. They would remember me as the father who did the bad thing and then killed himself.

Therapist: Is there a way of making any reparations to those you hurt? Can you do anything to seek forgiveness?

Sid: I tried to take back the decision I made, but it wasn't possible. Now I just have to live in this hell.

Therapist: It sounds to me like there's a part of you that is bothered by what you did. Not the part that wants to punish you, but the part of you that values something you ignored. There's something you ignored when you made this decision. What values are behind your remorse?

Sid: I ignored how I was really feeling and I ignored the feelings of my family. I suspected it was wrong, but I put those thoughts out of my mind. This decision made sense to me financially and that's what I based it on. I had no idea that it would make me feel so unstable and lost. I don't want to lose my family's love and respect.

Therapist: Do you know of anyone else who did something terrible and then tried to make things better?

Sid: Well, you read about financial wizards who broke laws and then went to jail and "found religion" or started charities when they were released, but I doubt their sincerity.

Therapist:	Sincere or not, they tried to make some positive change. What about really, genuinely sincere people who tried to make amends?
Sid:	My friend Calvin has made big changes. He's a recovering alcoholic. He lost a lot of money and was arrested on drunk driving charges. Then he joined Alcoholics Anonymous. I surely don't know all that Calvin did wrong, but I do know that he's not drinking now and is working the program, as they say. That includes making amends to people he wronged. He told me that when he began his recovery, he just tried to do the next right thing.
Therapist:	What do you think of Calvin's changes? Is there anything in his story that helps you figure out what to do?
Sid:	I've tried rumination and it wears me down. I can't find a way out if I'm busy condemning myself and thinking of suicide. I want to make amends, but that would take a long time.
Therapist:	It would take a long time of doing the right thing.
Sid:	Yes, but I would be taking responsibility. I would be accountable.
Therapist:	How would you feel about yourself then?
Sid:	I'd be paying a price, no doubt. It would be difficult and painful, but I want to be better to my family. I want to make up for my mistake.
Therapist:	How would you start? What behavior could you try as a first step to making amends?
Sid:	I could apologize to those I have hurt.

Behavioral experiments can be used to implement the values that lie behind the client's remorse. If Sid didn't have some good values, he wouldn't feel remorse. In this case, Sid ignored his own emotional needs as well as those of his family. His behavioral experiment might include working on better communication with his family along with expressing more empathy for their feelings. Work on his belief that lifelong self-punishment was necessary would follow. For other clients, reparation might include amends made to those who suffered, charitable gifts to relevant organizations or service to others in a meaningful form. Making amends, a principle that can be enacted in many ways, can help foster self-forgiveness. Sometimes a therapist needs to accept the client's belief that he has done something seriously wrong instead of trying to reduce guilt by looking at evidence that his transgression is not so bad.

Activating depressed clients

Clients who are depressed tend to have low motivation and energy. This can lead therapists to fall into Trap #3 and abandon or poorly deliver treatment methods that are likely to help a client with depression . Some of the common situations that trigger therapists falling into this trap are:

- Clients say they have no motivation or energy to try a new behavior, so the therapist sets low expectations for what can be accomplished.
- Clients say they have already tried a behavior and it doesn't work, and the therapist becomes argumentative or drops a potentially useful intervention.
- Clients say they don't want anyone telling them what to do, and the therapist becomes less active in proposing treatment steps.
- Client say "maybe" they will try a behavioral experiment, and the therapist assumes they have low motivation for change.
- Clients say they can't try a behavior because it is not them (don't have the skills, the task seems far-fetched, can't imagine doing it) and the therapist can't think of a different behavior to try.

Trap 3

When a client has low motivation or energy, therapists can tend to be inactive or skip therapy steps. As a result, the client experiences therapy as ineffective because the dose of treatment received is insufficient to be helpful.

It is helpful to remember that client inactivity is often fueled by hopelessness, a low sense of self-efficacy, and low self-esteem. Clients who are depressed often inaccurately predict failure or criticism. It is also possible they have disengaged from therapy tasks because they have not agreed with the rationale for behavioral assignments. Ask the client the following questions to identify reasons for reluctance:

- What are the advantages and disadvantages of being more active, doing a specific behavior, or trying a new behavior?
- What negative predictions are you making?
- Can your negative predictions be framed as hypotheses to be tested?

- What alternative outcomes are possible?
- What thoughts, feelings, or circumstances are preventing you from trying these activities?
- How could you manage these obstacles?

Keep in Mind

- Behavioral activation, like all behavioral experiments, begins with an experimental stance. You are discovering together what helps and what doesn't help.
- Rather than being discouraged by client reluctance to increase or initiate activities, use guided discovery to increase client curiosity and motivation to test out whether and which activities can help boost mood.

Daniel moved to town a year ago and works in a restaurant kitchen. He misses the friends he left behind. He moved from a rural area with local customs, culture, and social activities to a city where it appears to him that life is fast-paced, jokes are sarcastic, and people are cynical. Although he knows some people from work, he feels lonely most of the time. He is depressed and somewhat socially anxious. When he is more depressed, he feels quite disconnected from others. Because he predicts rejection, Daniel has difficulty leaving his apartment or inviting anyone to do anything with him. In this session, Daniel begins to describe what he wants to work on in therapy by telling his therapist how behavioral activation has failed.

Daniel: I've been to three other therapists and they all tell me the same thing: I need to go out more. I go out to bars and parties and nothing happens.

Therapist: What do you want to happen?

Daniel: I want close friends. I want a relationship with a woman. But I just don't fit in. I try to do what other people are doing, but I'm not good at it. I feel like I don't belong.

Therapist: Can you tell me about a recent time you went out? What happened?

Daniel: I went to a party last weekend. I didn't like the people there, so after about fifteen minutes I came home and watched television.

Therapist: What happened to make you leave so soon?

Daniel: The people there were just talking about themselves. It was hard to get their attention. I feel like I have to make an impression quickly or I'll be rejected. But that's when I get into trouble.

Therapist: What do you mean?

Daniel: The guys I see who are successful socially are somewhat aggressive. I see them in the bars being kind of rude and uncaring to women. I try to be assertive like that, but I need to drink a lot first to be that way.

Therapist: And then what happens?

Daniel: I make sarcastic comments and jokes. I get up in their faces. But it doesn't work. I don't get the positive attention that I want, and I feel hung over and more depressed the next day. It works for other men. What am I doing wrong?

In the Therapist's Mind

Although it is tempting to help Daniel see that his "in your face" style could be off-putting, it might feel like unhelpful criticism to be told what he's doing wrong right off the bat, especially since he painfully knows it's not working. Instead, it may be more helpful to find out what has been successful for him in the past by asking informational questions. I need to learn: *What are Daniel's strengths? What has been his prior experience with social interactions? What does he like to do?* To focus on improving his behavior at this early stage would support his assumption that there is a simple formula for successful social interactions. Indeed, this could sound like the message he learned in his previous therapy, *"Just do x, and everything will work out well."*

Therapist: Daniel, I can tell you're feeling stuck and discouraged. It's difficult moving to a new place and finding people to do things with. I wonder if you could tell me about your life before you moved here. What did you enjoy doing?

Daniel: I liked to play the guitar; I still do. I like to read. I like dark and gritty films and television shows. Before I moved here, I shared an apartment with four other guys, so there was always someone around to do things with.

Therapist: Did you have a lot in common with those guys?

Daniel: Not at first. We would just go to the bar together and play darts or pool. But over time, they became my friends. We weren't exactly alike, but that made it interesting. As we spent time living together, as we were around each other, we just kind of drifted into friendship. Eventually, we got to know each other pretty well.

Therapist: So, over time, as you spent free time around those guys, friendship developed just because you were always around each other?

Daniel: Yes, I guess that's right. Then they started coming to hear me play the guitar on open mic night at the coffee shop.

Therapist: You played guitar in front of an audience? What was that like?

Daniel: I liked playing the guitar for an audience, either alone or with other musicians. I would get lost in the music. I would never do that now; I'm too self-conscious.

Therapist: When you lived with these guys, did you ever have to talk them into going out?

Daniel: Rarely, but when I did I'd say, "Come on, it's no big deal. Let's go see what's happening, shoot some pool, just get a beer."

Therapist: And how did your friends respond?

Daniel: It worked. We'd go out, sometimes for a little while, sometimes for hours.

Therapist: What goes through your mind these days when you're about to go out?

Daniel: I think, "Here's another miserable night. I have to do this to fit in and have friends."

Therapist: And how does that make you feel?

Daniel: Terrible. I do not look forward to going out to another noisy bar scene.

Therapist: So the prospect of going out with your friends back home was no big deal, but the task of going out these days is . . .

Daniel: HUGE. It's do-or-die. Every time feels so important. If I don't fit in, I'll be rejected again.

Therapist: Those stakes sound pretty high.

Daniel: Yeah. I want my life to be easier like it used to be.

Therapist: What do you think would be the best way to do that?

Daniel: I don't know. I'm trying as hard as I can. I keep trying the same things over and over again—going to noisy bars and large parties where I can't talk to anyone. I'm not sure how I could do things differently.

Therapist: Well, so far you've told me some of the things you like to do and you've told me how just spending time with the same people on a regular basis can sometimes lead to having friends. So already you've come up with two important things that would be different about going out: doing something you like and being with the same people routinely.

In the Therapist's Mind

Oh no. I just drew a conclusion for him, rather than guiding Daniel's discovery. I could have made a written summary to help Daniel come up with this idea. We could have made two lists: one of behaviors (e.g., spend time with people on a regular basis, do things you enjoy) or principles (e.g., view going out as casual rather than as a test, remember that people's differences make them interesting) that worked in the past when Daniel had friends in his old town. Then we could have made a second list of behaviors (e.g., get loud and confrontational to get attention, drink) or principles (e.g., get noticed quickly) that guide his behavior now. Then I could ask Daniel, *What do you notice about these two lists? How might this information help you now?* I think I'll keep the forward movement right now but I want to help him make a summary soon.

Daniel: I'm not sure I have anything in common with people here. I'm really different.

Therapist: Do you think anyone is getting to know you?

Daniel: Well, not these days. I don't really let people know me. I was so shocked by the way people talk to each other here that I decided not to get hurt. I feel like I hide my true self and try to be as cynical as other people just to fit in, but it doesn't feel like the real me. Still, my feelings get hurt when I don't feel accepted. I know it's my sarcasm they're rejecting, but it feels like they're rejecting me.

Therapist: So your feelings get hurt even though you're trying to protect your real, likeable self. Would there be any advantage of showing your true self, of doing things you like with someone?

Daniel: I don't know. I just think of all the disadvantages: I would have to make the effort to find someone to do something with, they might not like me, and my depression could get worse. If I show my true self, then I might find out that people really don't like me.

Therapist: I see how risky that feels. (Pause.) Might there be any *advantage* to showing your true self by doing something you like?

Daniel: Well, I guess it would make it easier to live with myself. I could just be who I am. Some people have liked me in the past. I just take all this rejection to heart. I wish it didn't make me so miserable. I just don't know if I feel like trying anymore.

Therapist: Can you imagine a way to think about socializing that would help you feel better?

Daniel: If I could find a way not to take it all so personally, that would help. It's hard to bounce back from rejection.

Therapist: You would like to take things less personally, maybe see some other explanations for people's behaviors, and bounce back from rejection. Is that right? (Daniel nods.) Is there a part of your life that you feel satisfied with or even feel good about these days? (*Informational question* to see how he thinks when he's feeling good about something he does.)

Daniel: Sure. Work is actually something I feel pretty confident about.

Therapist: You told me that when you first started your job, your food prep was not going very well. Is that correct? (*Informational question* to see how he overcame obstacles doing something he likes.)

Daniel: Yes, right. Everything that depresses me now was depressing me then, plus my work was not going well. It was awful.

Therapist: It sounds very disheartening. What kept you going?

Daniel: Besides the fact that it was my job to keep going, I knew I could cook from previous kitchen work. You know, when I cook for myself, I experiment. Even when my cooking experiments don't go well, it's still interesting. I decided to take the long view and told myself, "This is just the natural occurrence of bad and good. I will have bad outcomes and good outcomes. Sometimes I have to find out what doesn't work before I come up with a good recipe."

Therapist: That's interesting.

Daniel: Yeah, when I cook for myself I don't always get exactly what I predict, but I can still learn something I can use in some way later on.

Therapist: So how would you summarize what you learned from cooking?

Daniel: Experimentation is part of getting to be a better cook. Not every recipe will turn out well, but I learn from every dish I try.

Therapist: Those are interesting ideas. Let's write them down. (Pauses while Daniel writes. Then points to his summary.) Can you think of a way these ideas might help you right now in terms of socializing?

Daniel: I guess I could try some things that worked in the past and steer clear of things that haven't worked so well recently.

Therapist: What would that look like?

Daniel: I know you want me to go out and be my "true self," but honestly, that's too much of a risk. I'd like to stay away from bars and parties for a while. There's a neighbor of mine who plays the guitar. We've talked about playing some together. I think I could do that.

In the Therapist's Mind

Even though Daniel is mind-reading my position, it is not worth a debate. It is exciting that Daniel has come up with his own behavioral experiment and knows it is his own idea. I'm going to follow up on that instead.

Therapist: Do you have a prediction about what will happen?

Daniel: I think if I am more low-key with my expectations and how I act then I won't feel so devastated by any rejection. I know how to play the guitar and I'll just view this as passing the time with someone. Maybe it could be tolerable or even pleasant.

Therapist: Can you imagine yourself playing guitar with your neighbor?

Daniel: I can now, but by the time the weekend comes I might feel too tired to knock on his door and ask him.

Therapist: Is there anything you could do to increase the likelihood that you'll invite him to play the guitar with you?

Daniel: I guess I could ask him tonight if he's free to play this weekend. Also, I could choose some music to play.

Therapist: And what if he says he's too busy?

Daniel: I could try again sometime. Plus, I could go to listen to music at open-mic night at a coffee house this weekend.

Therapist: Those sound like good experiments. Let's write them down and problem-solve anything that might prevent you from doing them.

Daniel was able to use his experience as a short-order cook to talk about principles he learned from experimenting with cooking: to see what works, to be able to use something from each cooking experiment, and to take the long view that ups and downs are to be expected. The therapist could have just as well asked about his guitar playing to identify principles he used to help himself when learning a new song or technique.

Keep in Mind

- Clients can be asked about any life experience they find rewarding, pleasurable, or satisfying in order to identify principles that have helped them get through difficulties.

- The principles, not necessarily the exact behavior, can be transferred to their current situation to help them feel more capable and resourceful.

Although it appeared likely that Daniel would do his behavioral experiment, he did not. He said he did not invite his neighbor to play the guitar with him because he felt too depressed. Daniel and his therapist completed a 7-Column Thought Record to see what prevented him from trying the experiment. As described in Chapter 2, Padesky's 7-Column Thought Record (Greenberger & Padesky, 2016; Padesky, 1983, 2020) guides the client through a process similar to Socratic Dialogue. It asks someone to provide a description of the situation, their moods, their negative thoughts related to one of the moods, information used to support these negative thoughts, a search for information they hadn't readily considered that does not support their negative thoughts, and then create a balanced thought or synthesis of the evidence provided before rerating their moods.

Daniel's therapist helped him begin to fill out a 7-Column Thought Record for the situation during the past week when he decided to stay home rather than ask his neighbor to play the guitar with him. Daniel reported he felt depressed, disappointed in himself, and discouraged. Compared to the time when he felt most depressed, he rated his depression in that situation at 75%. Daniel's most powerful or hottest automatic thought linked to his depression was "I can't make friends, so why try?" Other thoughts related to his mood were "He'll reject me" and "I am no fun to be with."

Therapist: Daniel, let's take a look at the thought you said made you most depressed this week. You said it was, "I can't make friends, so why try?" Is that right?

Daniel: Yes, it's useless.

Therapist: And is this the thought that prevented you from inviting your neighbor to play the guitar?

Daniel: Yes, I'm no fun to be with and I thought he would give me the brush off.

Therapist: OK. So this idea you can't make friends sounds like the hot thought then. How about circling that thought in your Thought Record? (Daniel circles his hot thought in *column 3* of the Thought Record.)

Therapist: I can see how that thought really discouraged you from trying. Now, what makes you believe this thought? What's the evidence that it is true?

Daniel: I haven't made friends so far.

Therapist: Okay, that goes in the column of evidence that supports your thought (*column 4*). Do you have any other evidence for that thought?

Daniel: Other people seem to know what to do.

Therapist: Is that evidence about your ability to make friends?

Daniel:	Not really. I can't think of any other evidence.
Therapist:	What about evidence that does not support the thought, "I can't make friends, so why try?"
Daniel:	Well, I should be able to make friends. (This is another automatic thought.)
Therapist:	That sounds like another thought that might make you feel discouraged. What about evidence from the past or present that suggests you can make friends?
Daniel:	I had friends before I moved here.
Therapist:	Okay. Let's write that in the column of evidence that does not support your negative thought (*column 5*). What helped you make friends in the past?
Daniel:	It took a while, but we did things I enjoy like play darts and shoot pool and listen to music.
Therapist:	Any other evidence that you can make friends?
Daniel:	Well, some people have asked me to do things with them lately, but I don't know if they will become close friends.
Therapist:	Oh, so some people have maybe wanted to be friends with you, or at least do something together.
Daniel:	Yes. (Daniel pauses as this new information registers.)
Therapist:	Let's write down who and what in column 5. (The therapist pauses while Daniel writes down the two examples as shown on Figure 3.1.) Have there been any other friendly gestures from people?
Daniel:	My neighbor always says hello. And people at work sometimes take a cigarette break with me. Shall I write those down? (The therapist nods and Daniel writes.)
Therapist:	When you look at these two lists: evidence that supports your thought and evidence that does not support your thought, is there a way of putting them together to help you? (*Synthesizing question*)
Daniel:	Well, I was able to make friends in the past by doing things I'm not doing now, things I enjoy doing. Plus, sometimes I don't always notice when people are trying to be friendly; that could be a problem.
Therapist:	When you reconsider the thought, "I can't make friends, so why try?", in view of this evidence, what do you think?
Daniel:	It might not be totally true. I guess if I give it some time and am willing to do things with people, I might make some friends here.
Therapist:	Let's capture that new thought in column 6. How would you say it?
Daniel:	I guess I had a defeatist attitude this week. I think my neighbor is a pretty good guy, so even if he can't play guitar with me, he wouldn't be rude about it. I could try again.

7-Column Thought Record

1. Situation	2. Moods	3. Automatic Thoughts (Images)	4. Evidence That Supports the Hot Thought	5. Evidence That Does Not Support the Hot Thought	6. Alternative/ Balanced Thoughts	7. Rate Moods Now
Tuesday night after therapy. I decided not to call my neighbor to play guitar together.	Depressed 75% Disappointed in myself 50% Discouraged 70%	I am no fun to be with He'll reject me I can't make friends, so why try?	I haven't made friends so far Other people seem to know what to do	I had friends before I moved here In the past it took a while but we did things I enjoy like play darts, shoot pool, listen to music Some people have asked me to do things with them lately My neighbor always says hello People at work sometimes take a cigarette break with me	It takes time to make friends and it's worth it to try again	Depressed 50% Discouraged 50%

Figure 3.1 Daniel's 7-Column Thought Record (adapted with permission).

Therapist: If you feel reluctant, what could you do to help yourself?

Daniel: I guess I could remind myself that it takes time to make friends and it's worth it to try again. That's kind of what I learned in the past when things went well.

Therapist: Why don't you add that idea to column 6 of your thought record? (Waits while Daniel writes the thought in *column 6* of Figure 3.1.)

Therapist: How are you feeling now?

Daniel: A little less discouraged and less depressed, more like 50%.

Daniel began therapy feeling frustrated by other people's suggestions about what activities to do to feel better. By identifying what he enjoys doing, he began to feel that change was under his control. Behavioral experiments became easier to consider when he designed them with the attitude borrowed from what he's learned as a cook: experimentation leads to new learning. Finally, learning to use a 7-Column Thought Record helped Daniel use guided discovery with himself. In these ways, he became more responsible for his progress and more prepared to recover from possible setbacks in the future.

When clients generate meager evidence to counter a hot thought

Completing a 7-Column Thought Record well enough that the client is able to generate an alternative or balanced thought that is believable to them on their own often takes weeks of practice. For more information on how to help clients develop these skills, see Padesky (2020). While clients are building these skills, therapists will be reviewing and helping clients fine-tune these thought records in session. Therapists can use questions and summaries to help clients learn how to construct more balanced thoughts that take into account all the evidence. In the following case example, the client did not believe her balanced thought because she had very little evidence to counter her hot thought, "I can't do this."

Roz had to write a report for the social service agency where she worked summarizing a survey done by the agency on people's needs in her community. She was overwhelmed by both the task and how destitute many people were. She felt incapable of writing the report and was pessimistic that it would have a positive impact on people's lives. She completed a 7-Column Thought Record at home, but said it made her feel worse because her balanced thought, "I CAN do this," was not believable to her. Of the two automatic thoughts on her thought record, "I can't do this" and "This report will do no good," she chose to work on the first with her therapist. She could not think of evidence that she was capable of the task. She had low energy and every time she thought of all that would go into the report, she felt incompetent and avoided writing. The more she procrastinated, the less capable she felt. Her therapist asks Roz for evidence that did not support her hot thought.

Therapist: (*Informational questions*) Roz, let's take a look at your balanced thought, "I CAN do this." How much do you believe that?

Roz: Not much, but I think that's what I should be thinking if I want to get the report written.

Therapist: 0%? 50%? How strongly do you believe it?

Roz: Maybe 5% at the most.

Therapist: Well, let's go back to the evidence and see whether there's a different view that could help you. Tell me about this report: what's it about, what do you have to include, how long is it supposed to be, all that. (*Informational questions*)

Roz: It's not that long. It's a list of statistics that I already have and some summary paragraphs about what the statistics mean. I should be able to do it, but I just can't.

Therapist: Have you ever written a report like this before?

Roz: Never. Tom in our office used to do it, but this year they asked me. I have no idea why, or how to begin.

Therapist: Do you think Tom would be willing to discuss how to prepare the report with you?

Roz: I don't know. I think he might be offended that they asked me rather than him. But, frankly, I don't know how to begin and he probably does.

Therapist: If Tom doesn't want to help you, is there anyone else who could give you some tips?

Roz: Our office assistant, Lucy, has seen dozens of these reports over the years. She could probably tell me what to include. Yet, even with that information, I feel exhausted just thinking about writing the report.

Therapist: Ok, so let me see if understand. You have never written a report like this before, but Tom and Lucy are familiar with such reports and might be able to guide you a bit. Still, it's hard to imagine having the energy for this project.

Roz: Right. Plus, I think I should want to write the report and I don't. I'm not that interested.

Therapist: I agree that it's hard to make yourself want to do something. Have you ever done anything you really hated to do?

Roz:	Yes, yard work. I loathe mowing the lawn and doing the weeding, but I do it.
Therapist:	How do you feel afterwards?
Roz:	Like I've won the lottery.
Therapist:	(Laughing.) What do you make of that?
Roz:	Well, sometimes the payoff comes at the end, I guess. Even something difficult can give a sense of satisfaction in the end I suppose. But yard work is not the same as writing a report. I have to think and be organized while writing a report.
Therapist:	Do you have any experience doing something in an organized way that was not enjoyable?
Roz:	(Thinks a minute.) I was in charge of my daughter's cookie sales for her scout troop. That was a real headache, but it turned out okay.
Therapist:	How did you manage to do it?
Roz:	Well, just like the yard work, I was systematic about it. I had various steps to go through: keep track of the orders, collect money, pick up the cookies at the warehouse, distribute the cookies to the scouts, and so on.
Therapist:	(*Summary*) Let's summarize what we've talked about. You don't have experience writing a report like the one you are writing now. However, you have experience doing difficult tasks that are not much fun, including tasks that require organization. Can we use any of this as evidence that doesn't support your hot thought?
Roz:	Yes, I see the connection. I don't have to love this report to work on it. I have done difficult things in the past—yard work, managing the cookie sale—by being systematic and going step by step. Also, perhaps Tom and Lucy can help me. (Roz lists these facts in the column of evidence that doesn't support the hot thought.)
Therapist:	What would be a balanced thought based on all the evidence in columns 4 and 5?
Roz:	This report is a real challenge, but perhaps Tom and Lucy can get me started. Also, I know how to be systematic even when I'm not especially motivated.
Therapist:	How much do you believe this balanced thought?
Roz:	About 70%.
Therapist:	And how much do you now believe the thought, "I CAN do it."
Roz:	About 50%
Therapist:	How can you use these ideas help you this week?
Roz:	I need to figure out a way to remember them.
Therapist:	Can you think of a way to do that?

Roz: (Quiet for a minute.) I'd like to write them on a card to keep in my purse. Also, I'd like to work on a way to approach Tom to ask for his help. I'm not afraid to approach Lucy.

In this instance, her therapist was able to help Roz find evidence that did not support her hot thought. Other times, clients can face situations when most of the evidence supports their hot thought. For example, perhaps the client has a hot thought, "I can't do this report" and they truly do not have the requisite skills or the ability to learn them in time. When all the evidence supports a hot thought, this means the hot thought is a problem that needs to be solved. In that case, an action plan is needed. Once an action plan is formed, the client will often feel better, as Roz did when she made her plan to speak to Tom and Lucy. Guided discovery does not rely on always discovering cognitive errors and correcting them. Solving problems is also a good strategy.

Hopelessness

Each of the following common occurrences in depression treatment can be linked to client hopelessness. In turn, each can trigger therapist hopelessness or contribute to therapist discouragement about the client's treatment prognosis.

- A client seems disengaged from therapy (e.g., does not do homework) and the therapist assumes the assignment was too hard or client motivation was too low and so does not explore their reasons for not doing it.
- A client misses sessions without an understandable external cause, and the therapist is resigned to that happening.
- A client asks, "What's the use?" and the therapist gives them reasons to try.
- A client frequently says, "I don't know," and seems disinterested in figuring things out, and the therapist loses motivation.
- A client focuses on self-harm and/or suicide in or outside sessions, and therapist anxiety begins to interfere with treatment

Following these types of therapy circumstances, therapists sometimes think, "How can I help someone who doesn't want to help themself?" and "If they don't do the homework, I can't be effective." These thoughts are warning signs of the fourth common trap in depression treatment, therapist hopelessness and disengagement.

Trap 4

Therapists become hopeless in the face of client hopelessness and lose motivation to stay engaged and collaborative, and to continue active problem solving.

Client hopelessness is to be expected when working with depressed and suicidal clients. Therapists can use guided discovery methods to actively engage clients in identifying and investigating the beliefs and behaviors that maintain client hopelessness, and also in exploring their own hopelessness. In this regard, Fennell provides some useful guidance (Kennerley et al., 2010, 71) and encourages therapists to hone the skill of decentering from their own hopeless cognitions in order to develop a stance of curiosity concerning their own mindset.

Keep in Mind

- Clients need to believe it is possible that their efforts and your efforts can help.
- The experience of therapy being helpful is more powerful than discussions of its helpfulness.
- Hopelessness can be chronic ("I am a complete failure") or acute ("There are current insurmountable problems that I cannot tolerate"). It is helpful to know which one you are dealing with, for chronically held beliefs can require patient use of guided discovery over time (see Chapter 6) and acute hopelessness may respond fairly quickly to problem-solving.
- Hopelessness is linked to suicide risk, self-harm, and therapy disengagement. Ask the client to put their hopelessness into words.
- Find out what types of evidence would be meaningful to the client in pursuit of harnessing hope (e.g., improve a concrete problem, demonstrate that change is possible, or reach a clearer understanding of what the problem is).
- Therapists can grow hopeless too, and these cognitions can be addressed using the very same strategies that we employ with clients.

Make a safety plan with suicidal clients

When clients are at risk for suicide it is important to develop alternatives to suicide as well as to make a safety plan for what they will do if they start thinking about suicide during the week. Safety plans are an evidence-based suicide prevention intervention (Stanley & Brown, 2012; Stanley et al., 2018). *Guided discovery methods* paired with more direct problem-solving are ideally suited to developing alternatives to suicide and making safety plans as the following case example illustrates.

Jamal has returned to college following a year-long medical leave after a suicide attempt. In the first few sessions, he told his current therapist about his attempt to kill himself as part of an assessment of his current risk. He had failed a course in the spring and then gone on a high-powered internship over the summer break. During the summer, he shared an apartment with a good friend from school, Roy. He found the internship exhausting and overwhelming, but thought that speaking up (e.g., talking to his supervisor to clarify instructions, admitting that he didn't know how to do something) was asking for too much help and would indicate weakness. He believed if he could not do his work completely on his own, then he was a failure. As his depression worsened, Jamal was less inclined to share his misgivings with anyone, including Roy. Drinking alcohol helped him numb out his emotions, but the next day he would struggle at work. He took an overdose of prescription medication after Roy left for work one morning, but was still alive and was found when Roy returned home that evening.

As further context, Jamal reported that his father has high and inflexible expectations for Jamal's achievement and demands he do very well in school. After gathering this information, Jamal's therapist decided that she wanted to get Jamal's agreement to collaborate in preventing another suicide attempt. She also imagined Jamal might want to have goals to manage his mood and decrease his hopelessness. However, she recognized it was important that Jamal collaborate in the formation of these goals.

In the Therapist's Mind

Working to prevent suicide and restricting access to lethal means are nonnegotiable, but the conversation must be reciprocal, especially since Jamal has felt coerced and powerless in the past.

Therapist: Jamal, the last time we met, we started setting some goals for therapy. We agreed to make a safety plan for when you're feeling suicidal.

Jamal: I haven't felt that way in a while. I think about it, but I wouldn't do anything. Why should I work on that now? I really don't want to think about it.

Therapist   (Providing a rationale.) I'm glad you're not feeling suicidal. Things are not so stressful now, but they might get stressful at some point in the future. Now is a good time, while your mind is clear and your mood is stable, to think things through and come up with some ways to keep you safe if you do feel suicidal. Let's write them down so that you can keep the safety plan with you.

Jamal: (Shrugs. Looks down.)

Therapist: How are you feeling right now?

Jamal: I don't know. (Therapist waits.) I don't really care. I don't know if I'll get better, so I might want to keep suicide as an option if things don't work out for me. If I work on a safety plan with you, I'll have to give up on suicide.

Therapist: It's hard to give up on suicide when you can't imagine another solution. What if we could come up with something else to do when you're feeling so awful?

Jamal: (Silence. Slowly shakes his head from side to side.)

Therapist: Jamal, it looks as though you're torn, like part of you wants to live and part of you wants to die. (Jamal nods.)

Therapist: (Writing.) What does the part that wants to die say?

Jamal: If I were dead I would stop being a disappointment to my father. That's the main reason. What's the point of living if you can't be a success?

Therapist: Do you have any other reasons for dying?

Jamal: Life feels too hard. And I'm sick of being depressed.

Therapist: Okay, I'm writing these down. Anything else?

Jamal: No, that's it.

Therapist: What about the other part of you? What does the part that wants to live have to say?

Jamal: Well, my dog needs me.

Therapist: Tell me about your dog.

Jamal: My dog belongs to the whole family, but she is really mine. She loves me best and I take the best care of her. I know what she likes to eat, I know her favorite places to go for a run, and I know how to train her. She kept me company when I was at home last year.

Therapist: You and your dog are close companions. You would stay alive to take care of her.

Jamal: Yes. Also, Roy has stuck by me. Sometimes I feel guilty that he's the one who found me, and yet he is still a good friend. He still likes me for some reason. I would not try to die on him again.

Therapist: Jamal, in addition to your solid connections to Roy and your dog, do you have any other reasons to live that are based on what you might want for yourself?

Jamal: Sometimes—rarely—I think I could do something with my life, not in computer science or medicine like my father wants, but something I want to do. It's hard for me to sort it out, because I'm so confused. I might as well be dead if I can't even decide what I want to do with my life. I have failed at everything my father wanted me to do. Every time I had a problem in school he'd tell me what to do and it didn't work. At this point, if you try to give me solutions I will dismiss you and if you agree that everything is hopeless, I will kill myself.

Therapist: Jamal, I am so sorry for what you've been through. Even in the depths of depression you have kept Roy as your friend and also taken care of your dog. I want to help you arrive at solutions that work for you. (*Empathic listening*) Could we look over the main points you've said so that we can both remember these important parts of your experience? (Jamal nods.) (At this point, the therapist shares the two written lists: reasons for dying and reasons for living.) Right now, part of you wants to die because life feels hard and you don't want to disappoint your father over your schoolwork. There's another part of you that wants to live. That's the part that feels close to Roy and loves your dog. It's also the part that wants to do something you choose with your life, whatever that thing is, still to be determined.

Jamal: Yes, to be determined by me. (Jamal relaxes a bit.)

Therapist (Continues with summary.) How do you think these lists can help us in therapy?

Jamal: I have no idea.

Therapist: Well, I'm wondering if we can make your life feel a bit easier by making a plan, like a safety plan, of things that could make you feel better when you're thinking about these reasons for dying. Would that help?

Jamal: I guess so.

Before evaluating any particular reason for dying, it helps to hear the whole list of reasons. Jamal's mood shifted rapidly from talking lovingly about his dog and his comradeship with Roy to expressing deep hurt and anger when his core belief "I am a failure" was triggered. This indicates that more than problem-solving might be needed to deal with his hopelessness over time. It could also help to begin identifying Jamal's strengths. Surviving a suicide attempt usually requires some wherewithal. Surely he exercised some strengths to accomplish that. Identifying strengths grounded in the reality of the situation conveys empathy and begins to help someone recognize their capacity to survive. His therapist can become more hopeful and Jamal might see himself as more resilient as Jamal's strengths are identified.

Finally, when constructing a safety plan, it is fine for the therapist to contribute to the list of alternative activities the client could do when having suicidal thoughts, both by asking questions and by offering suggestions based on knowledge of the client's life. Cognitive rigidity often prevents depressed clients from creatively constructing alternatives for themselves when they are having suicidal thoughts.

Client misses a session

As part of developing his safety plan, Jamal and his therapist worked on recognizing his personal warning signs of increased hopelessness and suicidal thinking. The need for this was apparent when Jamal missed a session without an understandable excuse. His absence also offered an opportunity for problem-solving.

Therapist: Jamal, can you tell me about missing our last appointment? I know on the phone you said you overslept. Is there anything else that got in the way of being here?

Jamal: (Looks down. Shrugs. Long pause.) I don't know.

Therapist: Is there anything I said or did that rubbed you the wrong way?

Jamal: No.

Therapist: Did something happen this week to upset you?

Jamal: I don't know. (Shrugs. Pause.) I got a call from the academic dean. Because I took a leave from school, the dean wants to work out a plan with me to check on my academic progress this semester. I have to go to her office every two weeks to review how I'm doing.

Therapist: How do you feel about that?

Jamal: I don't need her help. I can make it on my own. I signed up for extra courses this semester so I can get through school faster and show everyone I can do the work.

Therapist: So far, how are you finding the work load?

Jamal: I can't get it all done, but I need to.

Therapist: In the past, what happened when you couldn't get your work done?

Jamal: I got panicky, I started skipping classes, and then I gave up. It was hopeless. I don't want to feel overwhelmed like last time.

Therapist: Let me see if I understand the problem. It sounds like you're not sure how you'll get your work done. You want to do well, even take extra courses, but not get overwhelmed. (Jamal nods.) Let's look at the alternatives. What are some solutions that come to mind?

Jamal: I will just work harder. I used to cheat, but that just backfired and I felt stupid.

Therapist: Any other ideas besides working harder on your own without help?

Jamal: I can't think of any. I want to pass all my classes without asking for help. Smart people don't need help.

Therapist: Do you remember watching any students who did well ask for help to get their work done?

Jamal: Yeah, there was this girl in my computer science class who did well. She was very smart. Everyone knew her because she organized a study group and went to all the review sessions. Roy also did well in his courses. I envied his grades. I always thought he was just naturally good at writing, but he told me he got help at the Writing Center. He even went to meet with a couple of his professors when he had questions about lectures.

Therapist: That's interesting. So, as smart as they are, the girl from computer science and Roy both went to other people while studying. What do you make of that?

Jamal: Maybe they weren't so smart.

Therapist: That's a possibility. Anything else?

Jamal: Maybe even smart people can use help?

Therapist: When you look at Roy and the girl from computer science, how do your observations fit with your idea that you must work alone in order to succeed? (*Analytical question*)

Jamal: Well, I guess getting some help is okay if it worked for them. But I don't know if I have the time to go to review sessions and other things because I am so busy. I am taking so many classes. Maybe I should drop a course.

Therapist: Could we put some of their solutions, like going to meet with professors, going to review sessions, or being part of a study group on
the list of possible solutions?

Jamal: I don't think those solutions would work for me. I feel like you're
telling me I can't do the work.

Therapist: I want to list as many solutions as we can. Then we can look at the
advantages and disadvantages of each of them and you can decide
which ones you might be willing to try.

Jamal: Okay.

Therapist: (After a bit more discussion.) When you look at the list of solutions—
working harder on your own, getting help from review sessions,
asking the professors questions, being part of a study group, or
making a plan with the dean to drop a course if need be—which
solutions seem most useful to you?

Jamal: Working on my own or making a plan with the dean just in case my
schoolwork gets tougher.

Jamal and the therapist write down the advantages and disadvantages of the
two solutions that seem most viable to him. Working alone without help has
the advantage of making Jamal feel capable if all goes well, but the disadvan-
tage of making him feel like a failure if he starts to struggle. Working out a plan
with the dean has the advantage of potentially helping him get the work done
with reasonable expectations, but might make him feel less independent.

Therapist: What do you think of these two solutions when you anticipate
trying either one?

Jamal: I think I really want to try to do this on my own, but I could talk to
the dean about a back-up plan, like maybe dropping a course if
I need to.

Therapist: Can you see yourself talking to the dean about a back-up plan in
your meeting?

Jamal: Yeah, in fact the dean mentioned that when she saw how many
courses I'd registered for.

Therapist: How are you feeling about the meeting now?

Jamal: Still not crazy about having to do it, but I can go to it.

Therapist: Okay. Is it alright to get back to talking about hopelessness?

Jamal: If we have to.

Therapist: You know those panicky and overwhelmed feelings you were
talking about?

Jamal: Yeah.

Therapist:	They sound like warning signs that you are feeling worse.
Jamal:	Yeah, I had them before I took the pills. I started to have them this week too, when I knew I'd have to see the dean.
Therapist:	When you have these feelings, what's going through your mind?
Jamal:	I start criticizing myself and comparing myself to other people. I think I am a failure. I have that thought often, but when things are really bad, I just want to go to sleep and never wake up.
Therapist:	What do you end up doing these days when you're feeling hopeless?
Jamal:	I usually stay in my room. Sometimes I drink to get rid of the thoughts and feelings, but that just makes them worse. I think about the last time ...
Therapist:	Do you get any memories or images?
Jamal:	Yeah, I see myself in the apartment looking at the pills. That's all. It's like a freeze frame.
Therapist:	How do you feel in the image?
Jamal:	Mixed up. Sometimes I'm sorry I didn't die. I also feel guilty that Roy found me. Part of me never wants to go back to that place in my head. Sometimes in the image, I see myself throwing away the pills instead of taking them.
Therapist:	I can tell that this is painful to talk about.
Jamal:	I'm okay.
Therapist:	Okay. Let's take a look at what might help when you feel caught up in these thoughts and feelings. Is there something that you've tried that breaks the panicky feeling, like an action or another intense sensation?
Jamal:	Sometimes I run when I feel like I'm jumping out of my skin. Also, swimming helps settle me down.
Therapist:	That's good. Let's write these down. (Hands him a pen and a card.) What if you can't run or go swimming? Is there anything else you've found to help with those feelings?
Jamal:	Lifting weights. I can even do that in my apartment.
Therapist:	Sometimes an intense, but not harmful, experience can also help like taking a hot or cold shower.
Jamal:	I've never tried that. Holding a hot cup of tea sometimes works for me. It's intense, but also settles me. It gives me time to think of other things.
Therapist:	Are there other things you can do to soothe or comfort yourself?
Jamal:	I don't know what you mean.
Therapist:	Would it be comforting to look at photos of your dog?

Jamal: Oh, okay, yeah. I have them on my computer. I could also call my mother to hear how my dog is doing.

Therapist: Is there anyone else you could phone when you're down?

Jamal: I could call my uncle. He's my father's brother and knows how tough my father can be. He wrote me a letter after I got out of the hospital and told me he loved me and not to give up. I still have that letter.

Therapist: I'm glad you kept that letter. Is there anyone else you can think of to call?

Jamal: Roy. He's always awake. Plus, if he misses my call, he'll call me back. We text, but if I'm feeling really bad, I like to hear his voice. There are a few people who could distract me, but he's the one I'd call if I were in deep trouble.

Therapist: Let's add some extra people to the list just in case your friends and family aren't available. (They add the phone numbers of the psychiatrist on call at the hospital, a suicide hotline, and the therapist's work phone number.) How do you feel about having this plan for now?

Jamal: Sort of better. At least I have something to do when I feel really bad.

Therapist: Jamal, you've done a great job identifying warning signs when you're starting to feel overwhelmed and hopeless during the week. How will I know when you're feeling hopeless?

Jamal: (Shrugs and smiles faintly, but still looks down.) I won't show up for my appointment.

Therapist: What if we talk about something or I say something that upsets you in the session?

Jamal: I will do my usual shut down and not look at you or speak. When I feel that way, I just don't want to talk about anything upsetting.

Therapist: How would you like me to respond when you shut down? Do you want me to be quiet and give you some space until you're ready to talk or do you want me to "come get you" from wherever you are in your mind?

Jamal: If you could find me, that might work.

Therapist: So, I would interrupt your train of thought and ask you some questions to remind you of where you are. Maybe then we could find a way to take a look at the thoughts you're having and what triggered the hopeless feelings.

Jamal: Okay. Then I want them to go away.

Therapist: Okay. We'll find a way to manage the negative thoughts. In the meantime, do you think the actions you've written on your safety plan might distract you from the suicidal thoughts and help your mood?

Jamal: I don't know. I've never tried that before. I could try.

There are many places to intervene throughout this conversation: challenging reasons for dying and bolstering reasons for living, fleshing out a safety plan that includes activities Jamal can do when he feels suicidal at various times of day, and testing hopeless cognitions empirically, especially as Jamal begins to accomplish small goals. Each of these approaches is designed to shift the client from hopelessness to hope. Hope is conveyed in many ways, including having a safety plan itself, for it is a way out of the gridlock of suicidal thinking. A safety plan is expanded throughout the course of therapy as new activities and new ways of thinking are discovered. Other ways of harnessing hope include clarifying a problem, demonstrating that change is possible by doing a behavioral experiment, identifying client strengths and positive core beliefs, and imagining or achieving realistic, short-term goals.

Therapists often feel a sense of anxiety when working with suicidal clients. There is often a desire to shore suicidal clients up and keep them safe quickly. However, the therapist must also be aware of the client's level of energy and cognitive functioning and not be overly ambitious in terms of goals and assignments. Structure, concrete questions, summaries, and feedback help the client participate in the session. When a client's energy and interest are low, the therapist must make sure the client is invested in the goal they are working on. Short-term goals are usually the focus because effort, and often commitment, can be sustained only for short periods. Writing things down on a coping card is a tangible memory aid for assignments and for new learning.

Relapse Management

Depression is a recurrent issue for many people. Therefore, it is recommended that clients learn how to manage relapse (see Ludgate, 2009; Segal et al., 2018, for further descriptions of relapse management in CBT). This includes scheduling periodic booster sessions with the client following the end of therapy and having the client independently and regularly practicing CBT skills throughout the course of therapy as well as afterwards (Jarrett et al., 2008). Teaching clients to become their own therapists is an explicit goal of

CBT which is fostered when they learn the skills of identifying and testing automatic thoughts, testing and modifying underlying assumptions and core beliefs, and practicing behaviors that are congruent with new, adaptive ways of thinking. The continual emphasis on skills practice is thought to be one reason CBT treatment for depression has a lower likelihood of relapse than continuation on antidepressant medications (Cuijpers et al., 2013).

Depressed clients also can learn to become attuned to warning signs of relapse, such as changes in sleep patterns, social withdrawal, irritability, or the return of familiar negative thoughts. Common negative thoughts addressed in depression relapse management are all-or-nothing thoughts, such as thoughts about being in control versus being helpless. When dichotomous thinking is operating, any signs of low mood or old behaviors can be interpreted as proof that depression has returned and will likely get worse if the person does not implement a relapse management plan. As with other dichotomous thinking, efforts are made to have the client use less absolute language, see their current symptoms on a continuum of severity, or compare their functioning in several realms to how it was when they began therapy. An effective relapse management plan usually includes a list of personal warning signs that the target mood is returning, a list of skills learned in therapy that can help reduce relapse risk, and a specific plan for implementing those skills (Greenberger & Padesky, 2016).

Mindfulness, or remaining present in the moment without judging one's thoughts, can be incorporated into treatment once clients are in remission from depression (Segal et al., 2018). Further, having the client remember all the progress made and maintained so far can help restore a balanced perspective. Clients sometimes selectively focus on what's not going well, so the therapist can ask the client to shift attention to all they have learned as well as the resilience that comes from practicing skills again. Finally, since real life is full of problems to be solved, what may feel like the start of a relapse may actually be a sign that problem-solving is needed.

Recovery from a low mood

Selena made substantial gains in CBT for depression and was now having monthly booster sessions. She began therapy after moving to town to live with her boyfriend. She knew no one else in town, had no job, and did not know how to drive. She was isolated and alone during the day while her boyfriend was at work. In the course of her therapy, she found a job she could walk to, learned to drive, made friends of her own, and started exercising, even completing a short road race. These activities and focusing on issues of self-esteem helped change the way Selena saw herself. However, she became scared one week when her low mood returned. She predicted she was headed back into a major depression.

Selena: I don't know what's wrong with me. My mood has been low for a few days. I'm getting irritable with my boyfriend and with the people at work. I'm afraid I'm getting depressed again. After all the work I did in therapy, I can't believe I'm going back to the pits.

Therapist: Selena, it sounds like your mood has taken you by surprise. I can tell you're concerned. Can you tell me more about how you're viewing what's going on?

Selena: I thought I was well and in control of my mood. These symptoms mean I'm back to square one. I'm either in control or I'm depressed, and I don't want to be depressed. How can I get back in control?

Therapist: Let's slow down a bit so we can sort this out. First of all, what do you notice about how you're thinking about your situation?

Selena: (Pauses.) Well, it sounds like my old way of thinking, pretty black-and-white.

Therapist: Can we construct a new way of thinking about your situation?

Selena: I'm not sure. I feel like I'm either depressed or I'm not.

Therapist: Do you feel the way you did when we began working together?

Selena: No, I was really sad and lonely then.

Therapist: Is there anything else that was different?

Selena: Yes, a lot. I was sleeping a good deal because I had nothing to do all day. I wasn't sure I could find work and I felt dependent on my boyfriend for money and friends.

Therapist: Let's draw a continuum. (Draws a horizontal line on paper.) So, if we take those symptoms of depression when you were at your lowest as one end of the continuum, what would go at the other, optimal end of the continuum?

Selena: (Chuckling to herself.) I would never feel low. I would have my ideal job and I would solve problems easily. I would be in total control.

Therapist: What's so funny?

Selena: It's not possible to be in total control all the time. Life is not that easy or predictable.

Therapist: Well, given how you've been seeing things, where would you put yourself on this continuum today?

Selena: (She makes a mark on the continuum.) About half-way between how depressed I started out and what I imagine being all better and in control looks like.

Therapist: And it sounds like you're questioning your criteria for being "all better and in control."

Selena: It's unrealistic. It's just that I'd been feeling so good and I got scared when my mood started to get bad.

Therapist: Is there anything you can think of that might help you feel better?

Selena; Well, actually, I stopped doing my Thought Records because I was feeling good. It looks like my all-or-nothing thinking can still get to me if I'm not paying attention. Also, I haven't been exercising in the last couple of weeks and that usually helps my mood. I think I should get back to the gym.

Therapist: I'm wondering about this idea that any of us get "all better". What do you think of it?

Selena: I guess we're never done working on things. I know that I still have to watch my weight even though I'm eating better than I used to. My weight is a never-ending struggle. Just because I'm happy with my weight now doesn't mean I can forget about what I eat.

Therapist: That's a great example of managing a part of your life. How can you use that experience?

Selena: I guess I'm not done helping myself—with weight or with mood. I'm never in perfect control and I'm not where I used to be. I'm somewhere in the middle, and I can make things better; not perfect, just better.

One of the benefits of experiencing ups and downs over the course of therapy is that clients can learn how to recover from setbacks before therapy ends. This experience alone of recovery from setbacks demonstrates that a low mood does not necessarily predict a worsening depression.

For clients who have been suicidal, the suicide safety plan is one tool for relapse management. In addition, such things as thought records, coping cards with significant new perspectives written on them, and a list of mood-boosting activities can be used if signs of depression recur. Toward the end of his therapy, Jamal and his therapist discussed ways to respond to signs of relapse to depression. Their end-of-therapy plan and the methods Jamal was using to feel better formed a post-therapy plan for relapse management.

Therapist: Jamal, I know you have a notebook full of thought records and coping cards for difficult situations. I wonder if we could add to your resources by writing down some warning signs that your mood might be getting low and how you could respond to them.

Jamal: When I get overly self-critical, I know my mood is getting worse. Also, if I feel overwhelmed and panicky like I used to feel about schoolwork, that's a danger sign. If I don't want to see my friends and I think I have to solve all my problems alone, that's a real danger sign.

Therapist: Okay, let's write those down as warning signs and also write down what helps you at those times.

Jamal: Doing a Thought Record helps with the self-doubt and criticism. Also, I still have my safety plan that we made in the beginning of therapy, and when I do some of those activities, like look at photos of my dog, I feel better. One of the best things I can do is the opposite of what I feel like doing; so, when I feel like hiding, I call a friend so I'm not alone. (Writes a written summary of these ideas on his relapse management plan.)

Summary

A benefit of using guided discovery with depressed and suicidal clients is that clients arrive at new conclusions themselves as opposed to getting advice. This can help them feel more capable and hopeful. When energy and motivation are low or cognitive deficits (e.g., attention, memory, recall, creativity) are apparent, structure helps. Behavioral activation is a type of guided discovery that helps clients discover links between their activities and moods and learn what types of activities are most anti-depressant. Socratic Dialogue can be used to help test and reframe clients' negatively biased beliefs, to facilitate problem-solving, to recall other people who have modeled desired behaviors, and to remind a client of earlier coping or resourcefulness they have forgotten. Frequent written summaries during the session help consolidate information, written homework assignments keep track of what actually happened, and coping cards help clients remember conclusions generated in response to synthesizing questions.

For suicidal clients, a safety plan is constructed to manage future suicide crises. It contains a list of coping responses than can be tried instead of harming oneself. Constructing a safety plan combines guided discovery with more directive interventions. For example, both the client and the therapist actively generate the list of safe activities the client can do when feeling suicidal. As therapy progresses, the safety plan is regularly revisited. As client functioning improves, the client can be guided to play a greater role in editing and expanding ideas in their safety plan.

Relapse management focuses on identifying warning signs of depression and strategies that have worked to improve mood in the past. Preparing the client for the possibility of relapse is an important part of the end of therapy. A safety plan for suicidal clients is part of relapse management.

Reader Learning Activities

- Which of these traps are familiar in my work?
- Which of my clients fit with these traps?
- Which of the guided discovery methods illustrated might be helpful with them?
- What strengths do my depressed and suicidal clients have?
- How can I use guided discovery to make the most of their strengths?
- When do I fall into traps?
- What strengths do I bring to my work that will help me navigate traps?
- What do I need to learn or practice before I can try this out with these clients?
- How will I increase my understanding of these issues or my skills (e.g., reading, training, supervision or consultation)?
- How, specifically, will I make this happen?

References

Beck, A. T. (1967). *Depression: Causes and treatment.* Philadelphia: University of Pennsylvania Press.

Beck, A. T. (1976). *Cognitive therapy and the emotional disorders.* New York: New American Library.

Beck, A. T., Rush, A. J., Shaw, B. F., & Emery, G. (1979). *Cognitive therapy of depression.* New York: Guilford.

Beck, A. T., Ward, C. H., Mendelson, M., Mock, J., & Erbaugh, J. (1961). An inventory for measuring depression. *Archives of General Psychiatry, 4,* 561–571. https://doi.org/10.1001/archpsyc.1961.01710120031004

Cuijpers, P., Hollon, S. D., van Straten, A., Berking, M., Bockting, C. L. H., & Andersson, G. (2013). Does cognitive behaviour therapy have an enduring effect that is superior to keeping patients on continuation medication?: A meta-analysis. *British Medical Journal Open, 26*(3), e002542. https://doi.org/10.1136/bmjopen-2012-002542

Dimidjian, S., Martell, C. R., Addis, M. E., & Herman-Dunn, R. (2008). Behavioral activation for depression. In D. Barlow (Ed.). *Clinical handbook of psychological disorders* (4th ed., pp. 328–364). New York: Guilford.

Greenberger, D., & Padesky, C. A. (2016). *Mind over mood: Change how you feel by changing the way you think*. New York: Guilford Press.

Jarrett, R. B., Vittengl, J. R., & Clark, L. A. (2008). How much cognitive therapy, for which patients, will prevent depressive relapse? *Journal of Affective Disorders, 111*(2-3), 185–192. https://doi.org/10.1016/j.jad.2008.02.011

Jobes, D. A. (2016). *Managing suicidal risk: A collaborative approach* (2nd ed.). New York: Guilford.

Kennerley. H., Mueller, M., & Fennell, M. (2010). Looking after yourself. In M. Mueller, H. Kennerley, F. McManus, & D. Westbrook (Eds.), *The Oxford guide to surviving as a CBT therapist* (pp. 57–82). Oxford: Oxford University Press.

Ludgate, J. W. (2009). *Cognitive-behavioral therapy and relapse prevention for depression and anxiety*. Sarasota, FL: Professional Resource Press.

Padesky, C. A. (1983). *7-Column Thought Record*. Huntington Beach, CA: Center for Cognitive Therapy, Huntington Beach. Retrieved from https://www.mindovermood.com/workshe ets.html

Padesky, C. A. (1993, September 24). *Socratic questioning: Changing minds or guiding discovery?* Invited speech delivered at the European Congress of Behavioural and Cognitive Therapies, London. Retrieved from https://www.padesky.com/clinical-corner/publications/

Padesky, C. A. (2020). *The clinician's guide to CBT using Mind over Mood*. New York: Guilford.

Segal, Z. V., Williams, J. M. G., & Teasdale, J. D. (2018). *Mindfulness-based cognitive therapy for depression* (2nd ed.). New York: Guilford.

Shea, S. C. (1998). *Psychiatric interviewing: The art of understanding* (2nd ed.). Philadelphia: W.B. Saunders.

Stanley, B., & Brown, G. K. (2012). Safety planning intervention: A brief intervention to mitigate suicide risk. *Cognitive and Behavioral Practice, 19*(2), 256–264. https://doi.org/10.1016/j.cbpra.2011.01.001

Stanley, B., Brown, G. K., Brenner, L. A., Galfalvy, H. C., Currier, G. W., Knox, K. L., Chaudhury, S. R., Bush, A. L., & Green, K. L. (2018). Comparison of the Safety Planning Intervention with follow-up vs usual care of suicidal patients treated in the emergency department. *JAMA Psychiatry, 75*(9), 894–900. https://doi.org/10.1001/jamapsychiatry.2018.1776

Wenzel, A., Brown, G. K., & Beck, A. T. (2009). *Cognitive therapy for suicidal patients*. Washington, DC: American Psychological Association.

Wright, J. H., Turkington, D., Kingdon, D., & Basco, M. (2009). *Cognitive Therapy for severe mental illness: An illustrated guide*. Arlington, VA: American Psychiatric Publishing.

Young, J., Rygh, ,J. L., Weinberger, A. D., & Beck, A. T. (2008). Cognitive therapy for depression. In: Barlow (Ed.). *Clinical Handbook of Psychological Disorders*. (4th ed., pp. 250-305). New York: Guilford.

4
Guided Discovery with Anxiety

Gillian Butler and Freda McManus

> "Something terrible could happen, and I might not be able to handle it. What if the car breaks down and I'm stranded? Or what if one of the children had an accident? Or if I lost my job? Or if Mum got Alzheimer's and I had to look after her? I just feel so out of control and exhausted. Something horrible could happen at any time, so you're never really safe. Constantly worrying about everything that could go wrong spoils my enjoyment of nearly everything and stops me doing all sorts of things because they feel so scary. I really need to know that I'll be alright. Can you help me? Do you think I'm crazy? I sometimes think I'm completely mad."
>
> **—Client's description of her anxiety**

Understanding Anxiety

Anxiety is a universal emotion and a healthy response to perceived danger that has important protective functions. It becomes a problem when it is so frequent, severe, or prolonged that it interferes with people's ability to live their lives. Anxiety disorders, in general, are characterized by a *disabling overestimation* of threat, risk, and danger together with an *underestimation* of the ability to cope with such things. Anxiety is marked by heightened physiological arousal and by the effort made to protect oneself, predominantly using avoidance and safety-seeking behaviors. The experience of anxiety is thus both psychological and physiological, and it includes cognitive, somatic, emotional, and behavioral components.

These four components combine differently for different people, in different circumstances and in different anxiety disorders. While we all recognize the feeling of anxiety, we have many and various names for it: anxiety, fear, stress, worry, concern, angst, apprehension, and nervousness, among others. For these reasons clinicians need to gather information from their clients to define the particular type (or types) of anxiety from which they suffer, and to identify the ways in which the anxiety is experienced by that individual. In cognitive behavioral therapy, especially close attention will be paid to each person's thoughts and images, and guided discovery methods are ideally suited for this purpose.

Anxiety arises when thinking about the future: about negative things that could or might happen. Anxious thinking is therefore focused on perceived threats, risks, and dangers. What is perceived as a threat will depend both on how a situation is interpreted and on underlying assumptions and beliefs. Two kinds of beliefs are especially relevant: beliefs about the possible risks and dangers that may threaten us (what they are and how likely they are), and beliefs about our resources for coping with those anxiety-provoking events. Perceived resources can be internal capacities or external resources for problem-solving or support.

Resources include other people, escape routes, ways of minimizing the impact of an anticipated disaster, and available strategies for managing difficult or risky situations. If we think we can cope well with the threats and risks that we face, then we may feel more excited or challenged than anxious. Anxiety predominates when the perceived threats outweigh our perceived ability to handle them. Theoretically, susceptibility to anxiety is rooted in a sense of vulnerability, which is understandable if perceived dangers threaten to overwhelm our perceived coping abilities. As a result, anxiety occurs when "a person's perception of himself [is] subject to internal or external dangers over which his control is lacking or is insufficient to afford him a sense of safety" (Beck et al., 1985, 67).

Remember that anxiety is also a healthy and normal emotion that serves a useful function. Presumably it evolved to protect us from danger, and it still helps us to deal with stressful situations by prompting us to mobilize resources for coping with difficulties wherever these arise: at work, at school, in our relationships, or elsewhere. It is easy to understand how important it is for human beings to focus on threat detection and on sources of likely future harm. Mobilizing resources to defend against those threats, particularly in relation to threats of physical harm, is likely to keep us safer, and even to prolong life—if we suddenly have to take aversive action when crossing a busy road, for instance.

Shared features among anxiety and related disorders

The *Diagnostic and Statistical Manual of Mental Disorder*, 5th edition (DSM-5; APA, 2013) specifies eleven different anxiety disorder diagnoses including panic disorder, agoraphobia, generalized anxiety disorder, specific phobias, social phobia, separation anxiety disorder, selective mutism, and "unspecified anxiety disorder." Other disorders such as obsessive-compulsive disorder (OCD), illness anxiety disorder, and post-traumatic stress disorder (PTSD) also often include significant anxiety in their presentation. There is a wide range of symptoms occurring across these disorders that feature anxiety. Panic attacks can occur as a symptom in any of these disorders, just as binge eating can occur in the various types of eating disorder. The most common physiological symptoms reported to family doctors by anxious people are tension, headaches, insomnia, and fatigue. Common patterns of thinking include leaping to conclusions about the likelihood of negative occurrences and catastrophizing.

OCD and PTSD are both characterized by unwanted persistent thoughts, images, or impulses that are perceived as intrusive and anxiety provoking (Huppert et al., 2005). The repeated checking that is a hallmark of obsessive-compulsive problems may also occur in generalized anxiety disorder (GAD) (Mahoney et al., 2018). Intrusive thoughts and checking are also common in illness anxiety disorder, and similarly almost two-thirds of clients with panic disorder have at least one symptom of OCD (Torres et al., 2004). In addition, Dugas and Ladouceur have shown that many people who suffer from anxiety disorders find it difficult to tolerate uncertainty (e.g., Buhr & Dugas, 2012; Dugas et al., 1998; Hebert & Dugas, 2019). This is particularly prominent in GAD, as is the cognitive rigidity that has been extensively documented by Borkovec and colleagues (e.g., Borkovec et al., 1993; Borkovec & Newman, 1998). There is a lack of flexibility in the somatic, cognitive, and behavioral responses of anxious people—as if they are using their energies in an attempt to keep control so that they feel safer, and of course less vulnerable or at risk.

It is not that surprising that symptoms overlap across anxiety disorders as the disorders themselves are difficult to differentiate at a conceptual level. Consider the definitions of social phobia and agoraphobia. Social phobia is primarily defined as a fear of situations in which embarrassment may occur and agoraphobia is defined as anxiety about situations in which escape might be difficult or *embarrassing* (APA, 2013). People with GAD are prone to worry about a range of situations, which may well include social situations, fears of embarrassment, or anxiety about physical symptoms (as in agoraphobia). The high degree to which symptoms are shared across the anxiety disorders is acknowledged in DSM-5 and, as a result, extensive guidance is given on differential diagnosis and a series of "trumping rules" are provided to help clinicians make specific diagnoses.

There may also be common maintaining factors across anxiety disorders. For example, a seminal experimental study of 162 anxiety disorder clients by Arntz et al. (1995) demonstrated emotional reasoning (*ex-consequentia* reasoning: for example, "if I feel anxious there must be danger") across clients with simple phobia, social phobia, and panic disorder, as well as in a mixed anxiety disorder group. Similarly, data from information-processing tasks indicate that people with many different anxiety disorders pay selective attention to threatening external and internal stimuli, and that there is attentional avoidance of threat in specific phobia, social phobia, and generalized anxiety disorder (Harvey et al., 2004; Mansell et al., 2009). Although these information-processing tasks demonstrate selective attention to distinctive stimuli in individual clients, the process of selective attention to threat appears to be common across the anxiety disorders (Bar-Hiam et al., 2007). Interpretive and expectancy biases have also been found, demonstrating tendencies to interpret ambiguous information in a threatening way, and to expect that negative events are likely to happen. A variety of paradigms provide data that converge to demonstrate that common processing biases maintain different manifestations of anxiety (Cisler & Koster, 2010; Harvey et al., 2004; Hirsch & Mathews, 2000).

A common complicating factor is that many of the people who seek treatment for their anxiety have been anxious for many years and during this time they develop secondary problems. There is often overlap with features of avoidant or dependent personality traits, and other common secondary problems include depression (being anxious "gets you down"); emotions such as anger, frustration, and shame; low self-confidence; and low self-esteem. Anxiety tends to spread from one thing to another. Common secondary forms of anxiety are generalized anxiety (whatever your problem, you can worry about it) and social anxiety. This makes sense because anxious people often perceive others as more robust than themselves, and thus fear that others will judge them to be weak or inadequate or "stupid" because of their anxiety. The sum total of the problems faced by people whose anxiety is persistent or chronic, and by therapists working with them, may therefore be confusing and add to the uncertainty: "Whatever might happen next?" "Where should we begin treatment?"

Given that there are specific effective treatments for each of the anxiety disorders it is important for the clinician to assess and to understand the specific form(s) of anxiety from which each client suffers. Consistent with the points made above, this chapter emphasizes common symptoms, maintaining factors and secondary problems, and the use of guided discovery to resolve a range of clinical difficulties. The different models for the specific anxiety disorders will not be described in detail (cf. Bennett-Levy et al., 2004; Clark & Beck, 2011; Kennerley et al., 2017; Padesky, 2020). Instead, the general theory outlined above provides the basis for understanding the typical thoughts and beliefs, feelings, physiological responses, and behaviors involved. Examples will be drawn from the range of anxiety disorders, and recurring themes include the following:

- Difficulties in tolerating uncertainty about what the future might bring;
- Using overly self-protective and other unhelpful behaviors; and
- Rigidity in response to anxiety.

Common Traps Arising from Client Beliefs

Many treatment manuals are available to learn how to effectively treat anxiety and related disorders (cf. Clark & Beck, 2011; Leahy et al., 2012; Simos & Hofmann, 2013). Clinical practice is frequently more difficult (and more interesting) than one might suppose after reading about how to do it, or attending an expertly led practical workshop. Apparently straightforward methods turn out to be surprisingly difficult to apply well. For example, even though they understand the value of using guided discovery, therapists working with anxious clients can find themselves offering reassurance, or making directive suggestions, or explaining the meaning of the results of an experiment.

Viewing anxiety from the perspective of the client as outlined in the section "Shared Features among Anxiety and Related Disorders," there are three contexts within which therapists are likely to lapse into these generally unhelpful behaviors:

- When facing uncertainty, anxious people want to be "sure" that they will be OK and they often seek reassurance that this is so.
- When perceived threats, risks, or dangers loom large, anxious clients feel a pressing need to protect themselves so as to keep safe, and therefore they frequently ask for advice.
- When feeling anxious, people experiencing anxiety try to keep a tight hold on themselves for fear that letting go could have terrible consequences.

Common Traps in Working with Anxiety

Trap 1
Client has a high intolerance of uncertainty and the therapist offers reassurance.

Trap 2
Client has a high perceived need for self-protection and seeks lots of advice from the therapist who makes frequent directive suggestions for the client to stop avoiding and using safety-seeking behaviors.

Trap 3
Client is overly rigid in behavior and cognitive processing. The therapist inadvertently colludes with client by constructing homework tasks that reinforce the need to be in control instead of helping the client to tolerate more flexibility.

Therapists, who are of course also susceptible to anxiety, can easily be affected by the beliefs and behaviors of their clients that reflect these attitudes. So this section is organized around the three themes of (1) intolerance of uncertainty, (2) the perceived need for self-protection, and (3) rigidity in response to anxiety. We will address each of them in turn and describe common clinical challenges before illustrating how guided discovery can help resolve them.

Client intolerance of uncertainty

Trap 1

Client has a high intolerance of uncertainty and the therapist offers reassurance.

The desire for certainty in an uncertain world is bound to cause problems, as it is asking the impossible. One never can be sure that nothing will go wrong, or when something bad happens that one will cope well with it (see Butler et al., 2008, Chapter 9, for a detailed account of the effects of uncertainty). When doubts and uncertainties creep in, anxiety tends to follow along with patterns of anxious thinking. Feeling anxious makes disasters seem more likely, and when disasters seem likely, anxiety escalates (Butler & Mathews, 1983; Butler et al., 1995; Williams et al., 1997; Yiend, 2004). Then anxious people feel out of control, or fear that they might lose control and appeal to others for reassurance. As is illustrated in Example 1, even improbable disasters can seem likely to happen when people feel highly anxious.

Example 1: Something terrible might happen

Rebecca sought treatment for the panic attacks that had plagued her ever since she witnessed a violent assault on a train three years previously. Since the assault, she had avoided traveling by train and her journey to work by bus and on foot had become so tiring that she was considering a change of career. Rebecca was highly motivated to overcome her difficulties and participated actively in treatment, forming an excellent relationship with the therapist, and achieving a considerable amount of improvement in the first few weeks. The dialogue summarized below occurred after that, when she and her therapist were talking about whether she was ready to attempt a train journey.

Rebecca: If it wasn't crowded I might be able to do it.

Therapist: OK. What's the concern about it being crowded? How might that make it more difficult for you?

Rebecca: I just think I'll panic. One of those really bad ones that seems to come over me suddenly, just like a train in fact, and it goes on and on forever. I need to be sure that that won't happen before I can risk getting onto a train again.

Therapist: Yes. I can understand you feeling like that.

Rebecca: I'm worried that I'll do something mad and make a complete fool of myself.

Therapist: How do you mean? What would you be doing?

Rebecca: Well I'd lose it completely. I'd go mad. I don't know what I'd do … so mad that I wouldn't be able to get back to be myself again. Just out of touch and … inaccessible, and not knowing where I am or what to do [getting increasingly distressed] … I'd go completely psychotic. I'd have to be carted away, and probably tied down to keep me still and shouting … and … just crazy …

Therapist   But that won't happen. Panic attacks don't make people psychotic. It doesn't work like that. You've been so good at finding out so far that you have much more control than you think you have, and you know now that the panic doesn't go on forever. Think about all the things you have done so well in the past few weeks.

Keep in Mind

Socratic Dialogue is easier to maintain when clients are calm and responsive to questions asked but it is important to continue this form of dialogue into the inner storm of anxiety. Notice that Rebecca's therapist used the first two stages of Socratic Dialogue well at the start of this interchange and this seemed to help Rebecca talk in more detail about her fears. However, once those fears became more extreme, and Rebecca—in some distress—became immersed in imagery of what would happen if she went mad, the therapist empathized with her distress and started to offer reassurance. He said, "that won't happen," and provided reminders of information about panic attacks (they don't go on forever and are not linked to psychosis), and more reminders about Rebecca's recent successes. The last thing the therapist said here was "Think about all the things you have done so well in the past few weeks," but by this time Rebecca was so upset that she wasn't able to think clearly. She could not easily remember what she had achieved, let alone see the things she had recently done as achievements. The therapist's departure from Socratic Dialogue, however well-intentioned and accurate in content, interrupted a potentially productive exploration.

Below we continue the conversation, resuming at the point Rebecca begins to describe her anxious imagery in detail. Observe the difference it makes when Rebecca's therapist continues using Socratic Dialogue to guide her discovery.

Rebecca: Well I'd lose it completely. I'd go mad. I don't know what I'd do ... so mad that I wouldn't be able to get back to be myself again. Just out of touch and ... inaccessible, and not knowing where I am or what to do (Getting increasingly distressed.) ... I'd go completely psychotic. I'd have to be carted away, and probably tied down to keep me still and shouting ... and ... just crazy.

Therapist: Mmmmm ... That sounds terrifying—and really distressing to think about. I can hear how upsetting it is for you just thinking about doing it.

In the Therapist's Mind

The therapist moves from informational questions to empathic listening. The aim is to help Rebecca feel understood—to validate her feelings, and help her calm down sufficiently to be able to continue. What happens next, and the speed with which it happens, will depend on many things such as how upset Rebecca becomes and how easy she finds it to resume the work of the session. The following dialogue has been edited to make these main points clear.

Rebecca: I can see dreadful things happening to me, and I'm just so terrified of completely losing it.

Therapist: Mmm. Yes. No wonder that's so frightening.

Rebecca: I'm a real wimp. I'm really, really scared of going on a train again.

Therapist: Of course. Given these images you have, it makes sense that you feel that way. How about thinking it through together a bit and seeing if there are any ways we can make the prospect less terrifying for you?

Rebecca: OK. I'm not sure it will make any difference but I'll give it a go.

Therapist: What I'm wondering is what would happen if you did have another panic attack. What have you learned so far in therapy about your panic attacks?

Rebecca: Well ... I've been having them for 3 years, and lots of them each week ... and since I've been coming here I've actually had fewer attacks than before, but the bad ones do still happen sometimes.

Therapist: Let's write that down. (Begins making a written summary of Rebecca's learning to date.) And when you do have them, what happens to you?

Rebecca: It's awful. My heart thumps and races and I can't breathe properly and I can't think clearly. I get the shakes, and my stomach churns. It happens really quickly, and I think I'm going to pass out, or drop dead, or lose control or something horrible.

Therapist: And then what happens?

Rebecca: Well, that's kind of it—I feel dreadful. And when it's all over I'm completely exhausted.

Therapist: Yes. Quite worn out by it. So ... can you tell me a bit more about what makes you think that you might go mad?

Rebecca: It's because everything happens so quickly. I don't know where it might end if it went on and just kept escalating.

Therapist: And madness is your conclusion, so to speak?

Rebecca: Yes—even though you've told me about panic attacks, and I know you're right when you say that the symptoms always die away in the end. Maybe because I've had so many of them, the doubts still creep in. I do know I'm not going to go mad—I guess I'd have done it already if I was going to anyway. I just lose track of everything. As if I've lost my senses.

Therapist: I wonder why that might be?

Rebecca: I think it's because it all happens so fast, and I forget everything else—and because something dreadful always could happen again, so you never can know you'll be OK.

Therapist: Quite. I'm sure you're right there. It does happen very quickly, and the symptoms are so intense that everything else gets pushed out of your mind. And you're right that bad things could happen. What have you learned so far about your ability to manage the bad things? And about your ability to cope with the panic attacks?

Rebecca had learned much, and here the therapist is helping her draw on this knowledge to make it easier to keep things in perspective when Rebecca feels distressed. By making a written summary of what Rebecca says she has learned to date, the therapist helps create a memory bank that Rebecca can consult when she gets fearful. The discussion continued in a similar way, exploring her thoughts and feelings in some depth. The therapist's plan was to help Rebecca use the knowledge that she now had, and the evidence of her recent work, to rethink her catastrophizing thoughts, and to think more calmly about whether she was ready to experiment with getting on a train.

The discussion was a long one because there was much to cover—or rather to uncover. Examples included the links between panic and "madness" or psychosis, information about how anxiety in panic attacks increases rapidly and then plateaus and declines, leaving the panicky person feeling exhausted (and with their confidence shaken, but not psychotic), and all that Rebecca has learned about how to cope with panicky feelings, how to recognize patterns of catastrophic thinking, and what can be learned from facing things that have previously been avoided. They also reiterated what the benefits might be for Rebecca if she faced her anxiety and tested out her catastrophic predictions, rather than continuing to cope by avoiding difficult situations.

At the end of this session, after they had summarized her conclusions, the therapist asked Rebecca how she understood the moment earlier on when she had had the thoughts about going mad and had become so distressed. Rebecca's immediate response was that she felt embarrassed at how quickly she had slipped into the panicky way of seeing things, and she was worried that it might happen again. One further brief exploration was aimed at helping Rebecca make sense of her fears about going mad. This revealed that her family had no history of mental illness, that she had no specific risk factors for it, that she knew little about what it might look like in practice, and that she had suffered no alarming or weird experiences after taking non-prescribed drugs.

Rebecca thought, on consideration, that what scared her was the speed and intensity of her panicky reactions, triggered merely by thinking about being in a difficult situation—a "here and now" demonstration of the power of cognition but also an example of it not escalating out of control. Drafting a written summary of the information she now had about panic and about her more recent experiences encouraged Rebecca to continue to plan behavioral experiments, and to start thinking practically about how, and when, to travel by train once more despite being uncertain about what would happen when she did.

The general trap illustrated here is a common one that occurs in many forms of anxiety. In outline it takes the following form: the client says: "Something horrible might happen" and the therapist responds, "No, that isn't likely." This response cuts short the exploration that helps the client to rethink and re-engage with frightening situations despite being uncertain about what might happen. Typical thoughts that elicit such reactions might be, in social anxiety, "they don't like me"; in illness anxiety, "there's something seriously wrong"; in OCD, "I've put someone else at risk"; and in PTSD, "I'm not safe."

Keep in Mind

- Adopt a "Socratic attitude." Be genuinely curious about all aspects of the client's reactions: their feelings, interpretations, conclusions, the implications they draw about themselves, others, or the future, and so on. Using Socratic Dialogue often takes longer than reassurance or providing answers but it helps the client attain deeper understanding and greater confidence in alternative perspectives.

- Don't cut short an exploration because the client becomes distressed. Instead, listen empathically, validate the feelings, and continue to explore when the client is ready. Reassurance is far less helpful in practice than many therapists would like it to be.

- When the client becomes distressed it can be seen as an opportunity to access "hot" cognitions and find out more about what keeps the problem going.
- Written summaries of a client's learning experiences are important aids because people easily lose sight of things that they know, or have recently learned.
- Accept, and help the client to accept and live with the fact that outcomes are never certain.

Example 2: What if? Needing to be sure

Guided discovery is particularly useful when it helps clients to step back and evaluate their current strategy for dealing with the uncertainty that troubles them. Perhaps the clearest marker of uncertainty is the "What if … ?" question, and the following two examples illustrate different ways of responding with Socratic Dialogue when this attitude dominates a client's thinking.

Ted had engaged well in CBT for his illness anxiety and could use the techniques to deal with specific concerns when they arose. However, both he and his therapist were getting frustrated because he was finding it hard to generalize his new learning. Ted quickly slipped back into old habits of thinking, dominated by the uncertainty of "what if … ?" thoughts and by his old way of coping by searching for information to remove all possible doubt.

Ted:	The cancer worry seems to be better now but instead, because I've got this head cold, I've been thinking it could be a brain tumor …
Therapist:	Uh-huh. So I wonder if it would be useful for us to look at whether there is anything that you did, that helped with the concern you've had for the last few weeks about stomach cancer, that we could apply to this new brain tumor concern?
Ted:	OK. Well it did help a bit to do the thought record—not every stomach pain is cancer. And to ask other people about whether they ever got similar symptoms—indigestion and wind. And I think it just passed a bit with time, they usually do. But there is always another one … as soon as I hear about someone who's got something, or notice a symptom, then I'm off looking up what it might be.
Therapist:	And does that help?
Ted:	I don't know—sometimes it does, like if the symptoms are really specific. But with stomach cancer there aren't any really specific symptoms until it's very late on. So it could be just indigestion, or it

could be cancer. Same with a brain tumor—it might be a head cold, or it might be a tumor. But I just feel like I've got to know . . .

Therapist: Well perhaps we could try to use the thought record again for this concern and see if it helps?

At this point Ted and his therapist completed a written thought record, which did reduce the concern somewhat but, as predicted, another concern soon came up. Testing the likelihood of a specific fear on a thought record is not usually as helpful as identifying and working directly with thematic underlying assumptions that maintain anxiety (Padesky, 2020). Therefore, Ted's therapist decided to change tack and to work instead on Ted's need to be certain, and on the strategies that came into play when doubt crept in.

Therapist: One of the things you've talked about is needing to know if a symptom is a sign of a serious illness or not, is that right?

Ted: Yeah, I just feel like if I could know one way or the other, and be sure it wasn't an early sign of something serious, then I wouldn't be worrying about it all the time.

Therapist: Can we spend a bit of time thinking about that today?

Ted: Okay.

Therapist: It sounds like you have an assumption, "If I can know for sure it is not a sign of something serious, then I can stop worrying"?

Ted: That's right.

Therapist: Well I wonder if the "need to know for sure" might be one of the things that is actually keeping the problem going.

Ted: I don't know. It does feel important to know—and it takes up all my attention when I feel like that. Like I just have to find out for sure one way or the other and then I can at least plan for it and do my best.

Therapist: So what would you do if you did know for sure that it was a serious illness? What would that be like?

Ted: Well it would be awful but at least I'd have some time—I could prepare my family. Start making arrangements . . . get things in order . . . at least I'd know what the likely picture was.

Therapist: And would that be better?

Ted: I think so . . .

Therapist: It sounds like you're saying you'd feel better if you could only know exactly what was going to happen in the future? Even if it's bad news?

Ted:	Yeah, I've always liked to be in control. I do like to have a plan, to know where I'm going and make a plan for it. But that's really difficult to do with health—you just don't know what's going to happen or when.
Therapist:	Would it really be better if you did? Can you tell me a bit about how you imagine that to be?
Ted:	Well I'd be gutted but at least I could tell my wife and get things in order with her and the kids. Have a chance to make my peace and say my goodbyes. Let people know what they've meant to me.
Therapist:	So it sounds like you're saying you'd prefer to know exactly what was going to happen to you in the future and when? Even when you were going to get sick, and when and how you will die?
Ted:	I guess … I'm not sure. I had thought so but I'm not so sure now! Maybe I wouldn't like to know exactly when I was going to die— might be a bit morbid to feel like you knew exactly how many days you had left, and when you were going to start suffering.
Therapist:	So are you saying some uncertainty about the future is helpful? Would it be better, for some things, not to know?
Ted:	I guess it would be a bit weird to know everything that was going to happen.

From this discussion the focus of the work shifted onto the ways in which Ted might cope more effectively with his doubts and fears. He started to explore the ideas that maybe it could be better not to know everything in advance, and that maybe he could achieve some of the things that he had thought certainty would give him (like relief from preoccupation with his health) while retaining the benefits of uncertainty. He decided to try to tell the main people he cared about how much they had meant to him even though his death wasn't imminent, and also to have a general discussion with his partner about practical arrangements in the event that either of them should die unexpectedly.

After doing these things, he was more able to focus on developing realistic standards for symptom monitoring and for getting symptoms checked out: standards that were not driven by his need to be certain. Ted and his therapist worked on devising a more general strategy, phrased in his own words, that would enable him to tolerate a greater degree of uncertainty and at the same time to seek medical consultations only so as, in his view, to promote good health. Ted made a written summary of this and kept it on his mobile phone so that he could refer back to it during anxious moments.

Keep in Mind

- Ted's therapist helped him speak openly about "what if…?" the antici-pated disaster did happen. Sometimes this is hard to do and it must, of course, be done sensitively and in the context of a respectful working alliance. It can seem obvious, or feel cruel, but unless therapists are prepared to directly enquire about the worst that could happen, in-cluding before and after death, underlying fears are hard to discern. Exploration of alternative beliefs requires knowing the specifics of anxious thoughts and images.

- It is essential to take the uncertainty, and the distress that goes with it, seriously, in order to find out exactly what is making the client feel vulnerable.

- It can be helpful to clarify links between "what if … ?" assumptions and the behaviors, or strategies, that go with them.

- Making, or rehearsing, a plan for dealing with potential worst-case sce-narios can help to increase a client's coping resources and their confi-dence in using them.

Example 3: Endless worry

People who suffer from generalized anxiety disorder are characterized specif-ically by their intolerance of uncertainty (Hebert & Dugas, 2019). Worrying can seem endless, as one worry leads to another. Therapists often observe that if they put the fire out in one place, it only pops up in another. It is easy to fall into the trap of taking each of the worries in turn, and focusing on dealing with each one separately. Therapists who do this use Socratic Dialogue to ex-plore what each worry is specifically about, whether the feared outcome is likely to happen, how bad it would be if it did, how other people might deal with this particular worry, and so on. These methods can certainly make people feel better temporarily, but usually the worry returns (as in Ted's case in Example 2), sometimes with the same focus, but often with a different one.

Instead, it is useful to work on the process of worry rather than on the con-tent (Nordahl et al., 2018). In practice this is sometimes difficult to do, espe-cially if the therapist wants to introduce this idea Socratically. It is only too easy to get sidetracked by a particular, pressing worry, the "concern du jour." It is difficult to step back sufficiently to help clients to think about the process of worrying—about the pattern of thinking that has become habitual to them—rather than focusing on current, here-and-now concerns. It is also sometimes difficult to find the right language to introduce the idea in a way that makes sense to your client that it will be more useful to think about the process than the content of the worry.

The following example illustrates how one therapist succeeded in doing this with a man who suffered with GAD and who described himself as a lifelong worrier. The client, Dave, was the owner and manager of a small hardware store whose business was threatened by economic recession. He was nearly 60 when he started therapy and the following dialogue occurred during the eighth session after he had learned to use CBT methods for dealing with specific worries. Earlier in this session his therapist was feeling her way through, trying to find a way of getting Dave to step back and think about the worrying itself. Instead of responding to what she says, Dave continued talking about a particular concern and how this affected him during the past week.

His therapist tried to help Dave reflect on the process, and when he did not respond she said, "It suggests to me the problem is the worry, not the content." This comment could be drawn from a textbook, and it may not be surprising that Dave did not really respond to her comment but continued describing his worrying. Later on she found a more productive—and a more Socratic way of coming back to this point. The dialogue below illustrates how she did this. It begins with Dave talking about a particularly distressing bout of worry from the previous week. Notice how his therapist tries to turn his attention towards the process of worrying while not asking for more details about the content.

Dave:	… that worry lasted a complete week—I couldn't stop. It's exhausting. It's just the way I am. But I so much want a break from it …
Therapist:	What does that tell you about the nature of worry?
Dave:	That I'll pick up on anything … fester on it.
Therapist:	Do you need to worry? What does it tell you about that?
Dave:	I'm not sure … seems like it's a bit of a habit.
Therapist:	I wonder if the problem is the worry, not the actual content of each worry. What do you think?
Dave:	I analyze each situation until I'm blue in the face—it makes no difference. How can I tell whether it's just a worry or an actual problem? That's what got to me …
Therapist:	If it was a real problem, would worry help?
Dave:	No. It's the feeling that I have. Then I have to worry.

In the Therapist's Mind

There seem to be two issues here: (1) is worry useful? and (2) how can you differentiate real problems from worries? At this point the therapist strives to get Dave to focus on the process of worry rather than getting sidetracked into the second issue, which can be discussed at another time.

Therapist:	What do you think about whether worry is useful?
Dave:	I do believe that I need to worry to solve problems—or I'd be fooled into thinking I was OK when ... something bad or negative could happen.
Therapist:	Why does that matter?
Dave:	Fear—not letting my guard down. Some bad thing could happen.
Therapist:	What's the worry doing to prevent that?
Dave:	Making sure—checking. It keeps me more on my guard. It gives me a safety net.
Therapist:	What might it be protecting you from?
Dave:	Things going wrong. I'm so frightened all the time of something going wrong.
Therapist:	So it makes sense that you worry—if it protects you. Do you think the worrying does stop things from going wrong?
Dave:	No, not really. And in the end it gets me down. I just get depressed, so more things go wrong.
Therapist:	The worry seems like a process you go through automatically?
Dave:	It's like punch bag man—you hit it, and it always pops back up ...
Therapist:	So the worries always come back ... Seems like the worrying is a bit like a bully?
Dave:	How so?
Therapist:	A bully needs a victim—like a parasite needs a host ... The worry could be like a bully that forces you to give it air time. A bully threatens you: "If you don't pay me I'll come back and beat you up," and the worry does the same thing: "If you don't pay attention to me then something bad will happen ... ?"
Dave:	Oh yes!
Therapist:	What do you think of ...
Dave:	I need to be stronger before I can stand up to the bully.

Therapist: What do you think of the analogy?

Dave: Yes—you're waiting to be stronger, but getting weaker with the worrying—it grinds you down. As long as I keep doing it—worrying—it's not serving any purpose—it's making me worse.

Therapist: How much do you believe that?

Dave: 100%! Actually worry is worthless.

Therapist: So has worry ever stopped things going wrong?

Dave: Not a lot—but it must have done sometimes.

In the Therapist's Mind

This therapist considers exploring Dave's last comment in detail but that would risk losing the thread of the discussion. Therefore she decides to follow the new metaphor through rather than take a sidetrack to hear about times when worrying has apparently been useful.

Therapist: A victim needs to stop giving the bully money before he feels strong.

Dave: I need to take a risk and say, "I don't need to worry." That's a completely new idea for me ... that worry doesn't stop it from happening ... just makes you worse.

Therapist: So what do you need to do differently?

Dave: Try it out? ... Not worry for just for one week ... take a risk that things won't go wrong.

Therapist: Something might go wrong—we're testing this out.

Dave: I'm ready to try. It's like saying I'm going to jump off the cliff this week and just not let myself worry about things.

Therapist: OK ... so when worries pop back, how would you like to respond?

Dave: Something mental to do instead—Sudoku or something? Something that involves the mind and body—so that I can take the risk of not going there.

Therapist: So you're going to try not to get involved in the worrying?

Dave: Yes, I'll try that.

Therapist: What are you going to do if you get caught up in it?

Dave: I've got to walk away. It's just an experiment this week—it's not going to put me in grave danger in one week is it?

In the Therapist's Mind

His therapist considers three main options at this point: to provide the reassurance that Dave is asking for, to comment on and help him to understand his need for reassurance, or to summarize the decision made. Providing reassurance would fall into the trap of trying to satisfy Dave's anxiety about uncertainty. Instead, she decides it will be more helpful to carry on with the Socratic Dialogue and make a summary because the session is nearing a close.

His therapist asked Dave to make a written note of the homework task because it was important to ensure that he was clear about exactly what he was going to do during the next week, and what the purpose of that was. This strategy also helped to keep the new idea about the value (or uselessness) of worry in mind and encouraged him to continue thinking it through as he tested it out by changing his behavior. Making a summary and written homework plan was a wise decision. It anchored the clarity of this session. There are likely to be plenty more opportunities to come back to the theme of reassurance-seeking.

In this session, Dave explained to his therapist that he believed that if he did not worry then something might go wrong. This fits with the idea that worry reflects a sense of vulnerability, and that each person's idiosyncratic sense of vulnerability will determine what they worry about. The Socratic question that elicited Dave's explanation in this context was: "What might it [the worrying] protect you from?", but the sequence of questions leading up to this one probably helped Dave to tune in to the meaning of worry for him. Other common meanings clients often report include not being able to cope, being rejected, and getting hurt in some way. Use of Socratic Dialogue helps guard against therapists jumping to conclusions about why someone worries and it also gives the client time and space to uncover relevant idiosyncratic meanings.

Keep in Mind

- Avoid using jargon or technical language—use the client's language. Notice how the client starts to reflect on the process after being asked, "What do you think about whether worry is useful?"

- Step back from the pressure of considering or testing out the likelihood of specific worries.
- Use metaphors that make sense to the client. These can demonstrate that the therapist understands. Check out whether the metaphor fits the client's experience. If clients use helpful metaphorical language, adopt their language rather than using your own metaphor.
- The client may appear suddenly to get the point and (as in Dave's case) go for it 100%. Check out whether this is all-or-nothing thinking or a sign of compliance with the therapist's ideas. No matter the degree of client belief, follow up with a behavioral experiment. Review the results of these experiments with Socratic Dialogue so client learning opportunities are maximized.
- When planning an experiment to test out a new idea, think about what might go wrong. Define and ask the client how they want to handle difficulties with experiments so they don't abandon them.
- Listen to the individual's sense of vulnerability and express empathy.

The perceived need for self-protection

Protecting yourself seems sensible if you are in danger, or even if you perceive yourself to be in danger. However numerous experimental studies have confirmed the role of avoidance and/or safety-seeking behaviors in maintaining anxiety (e.g., McManus et al., 2008; Salkovskis, 1991; Salkovskis et al., 1996). Further studies have also demonstrated reductions in anxiety when these behaviors are changed (Blakey & Abramowitz, 2016; McManus et al., 2009; Salkovskis et al., 1999). However, encouraging clients to stop avoidance and safety-seeking behaviors is difficult because the perceived danger so often feels to the client like a real one. Of course if the danger (threat or risk) is not real, then self-protection is unnecessary. But many clients do not know this at first, and feel extremely vulnerable if they stop protecting themselves. One of the main purposes of behavioral experiments is therefore to help clients learn that they will be alright without using safety-seeking behaviors or avoidance, and that these behaviors contribute more to the maintenance than to the resolution of their anxiety.

Trap 2

Client has a high perceived need for self-protection and seeks lots of advice from the therapist who makes frequent directive suggestions for the client to stop avoiding and using safety-seeking behaviors.

Therapists can easily fall into the trap of persuading clients to reduce those self-protective behaviors that clearly keep the anxiety going. But persuasion can have the unwanted consequence that "successes" are attributed to the good work of the therapist, or to chance, rather than to the client's own efforts. Successes are readily discounted by people with persistent anxiety disorders, especially when self-confidence and self-esteem, are low. Examples 4 and 5 illustrate ways therapists can use Socratic Dialogue instead of persuasion to help clients test out the value of self-protection beliefs and strategies.

Example 4: Taking a risk

The dialogue below demonstrates how difficult it can be to reduce avoidance and safety behaviors when a client has relied on these strategies as a means of managing his anxiety effectively. Carson was seeking treatment to overcome social anxiety that he felt was holding him back both professionally and socially. After a few sessions the therapist realized she was becoming too didactic and getting drawn into arguing with Carson about the utility of reducing his avoidance and use of safety behaviors. On noticing this she decided to "pull back" and ask Carson to reflect on the advantages and disadvantages of trying a different strategy, rather than continuing to try to convince him of what to do. This led to the following discussion:

Therapist: It feels a bit like we have reached an impasse with you thinking the best way forward is to use lots of safety-seeking behaviors to manage your anxiety, and to avoid the situations where you can't stop the anxiety from escalating, and me trying to convince you to try a different approach. Does it seem that way to you too?

Carson: I guess so.

Therapist: I wonder if we could spend a few minutes talking about that?

Carson: Sure.

Therapist: I can see why you feel that the safety-seeking behaviors have really helped. After all, they've got you this far.

Carson: I know.

Therapist: And it sounds like you have some pretty grave fears about how awful things would be if you didn't use them?

Carson: Yeah ... I think if people saw the real me it would be a hundred times worse. If I didn't try to hide the anxiety then I think I would come across as a total fool, and my colleagues would lose all respect for me. That would have lifelong consequences for my career. If I didn't prepare for conversations, I literally would just dry up and it would look like I was really weird, or there was something pretty seriously wrong with me.

Therapist: So I can see it must be pretty terrifying to even consider doing something different. And I have to recognize that these strategies have got you this far in coping with a pretty difficult problem.

Carson: Yeah, they have. On the other hand, I'm still not where I want to be...

Therapist: I know. I guess we know how things are when you do use the safety-seeking behaviors and avoidance strategies, but we don't know much about what the alternative might have been.

Carson: Yeah, I just can't help imagining it would be worse.

Therapist: I guess there aren't any guarantees that it won't be, which makes trying to make changes pretty scary. However, using those strategies hasn't gotten you where you want to be. (Pause.) Do you feel that you have given your current method for managing the problem—protecting yourself whenever you can by avoiding or using safety-seeking behaviors—a pretty good shot? Have you given that strategy a fair try in seeing if it will get you to where you want to be in terms of your social anxiety?

Carson: (Laughs.) Oh yeah, I think you could say that...

Therapist: How do you know you've given it a fair shot?

Carson: Because this is what I've been doing for the last 15 years. I've found more and more complicated ways of avoiding and protecting myself to keep people from finding out what I'm really like. So it's like a really complicated series of maneuvers now whenever I go into any social situation.

Therapist: So you've given avoidance a fair try to see how far it gets you, but it hasn't really gotten you to where you want to be?

Carson: I guess not—if it had I wouldn't be sitting here...

Therapist: So can you see any advantage in giving a different strategy a try?

Carson: I guess so. There is a chance it might work better.

Therapist: OK. How long do you think you would have to do something different if you were going to give it a "fair shot"?

Carson: Well, I don't think it needs to be for 15 years, maybe I could try it for a few weeks and see whether there are any benefits then?

Therapist: That makes sense. Is there anything you could do in those few weeks, or any way of approaching it that would maximize the chance of giving a new strategy a "fair try"?

Carson: Well maybe to stop questioning whether it is going to work because that undermines my motivation to try it. Maybe just treat it as another experiment—set a date to review how well it works, and between now and then give it as much of a go as I can?

Therapist: That sounds like a good plan—how could we go about putting it into action?

Notice that Carson hasn't actually been convinced that it is better not to avoid or use safety behaviors. All that has happened is that he has agreed it is worth trying a different strategy for managing his social anxiety. And he seems more motivated to give a new strategy a fair trial rather than being pushed down that route by the therapist. Here it was as much the therapist's Socratic attitude—accepting that we really don't know what will work better or worse for him—as much as the use of Socratic questions, that enabled them to regain their collaboration in tackling Carson's difficulties.

Keep in Mind

- Make sure clients understand exactly what words like "avoidance" and "safety-seeking behaviors" mean. Using specific examples from that client's experience is essential.

- If possible, validate what the client is trying to do (feel better) but not the way that they are doing it (using self-protection).

- Make it clear that you are not asking them to try harder—they are probably already putting in maximum effort—but to try *differently*.

- Make sure they are clear about what to do instead, about exactly what the alternative method is to involve.

- Work on something specific, then generalize to other issues.

- Accept (and ask for) doubts and reservations and encourage behavioral experiments to test these.

Example 5: Four aspects of homework

CBT theories of anxiety tell us that all types of safety-seeking keep anxiety going, and decades of research (half a century of it by now if one counts early work on methods of exposure) show that the most effective way to build confidence and to reduce all types of anxiety is to face the fear. Therefore, behavioral assignments to approach situations that evoke anxiety, usually taking the form of behavioral experiments (Bennett-Levy et al., 2004), form an essential part of treatment. These should be placed in a cognitive context, and constructed so as to make it possible to confirm or disconfirm beliefs. This means finding out what clients are thinking, and developing hypotheses about underlying assumptions and beliefs. Incorporating this information into the construction of homework assignments helps make those assignments maximally effective.

Socratic Dialogue is essential to capture learning from these experiments. Be alert to the many times in the process of debriefing homework when even experienced therapists are tempted to tell people what to do, or to explain to them what it all means. Instead of illustrating these difficulties using one extended example, in this section of the chapter we provide four short sections of dialogue which deal with difficulties that arise at different stages in the development and debriefing of homework.

Deciding what to do next

Anja's longstanding dental phobia meant that she had not had a check-up with a dentist for seven years. Consequently, she was suffering from intermittent toothache. Her main fear was about choking. She had numerous thoughts and images about choking and about what would happen if she did. During therapy she practiced with her partner at home, opening her mouth as if for an inspection, and letting him tap her teeth with a toothbrush, and then with a fork. She and her partner invented various other experiments, all of which contributed to building her confidence. Anja and her therapist then talked in more detail about her fear of choking and about explaining this to a dentist. They summarized this part of the work as follows:

Therapist: So you were saying that you would feel a lot better if the dentist knew how you felt and if you were able to explain to him that you might need to take a breather, or to ask for a break if things got too scary. Is that right?

Anja: Yes—and also that this would be just like doing another experiment like the ones I did at home, only this time it would be rather more difficult. I want the dentist to know what really bothers me too.

Therapist: So why don't you make an appointment just for a check-up before we next meet. Could you do that?

Anja: I'm not sure this is the best week because I have a lot of work due.

It is easy to get carried away with someone's enthusiasm and motivation, and to make what seems like an obvious suggestion. It is also tempting to do this when someone is, unlike Anja in this case, unable to think for themselves what to do next. However, as described in Chapter 2, giving the client a suggestion is likely to elicit a "Yes, but ... " response including thoughts about what is wrong or premature about the suggestion.

Keep in Mind

Turning a suggestion into a question quickly re-establishes the collabora-tive spirit of Socratic Dialogue. People are more likely to act on decisions they have made themselves than on suggestions made to them by others. "What" and "how" questions are good for eliciting ideas and suggestions from the client. For example:

- What would you like to do in the next week to take this forward?
- How exactly could you find that out?
- It sounds like you've done really well—what do you think the next step might be to keep building on the changes you've made?

Invitations can also work well:

- Shall we think together about what to do next?

It is important for therapists to develop their own Socratic Dialogue style, and to expand their repertoire of questions, so they are well prepared to resist the temptation to make suggestions.

Providing reassuring answers to questions

Miriam had obsessional worries about cleanliness. She feared that she would cause her small children, ages 3 years and 18 months, to become ill if she did not keep the house spotlessly clean. The amount of time she spent cleaning was increasing and was starting to interfere with her ability to look after the children. She had help from her mother and partner and so, while they were in the house, she devoted all her time to washing and cleaning. Miriam was deeply ashamed of her problem, and sought help reluctantly. She believed others would despise her, and think that she did not love her children.

Miriam understood the reasons why her treatment would involve doing some of the things that she feared (the rationale for exposure and response prevention). Even so, she consistently struggled to carry out behavioral exper-iments she agreed to do at home such as not washing clean clothes that had merely fallen on the floor, or playing with the children for half an hour without cleaning. When discussing this she became tearful, and said:

Miriam: It feels so dangerous. I'm so frightened that they will get ill.

Therapist: Shall we think about the amount of clothes washing you do? Tell me a bit more about that.

Miriam:	I'm doing half a dozen loads in the machine every day, and some stuff by hand too.
Therapist:	How much do you think you should be doing?
Miriam:	Mum says one load a day would do—and she gets so cross with me... for instance when I change the children's clothes after they've got them messy, or when they've been playing on the floor.
Therapist:	What do you think?
Miriam:	I know I'm doing too much. I just can't do what others expect.
Therapist:	What makes that so hard for you?
Miriam:	As soon as I've noticed something's dirty I start to think about one of them lying ill in a hospital bed with drips and everything... and it being all my fault because I could have prevented it if only I'd taken a bit more care .... I'm never sure I've got things clean enough. How do I know what's enough? How can I tell they'll be safe if I let things go?
Therapist:	By thinking about what others do, and about what you used to do before this all started. They'd be perfectly safe if you cut down your washing by half, or even more than that.

Notice the change in tone at the end when the therapist stops using Socratic Dialogue. These last points were, in this case, hardly heard by Miriam. She went on talking about being ashamed of being such a bad mother, about her fears of harming the children, and about her embarrassment about having to rely so much on others. When clients ask the therapist direct questions it is of course tempting to answer them: "How do I know what's enough?" "How can I tell they'll be safe if I let things go?" But instead it is more useful to continue on with Socratic Dialogue and invite your client to reflect on the questions, or on their fears, or on their reasons for their fears.

For example Miriam's therapist might have said: "I wonder how others know when they've done enough? Or how they get the balance right for them and their child?", or "Have you found that doing more washing makes you feel safer?" Or "How does it affect you if you think about them not being safe? What comes into your mind? How does it affect your worrying?" Reflections are also useful: "It sounds as if doubts creep in. Shall we think more about why that is?" or "It sounds like you are terrified that you will be responsible for them becoming really seriously ill if you don't clean everything to the nth degree?" The type of question that will be useful here will depend on the precise context, and on whether the client is ready to consider underlying assumptions and beliefs. The main point is that attempting to provide direct answers to such questions, rather than remaining Socratic, tends to end the reflective process and therefore to interrupt the work of therapy.

Reviewing progress

Haley was a nonbinary client who experienced agoraphobia and had not been out shopping alone for years. Their children shopped on their way home from school, and Haley was prompted to seek help when their last child was about to leave home. Haley made good progress in therapy in the first few weeks, and was surprised to discover that they could walk to the local shop on the corner of the road without too much difficulty. Before long Haley did this every day, and in reviewing the work their therapist commented: "You have done really well. What would you like to do next?" Haley decided to go with a neighbor to a nearby shopping center.

Again Haley completed this homework assignment. Rather than using Socratic Dialogue to debrief this experiment, their therapist said: "Well done. That's excellent" and swiftly started to plan what to do next. But the therapist had jumped to conclusions too quickly. Haley did not yet know what to expect by way of progress, and did not want to disappoint their therapist, or to reveal how panicky they had been. In fact, they had avoided doing anything alone during this last assignment, and was now finding it hard to continue with regular trips to the local shop. Some examples of Socratic questions the therapist might have asked when hearing about the apparently successful trip to the shopping center are the following:

> *What did you do?*
> *How do you feel about having done that?*
> *What was the hardest thing about what you did?*
> *How much were you able to do when you were there?*
> *How did it go, from your point of view?*
> *Was it easier or harder than you expected?*

The point of these informational questions is to discover more about the client's perception of and reaction to the recent experience. Without this detailed information it is difficult for both parties to work closely together, and to plan the next steps in ways that link the behavioral and cognitive aspects of treatment closely together. The more closely linked they are, the more effective client learning is likely to be.

Debriefing homework

When Rafael was 13 he came home from school and found his father dead in the sitting room. That morning, so far as he knew, his father had been perfectly well, and ever since then Rafael had worried that he too might unexpectedly become seriously ill and die suddenly. Rafael came for treatment when he was 45, the age at which his father died. His anxiety had escalated over the previous year and he was no longer able to work. When therapy started he was depressed as well as anxious.

When his family were out, Rafael spent much of the day checking himself over physically and mentally to make sure that he was OK. His main thoughts, consistent with his underlying belief, were about having something serious, and potentially life-threatening, wrong with him. His main assumptions dictating his behavior were phrased in pressurizing words: "I need to get this checked out", "You should always see the doctor quickly if you don't feel right", "I must see a specialist as soon as I can".

Therapy focused on using experiments designed to test out Rafael's assumptions. In the dialogue below Rafael and his therapist are talking about the results of an experiment to find out what happened to his symptoms when he delayed seeking medical advice.

Rafael: I did it! I managed a whole week without ringing the GP—and I'm still here to tell the tale.

Therapist: That's fantastic. You sound really pleased about that.

Rafael: Yes I am. It really made a big difference—what we talked about, and planning a proper test helped me to calm down, and not get so caught up in the terrible thoughts and the checking.

Therapist: Tell me more about it. Did you have any worrying symptoms?

Rafael: Yes—lots. I had a bad headache on Tuesday, and got really worried about it. But I went through the ideas we had written down after last session, and managed to hang on all day without ringing my doctor.

Therapist: What happened to the headache?

Rafael: By morning it had gone. That was the first symptom I had—and I think I was lucky because we watched football quite late that night and it was a great. That helped to take my mind off it and I slept much better. But later in the week I had quite a lot of other worrying symptoms—I've written them all down here. But I just kept in mind the idea that if I managed to resist checking up on them or going to the doctor then I'd be able to find out if they would naturally die away.

Therapist: And did they?

Rafael: Yes—every single one of them.

Therapist: So what do you make of that? What does it tell you?

Rafael: That it was a good experiment to do. I'm not sure I could do it again though, or keep it up much longer, but it did help.

Therapist: What's the most important thing to hang on to?

Rafael: It really helped to watch football, and to have my son with me doing that.

Therapist: And what else did you learn from it?

Rafael: I felt I'd been so foolish. I've been an idiot really.

Therapist: I don't think you have. Let's think it through together. You're saying that the experiment went really well, and you certainly came in today sounding really pleased with what you have been able to do. I think that proves you don't need to ring the GP so often. And it shows that you don't need to ask for medical advice every time you get one of these symptoms. That's because they don't mean that there's something seriously wrong with you at all. In fact they are perfectly normal mild symptoms that don't even last very long. Is that fair?

Rafael: . . . I suppose so . . . (speaking with some uncertainty).

Towards the end of this dialogue the therapist attempts to encourage Rafael to think about the meaning of his behavioral experiment, but Rafael first focuses on something specific to the particular situation: "It really helped to watch football . . . ", and then talks about his feelings, in a somewhat disparaging way: "I felt so foolish. I've been an idiot really." After having done a good job on the first two stages of Socratic Dialogue (informational questions and empathic listening) the therapist skips over the last two stages of Socratic Dialogue. Instead of making a written summary with Rafael of what he learned and then asking him an analytical or synthesizing question to link his experiences with assumptions they were testing, she draws conclusions for him.

Of course the conclusions stated by his therapist are ones we want Rafael to generate. Reading the dialogue, we might also think that the conclusions are justified on the basis of his new observations, or even that Rafael himself has already come to these conclusions although he has not yet said so. But if we are going to be able to help Rafael evaluate his assumptions and his beliefs, then he needs to be doing the rethinking for himself, and of course his thought processes might be quite different from those of his therapist. In particular, he might have his own reservations about the implications of what he has just done.

His therapist could have continued this discussion while maintaining a Socratic approach. For example, she could find out what Rafael is thinking about why the symptoms died away, what kinds of symptoms they were, or what would happen if he had those symptoms again—and if they were worse, stayed with him for longer, and so on. They could discuss Rafael's understanding of how his new observations fit with his previous assumptions. It could be useful to ask: "Do you remember what you said earlier about what you *should* do when you have a headache?", and then find out whether his recent experiment's results fit with that assumption. Since assumptions tie in so closely to behaviors (e.g., if you think you should get your symptoms checked, then you are likely to make an appointment with a doctor), then it is also important to help Rafael, if the old assumption turns out to be questionable, draft a new assumption and identify new behaviors that might fit with that.

Well-constructed experiments also have implications for underlying beliefs. We know that Rafael's experience with his father's quick and unexpected death was his good reason for believing that he could have something serious and life-threatening wrong with him. Of course the results of one week's experiments are hardly likely to change a strongly held underlying belief, especially for someone with Rafael's history. Socratic Dialogue helps a therapist prompt the client to recognize the old belief, and its effects on him, and begin to build up a body of evidence that might help draft a new belief. One way of doing this is illustrated in the dialogue below.

Rafael: I felt I'd been so foolish. I've been an idiot really.

Therapist: What makes you say that?

Rafael: For years and years I've been giving other people control over my life.

Therapist: I'm not sure I know what you mean by that.

Rafael: Well, what I'm thinking is that I've let everyone else be the judge of what's going on inside me—as if only doctors could be the experts. As if seeing them was the only way of knowing whether I was really ill. I just assumed I would never be able to find stuff out for myself.

Therapist: What sort of stuff do you mean?

Rafael: Like whether I need to take my symptoms seriously. It's amazing to discover that ones that really scare me can just disappear if I don't think about them all the time.

Therapist: Right—I really agree. So what might you say to yourself when the next one comes along, instead of thinking "only doctors can be experts?"

Rafael: Don't be an idiot. Do something to take your mind off it and see if it passes.

Therapist: OK—but how do you know that's the right thing to do?

Rafael: I'm not sure.

Therapist: You said something about discovering you could find stuff out for yourself . . . is that something you really believe?

Rafael: It really hit me in the face just now—but I'm not sure I'll be able to hang on to the idea if things get difficult. I think I should try to find out first and only go to see doctors much later.

Therapist: As if you could become the judge of what is going on inside you . . .

Rafael: Yes. I should trust myself more, and my body too. Trust my body to put the simple things right. I should give it a chance and discover how to use my own judgment.

Therapist: That sounds like really important learning. Maybe we should write that down in our session summary so we don't forget it.

More experiments and discussions with Rafael will be needed. However, this dialogue has provided a context within which it is much easier to address the doubts and reservations that will inevitably arise as Rafael works to change his beliefs as well as his behavior.

Keep in Mind

When debriefing homework:

- Use "What?" and "How?" questions.
- Resist the temptation to make suggestions. They are less likely to be acted on than ideas coming from the client. Vague ideas can be refined during discussion.
- Don't take homework reports at face value. Find out as much as you can about what happened, remembering that clients may have found things harder than they like to admit, or be discounting successes.
- Resist the temptation to draw conclusions for the client. Instead, explore the ways clients interpret the results of their homework. Make written summaries of useful ideas generated by the client so they are not forgotten.
- Help clients consider how evidence collected during homework assignments fits with or contradicts old assumptions and beliefs.

When appropriate, use this evidence to draft new assumptions and beliefs.

- Remember that clients may have reservations about drawing conclusions that seem obvious to the therapist.
- Ask the client for their suggestions as to what the best next steps might be, or how they might resolve any remaining uncertainty.

Rigidity in response to anxiety

It is understandable that people want to try to keep a tight hold on themselves after an experience of being seriously frightened or a long period of experiencing anxiety, especially if there is a belief that you can keep fear and its alarming symptoms at bay. People sometimes develop rigid habits and routines designed to prevent anxiety. Clients can feel excessively anxious about changing these habits. When they attempt to make a change, feelings of being out of control seem to be on a hair trigger. Therapists can then fall into the trap of constructing homework tasks that inadvertently reinforce the need to be in control instead of helping the client to tolerate more flexibility. One way out of this difficulty is illustrated in the next example.

Trap 3

Client is overly rigid in behavior and cognitive processing. The therapist inadvertently colludes with client by constructing homework tasks that reinforce the need to be in control instead of helping the client to tolerate more flexibility.

Example 6: Letting go of control

Cecil suffered from lifelong illness anxiety and OCD. He had recently retired from a successful military career. Since retiring Cecil had more unstructured time. His rituals expanded to fill the time available. His wife prompted him to seek therapy. It was clear that Cecil's obsessional routines were placing significant strain on his family relationships. The first few sessions concentrated on reviewing the history of the problem and drawing up a hierarchy for exposure and response prevention. The excerpt below begins with the therapist and Cecil reviewing his progress with exposure and response prevention.

Cecil: It's gone very well. I've been able to leave things out of place every day and one day I even left the kitchen in a complete mess for 3 hours.

Therapist: That sounds great. How was it to do that?

Cecil: I was surprised it didn't really make me that anxious. Things that normally cause me to blow up haven't really bothered me so much.

Therapist: What do you make of that?

Cecil: Well I think it is OK because I know that in exactly 2 hours and 59 minutes I'm going to get in there and sort it out, so it's not the same as when my wife leaves a mess.

Therapist: How do you mean?

Cecil: Well this week my daughter visited and it drove me up the wall— she kept putting things back in the wrong place, like the towels that are guest towels she left in the main bathroom. I just flipped and started shouting at her and then everyone was upset and she said that I didn't want her there.

Therapist: So how is it different when your daughter does that compared to when you have purposefully left things in the wrong place?

Cecil: Well I guess it is the control—when I've done it I at least know where it is.

By retaining a sense of curiosity about Cecil's experiences during the week, his therapist's Socratic questioning uncovered that the previous homework assignment was somewhat misguided as it focused on exposure to things being out of place, but had not involved exposure to his core cognitive element of not being in total control of his environment.

Cecil and his therapist worked together to draw out a formulation of his current difficulties which put his desire to be in control of his environment in a central role in the maintenance of his problems. This revised formulation made better sense of why he was able to create mess himself, but became extremely upset, anxious, and angry if someone else interfered with his environment. Further exploration of Cecil's history made sense of how his need to be in control of his environment had developed and he was able to see that that strategy had more disadvantages than advantages at home.

Subsequent therapy tasks concentrated on more cognitively oriented behavioral experiments designed to test out the consequences of not being in control. Cecil experimented with situations that he found distressing, such as tolerating his wife reorganizing some cupboards. He also tried acting spontaneously in positive ways by, for example, deciding to go out for the day because a last minute invitation came along, or because it happened to be good weather, rather than planning everything in advance.

Keep in Mind

- Work with your clients to develop a longitudinal formulation of their beliefs and consider how well their beliefs work for them in their current environment.

- Make sure to stay curious and explore the meanings behind both progress and lack of progress in therapy.

- Engage your clients in working creatively to overcome blocks to progress.

- Search for ways of increasing flexibility so your clients will be able to adapt to new situations.

Common Traps Originating in Therapists' Beliefs

Previous examples have illustrated common traps that arise when working with people who struggle with anxiety and how guided discovery can be used to alleviate these difficulties, keeping in mind anxiety treatment principles. In this section we show that sometimes therapists' beliefs such as "She's too fragile" or "He's not ready for this yet" can also interfere with therapy progress.

Recognize these Traps?

Trap 4
Colluding with avoidance for fear of being unkind.

Trap 5
Colluding with avoidance due to fears the client's vulnerability might be real.

Successful therapy necessarily involves a focus on client anxiety and perceived sources of threat. This exposure is often difficult and upsetting for clients with high levels of anxiety. Therapists who work with anxiety sometimes find it challenging to know how to tolerate and respond to appropriately high levels of affect in the room. For most therapists, it runs against the grain to do anything that causes the client to feel worse, even if only temporarily. To the degree this type of therapist discomfort reduces a client's exposure to effective treatment interventions, therapist avoidance of client discomfort can reduce client benefit from treatment (Farrell et al., 2013; Waller, 2009). For example, the evidence base for the treatment of PTSD suggests that therapy should involve exposure to all specific traumatic images (Bryant et al., 2008; Cusack et al., 2015; Foa & Rothbaum, 1998; Foa et al., 2007; Watkins et al., 2018) and that therapists often avoid doing this (Becker et al., 2004; Farrell et al., 2013).

Fear of being unkind

> **Trap 4**
>
> Colluding with avoidance for fear of being unkind.

Example 7: Fear of being unkind

Julie had been assaulted and raped on her way home from a party when she was 18. During treatment for PTSD three years later she agreed to engage in a detailed reliving exercise designed to identify the main cognitive themes involved. The intention was to identify "hot spots," or the worst (most emotional) moments of the traumatic experience (see Foa & Rothbaum, 1998; Grey, 2009), and an extra-long therapy session had been planned to leave sufficient time for this. Julie became extremely distressed when describing details of the rape. She cried out, opened her eyes, sat up suddenly, and said she was unable to continue. After a pause, and some comforting words, she calmed down and said she was ready to start again. Her therapist said:

Therapist: OK. This is really painful stuff. Probably the worst bit of all. Take a deep breath. Let's stop and think together about what we should do now.

Julie: I really don't want to talk any more about that bit today.

Therapist: I'm not surprised. Can you think back and tell me how you feel about the first part of the reliving exercise, before you got to the worst bit?

Julie: I didn't realize until we went through it in detail how powerless I felt.

Therapist: That seems really important. Let's write that down. You have told me before that you managed in the end to get away, and to call for help. Is that right?

Julie: Yes.

Therapist: So you found the power to get away. How did you do that?

Julie: I can remember exactly ...

Therapist: How do you feel about us exploring "finding the power"?

Julie: That would be good, I think. Finding that power is what made the difference.

Therapist: We could do that in reliving, so that we get a really good idea of how you managed to get away. We could start from the point when you found the power to escape. Are you ready for that? Could you do it if we started from the point when you are about to get away?

Julie was able to resume the reliving and to describe the rest of the traumatic experience in detail. When the session ended she had learned something important (about the feeling of powerlessness). She left with a sense of achievement, and follow-up work focused on her thoughts and feelings about being powerless, predominantly using cognitive restructuring techniques. Both Julie and her therapist were reluctant to talk further about the worst part of her trauma, which remained unexplored.

Theoretically, avoidance will limit Julie's recovery. Collusion with avoidance is understandable, but ultimately not helpful to her, and of course the therapist may resolve this issue in supervision, or through peer case discussion. Self-reflection, though, is always available when supervisors and colleagues might not be. Here is a list of Socratic questions therapists can ask themselves during the process of self-supervision:

- What went well in this session? What went less well?
- If we continue in this way will the client be likely to make lasting changes?
- What does the literature tell me about effective methods for this problem?
- Theoretically, what should I be doing with this client?
- What are likely to be the limitations on progress with this person if I follow evidence-based guidelines? If I don't?
- How do I feel about the work with this client? Is there anything I am avoiding doing?
- Is there anything I dread talking about with this person?
- Is this client strong enough (e.g., to complete the reliving exercise)?
- How does it feel to me to upset someone who has already been hurt?
- What would an ideal therapist do here?
- If I were the one in treatment, what would I want my therapist to encourage me to do? Could I handle this, even if it is difficult or uncomfortable?

This list of questions can be elaborated, of course. The point is that the Socratic questions are extremely helpful when reflecting on the work of a session. Answers to such questions also can help identify assumptions so they can be tested. A therapist who is thinking, "If I push this person, then they will become too distressed to continue our work," is less likely to help someone to face their traumatic intrusions than one who thinks, "If we complete this reliving exercise, then recovery is more likely."

Fears the client's vulnerability is real

Trap 5

Colluding with avoidance due to fears the client's vulnerability might be real.

CBT for anxiety disorders requires exposure to core concerns, triggers, and associated situations and feelings. Therapists are typically concerned about what their clients might do when they feel severely anxious. Can they be certain, for instance, when their client with OCD experiments standing next to an open window holding her baby that she will not do as she fears and actually throw the baby out of it? Can they be sure that the client will not have a heart attack if they bring on a panic attack in the session? Will the anxious driver also be a safe one? Therapists can use the same methods of guided discovery to explore their own fears, either during sessions or outside them. This exploration is often a necessary step for resolving therapy difficulties.

Example 8: The vulnerability might be real
Mark had an extensive family history of heart failure. During his treatment for severe panic disorder it was thus understandable that he was reluctant to engage in any therapy tasks that he thought might bring on a heart attack. Through discussion with his physician and research on the Internet, Mark learned that there was no evidence that there was currently anything wrong with his heart. He also learned that not all heart conditions were detectable. He understood that, in rare circumstances, exertion could be dangerous to those with a pre-existing condition. The therapist recognized they had reached an impasse when both of them became too frightened to test Mark's fears about whether any exertion or stress could indeed provoke a heart attack.

Therapist: It seems that we have a good understanding of what keeps your panic attacks going. You have the idea that there might be something wrong with your heart and that if you let any anxiety escalate, or exert yourself physically, this could bring on a heart attack. Feeling stressed or taking exercise is really frightening, so you avoid those things.

Mark: Yeah, I don't feel that I have much choice. As soon as the panic starts I just have to get out of the situation. If I don't, that might be it.

Therapist: It sounds as if you live every day feeling as if you've narrowly escaped death?

Mark: Pretty much!

Therapist: Normally the way forward would be to see if your fears were realistic—to try and test out whether those panicky sensations really were signs of a heart attack. Do you think there is any way we could do that?

Mark: No, definitely not. I really don't want to take the risk.

Therapist: I do understand that, and so I want to think how best to help.

In the Therapist's Mind

At this point Mark and his therapist felt stuck. His therapist decided to return to basics and look at Mark's evidence for his belief that his heart may be especially vulnerable. It turned out that the men in his family who had died of heart failure were mostly in their 50s, while Mark was only 34, and so far he had a clean bill of health. So the therapist tried to engage Mark in problem solving about how they could take the work forward.

Therapist: So can you sum up what we have learned about your family history of heart disease for me?

Mark: Well most of my uncles who died did so when they were in their fifties—quite a lot older than me, and I could go the same way.

Therapist: Yes—we have to acknowledge that you could have inherited a real vulnerability even though there's every sign that you're well now.

Mark: Yes.

Therapist: How do you understand this vulnerability? Can you tell me more about that?

Mark:	Well I guess I really am more vulnerable than other people, so I don't want to do anything that could be dangerous.
Therapist:	Uh-huh.
Mark:	It just feels way too scary to let the feelings escalate and take the risk that I could die ...
Therapist:	I can understand that. For a long time you've thought that your heart could suddenly give out, and you say you have avoided any situations that would put it under stress, so it would be pretty scary to act against that.
Mark:	Yes, but I don't want to carry on like this either—I feel like I'm living a half-life. In order to stay alive I'm sacrificing living life to the full ... there are so many things I can't do because of the fear.
Therapist:	So it sounds like you are keen to try to find a way around this and get the other half of your life back?
Mark:	Yes.
Therapist:	But to also try to minimize the risk of putting stress on your heart?
Mark:	Exactly. But I guess I've got to put my heart under stress if I want to get the other half of my life back?
Therapist:	To some degree yes, but I was also wondering if there was some way to go about that that might make it a bit easier for you.
Mark:	Well I guess it would be easier if we had a full team of paramedics on call in case anything did go wrong. (Laughs.)
Therapist:	(Laughing too.) But would that really be helpful? What would you learn from that?
Mark:	I'm not sure ... perhaps something about how important it is not to put myself under stress and strain unless I'm sure I'm safe.
Therapist:	OK. And my fear is that that would leave you feeling just as vulnerable in the end. Instead let's think about how fit you now are. How much exercise do you take?
Mark:	Hardly any. I'm certainly less fit than I was even a year ago. Even carrying the shopping I stop and rest if I get out of breath.
Therapist:	So do you think there's a possibility that being relatively unfit has made your sense of vulnerability even worse?
Mark:	I've thought about that myself. I think it has.
Therapist:	What would you feel about checking out with your doctor whether an exercise program might help you? And find out what kind of program. Should you start gently or what would help keep you physically in good shape?

Mark: I know it would help to be fitter—and it would give me a better chance of surviving if there really was a crisis. But I get really scared when I get out of breath. I'm not sure I could manage an exercise program. But I will talk to the doctor.

Therapist: And would you give me permission to talk to your doctor too? If all of us agree, then you and I could work out the kind of program that would build your confidence and make you fitter at the same time. Meanwhile, could you start by keeping a record of the exercise you take this week?

Mark and his therapist have taken a long time to get to this point, and it will take even longer to work out the details of a program that he is able and willing to engage in. However, this is time well spent in the circumstances, and illustrates how important it is for therapists to take such fears seriously if the client is to remain motivated.

Furthermore, it may be anxiety provoking for both Mark and his therapist to drop all safety-seeking behaviors during experiments or exposure tasks. Even so, all is not lost if the client is unwilling to drop all safety-seeking behaviors immediately—Rachman et al. (2008) conclude that there is sufficient theoretical justification, experimental evidence, and clinical observation showing that the judicious use of safety-seeking behaviors, especially in the early stages of treatment, can be facilitative, and does not necessarily prevent disconfirmatory experiences. During the session excerpted above, Mark's therapist was able to use Socratic Dialogue to (1) explore the evidence behind problematic beliefs, (2) gain new information about the problem, (3) help Mark synthesize new information into his pre-existing beliefs, and, most importantly, (4) overcome the "block" they mutually had reached in testing out his beliefs.

Fine-tuning Socratic Dialogue

One of the many advantages of using Socratic Dialogue is that it helps people learn and it helps people to remember what they have learned. Written summaries and notes made when listening to a recording of therapy sessions also help with this. When clients are encouraged to find out more about their lives and then draw their own conclusions, this learning is likely to be more memorable for them. However, there are some situations when using Socratic Dialogue or other methods of guided discovery elicit unhelpful responses, or when they appear to inhibit learning and interfere (temporarily) with progress. Four of these are described next, together with ideas about how to "fine-tune" the methods when such difficulties arise.

Avoid questions that unhelpfully amplify worry

Socratic Dialogue can be useful or problematic depending upon whether the questions asked and the summaries made are consistent with the conceptualization of a particular anxiety issue. For example, some clients are superskilled and well-practiced at identifying possible negative outcomes to future events. The most skilled of all are probably those with GAD whose thinking is focused on the terrible things that might (but also might not) happen. These experts in worrying repeatedly ask themselves, and others, "What if … ?" Asking a standard Socratic question such as "What might happen then?" can amplify and expand the process of worry. This can be helpful when the goal is to learn the most catastrophic outcomes feared by the client. A person who worries will respond to "What might happen?" with increasing numbers of potential disaster scenarios.

However, in the treatment of worry, Socratic Dialogue is more usefully employed to refocus the process of worry on ways of coping with fears and the search for specific solutions rather than on the content of worries. Thus, more helpful Socratic questions ask, "What could you do when that catastrophe happens? How could you cope? What resources could help you?" This was illustrated in Example 3 earlier in this chapter.

When clients avoid affect

Guided discovery may not bring with it the expected advantages when someone avoids affect. People who habitually avoid the experience and/or the expression of emotion, and try not to let their feelings show, often do this because they are frightened of having feelings, talking about feelings, and/or provoking feelings or the expressions of feelings in others. Avoidance of affect may coexist with an inability to distinguish thoughts, feelings, and behaviors accurately. It may also be associated with degrees of alexithymia, which makes it hard to name feelings or even to recognize them (for more detailed accounts of avoidance of affect and its treatment, see Butler et al., 2008; Butler & Surawy, 2004; Padesky & Beck, 2014).

When working with clients who avoid affect, it is important to come to some understanding about why this might be. Sometimes these clients' early experiences have involved neglect or emotional abuse and the sense that they are not valued by others but instead are more likely to be criticized or humiliated by them. These clients can become distressed or withdrawn when questioned about their feelings, or when trying to describe their reactions to difficult experiences. Focusing more than usual on the second stage of Socratic Dialogue, empathic listening, is often helpful. One might, for instance, say, "That sounds alarming," or "You look sad when you say that," or "I can see that that makes you uncomfortable," or "Underneath you sound a bit hopeless." An emphasis on empathic listening can be very effective in these cases and allows the therapist to maintain a Socratic attitude throughout.

People who avoid affect also benefit immensely from the third stage of Socratic Dialogue, summaries, which prompt them to reflect on the work that has just been done rather than quickly pushing it out of their mind. Helpful questions to summarize learning in a session or to encourage a client to reflect on its potential value include "What will you remember about our discussion today?" and "What's the most important part of that for you?" Once a summary is written, a helpful analytical question (fourth stage of the 4-Stage Model of Socratic Dialogue) is "How would you like to take this forward during the week?" Written summaries and analytical questions are especially important for clients who are prone to avoid thinking about issues between sessions.

When clients lack confidence

Some clients who are seriously lacking in confidence and those who are habitually reticent may work very hard to please the therapist and be reluctant to volunteer their own opinions. This can present problems for them in answering Socratic questions. They may respond to open questions with "I don't know" or "What do you think?", or even with silence. Therapists need to be comfortable with silence, willing to take things slowly, waiting perhaps for a response to be formed. Socratic Dialogue can help if the therapist uses questions to draw the client's attention to information that is outside of current awareness, e.g., "What has worked for you before in similar situations?" or "What might you advise someone else to do in this situation?" or "What ideas do you have about what the range of possible responses might be?" If these questions are met with a blank stare, the therapist can offer a number of suggestions and ask clients to choose among them.

Alternatively, therapists can address this process issue directly, using Socratic Dialogue to guide the client to examine their thoughts, feelings, or behaviors, including what is in the client's mind when they find it hard to respond.

Therapist: Could we take a moment to think together about how therapy is working for you?

Joe: Uh—um ... Yes.

Therapist: I've noticed that sometimes it seems hard for you answer the questions I ask, or to think what to say. I feel I put you on the spot, and make you feel uncomfortable.

Joe: (Slowly.) ... Often I don't know what to say. I can't think of what's the right thing to say. And I'm not sure how to say it right ...

Therapist: When you do try to tell me more about yourself, and about how you feel, it is much easier for me to think about how best to help.

Joe: ... but sometimes I just go blank.

Therapist: How do you feel then, when you go blank?

Joe: A bit stressed really ...

Therapist: Do you know it would really help me to know that at the time? Do you think you could let me know when you're feeling stressed?

Joe: OK.

Therapist: If you could do that then I would know to give you more time, or not to keep pressing you so hard. We could work together to find a way of coping with feeling stressed. How do you feel about that?

As usual, guiding discovery takes time. If, in the future, Joe is able to identify a moment when he feels "stressed," his therapist can help him identify additional thoughts and feelings then. This may lead to behavioral experiments in session to test out beliefs about how it feels to express an opinion and whether the therapist responds in ways he expects or fears.

When a client has limited experience of not being anxious

Guided discovery can be especially challenging to use effectively when working with someone who has a long history of feeling anxious. People who have lived with chronic anxiety may present for treatment with complex, long-standing problems originating in early childhood. In addition, sometimes people who have grown up in circumstances filled with violence or emotional abuse may continue to remain hypervigilant for signs of rejection, violence, or abuse so that they live with high levels of anxiety even when their situation has changed. Asking people who have lived with anxiety most of their life to think about other ways of seeing things or of other ways of coping with difficulties may meet with silence. It is as if there is no alternative set of information to draw upon.

Normally with Socratic Dialogue we use questions to draw attention to something within the person's realm of knowledge, but currently outside awareness. When the realm of knowledge is one-sided, or one-dimensional, there may be little else to draw attention to.

When this is the case, some clients benefit from learning how to use relaxation exercises or simple meditation exercises. This then gives them a non-anxious experience to draw on, an experience that might be taken forward in a behavioral experiment.

With people who have experienced chronic anxiety, it is also very helpful to look for alternative interpretations of present-day experiences. By focusing first on understanding what is in the client's knowledge and awareness, the therapist can help the client focus on information that suggests dangers may not be as great as imagined and that coping might be more effective than the client believes. Small behavioral experiments, first in the office and then outside therapy, with clear predictions in advance for what "anxiety predicts" and what an alternative belief predicts are quite helpful. It can be useful to interweave relatively didactic moments with more Socratic ones (be they behavioral or verbal). For example, a therapist could explain to a young adult starting a new job what might be expected of them in their new work setting. Next, they could reflect together on how to use this information in a behavioral experiment and consider what various outcomes might mean.

Summary

In this chapter we have illustrated many ways of using Socratic Dialogue and other forms of guided discovery when working with people who suffer from one (or more) anxiety or related disorders. We have focused on some of the more common problems that arise in normal clinical practice, and our examples illustrate many different types of anxiety. Remember that these most common problems arise in most of the anxiety disorders, and therefore the points made by the examples, and the Keep in Mind boxes at the end of each of them, apply generally. The traps addressed are listed in Box 4.1, and this list can be used to find relevant ideas when problems arise in practice.

We think that the examples described in Box 4.1, "Summary of Traps Addressed," link closely with the theoretical ideas with which this chapter began. When applied in clinical practice the methods illustrated exemplify the main principles in the following "Keep in Mind" box.

Box 4.1 Summary of Traps Addressed

Common traps arising from clients' beliefs
Trap 1: Intolerance of uncertainty; therapist falls into reassurance trap

1. Something terrible might happen

2. Needing to be sure

3. Endless worry

Trap 2: The perceived need for self-protection; therapist becomes too directive

4. Taking a risk

5. Four aspects of homework

    Deciding what to do next

    Providing reassuring answers to questions

    Reviewing progress

    Debriefing homework

Trap 3: Rigidity in response to anxiety; therapist colludes with desire to stay in control

6. Letting go of control

Common traps originating in therapists' beliefs

7. Fear of being unkind

8. A client's vulnerability might be real

Keep in Mind

- Make sure you understand the reasons for using Socratic Dialogue in relation to anxiety, and therefore also understand when to use other guided discovery methods as well.
- Develop your own style of being Socratic rather than modeling yourself on someone else. The variety of examples provided in this chapter is intended to illustrate that there is no single right way.
- Work on the process of worrying more than the content. As therapy progresses, shift more attention to the processes that maintain anxiety.
- Use Socratic Dialogue to clarify personal meanings, especially those that link to personal vulnerability.
- Use action methods of guided discovery, especially behavioral experiments. When new ideas or perspectives come to mind, behavioral experiments provide a source of new data and a means to compare anxious beliefs with alternative perspectives.
- Calculating probabilities is only rarely helpful. Images of an air crash, however unlikely to happen, are still likely to frighten a client. It is the personal cost of danger that matters to the client. Socratic Dialogue can help a client assess that cost and figure out ways to mitigate and cope with it.

Although therapists using cognitive-behavioral methods may read the same literature, apply the same theory, and in general use the same methods, we all have different personalities and different clinical styles. Therefore, we hope readers consider the ideas in this chapter as food for thought, rather than rules. Best use of the principles discussed requires each clinician to consider how to adapt these concepts to their own circumstances and the cultural contexts relevant to them and their clients.

Reader Learning Activities

- Reread the clinical examples. Thinking about the clinical difficulties described, consider how you would use guided discovery in each type of situation. Mentally role-play the words and/or experiments you would use to identify, explore, or test your clients' beliefs.

- Listen to a recording of yourself in therapy with a client who experiences anxiety. Ask yourself how Socratic the process sounds. Think about how to make the interactions more Socratic. Identify any statements you make and ask yourself whether you could have enabled the client to access that information themselves by using questions.

- Think about the advantages and disadvantages of your particular style for work with people who suffer from anxiety. How can you develop and make the most of your style?

- Devise your own list of Socratic questions for self-supervision. Use the questions on p. 180 as a starting point.

References

American Psychiatric Association. (2013). *Diagnostic and statistical manual of mental disorders: DSM-5* (5th ed.). Washington, DC: American Psychiatric Association.

Arntz, A., Rauner, M., & Van den Hout, M. (1995). "If I feel anxious, then it must be dangerous": Ex-consequentia reasoning in inferring danger in anxiety disorders. *Behavior Research and Therapy, 33*, 917–925. https://doi.org/10.1016/0005-7967(95)00032-S

Bar-Hiam, Y., Lamy, D., Pergamin, L., Bakermans-Kranenburg, M. J., & Van Ijzendoorn, M. H. (2007). Threat-related attentional bias in anxious and non-anxious individuals: A meta-analytic study. *Psychological Bulletin, 133*, 1–24. https://doi.org/10.1037/0033-2909.133.1.1

Beck, A. T., Emery, G., & Greenberg, R. (1985). *Anxiety disorders and phobias: A cognitive perspective*. New York: Guilford Press.

Becker, C. B., Zayfert, C., & Anderson, E. (2004). A survey of psychologists' attitudes towards and utilization of exposure therapy for PTSD. *Behavior Research &Therapy, 42*, 277–292. https://doi.org/10.1016/S0005-7967(03)00138-4

Bennett-Levy, J., Butler, G., Fennell, M., Hackmann, A., Mueller, M., & Westbrook, D. (Eds.). (2004). *Oxford guide to behavioural experiments in cognitive therapy*. Oxford: Oxford University Press.

Blakey, S. M., & Abramowitz, J. S. (2016). The effects of safety behaviors during exposure therapy for anxiety: Critical analysis from an inhibitory learning perspective. *Clinical Psychology Review, 49*, 1–15. https://doi.org/10.1016/j.cpr.2016.07.002

Borkovec, T. D., Lyonfields, J. D., Wiser, S. L., & Deihl, L. (1993). The role of worrisome thinking in the suppression of cardiovascular response to phobic imagery. *Behaviour Research and Therapy, 31*, 321–324. https://doi.org/10.1016/0005-7967(93)90031-O

Borkovec, T. D. & Newman, M. G. (1998). Worry and generalised anxiety disorder. In P. Salkovskis (Ed.), *Comprehensive clinical psychology* (vol 6, pp. 439–59). Oxford: Elsevier.

Bryant, R. A., Mastrodomenico, J., Felmingham, K., Hopwood, S., Kenny, L., Kandris, E., Cahill, C., & Creamer, M. (2008). Treating acute stress disorder: A randomized controlled trial. *Archives of General Psychiatry, 65*, 659–667. https://doi.org/10.1001/archpsyc.65.6.659

Buhr, K., & Dugas, M. J. (2012). Fear of emotions, experiential avoidance, and intolerance of uncertainty in worry and generalized anxiety disorder. *International Journal of Cognitive Therapy*, 5(1), 1–17. https://doi.org/10.1521/ijct.2012.5.1.1

Butler, G., Fennell, M., & Hackmann, A. (2008). *Cognitive-behavioral therapy for anxiety disorders: Mastering clinical challenges.* New York: Guilford Press.

Butler, G., & Mathews, A. (1983). Cognitive processes in anxiety. *Advances in Behaviour Therapy and Research*, 5, 51–62. https://doi.org/10.1016/0146-6402(83)90015-2

Butler, G., & Surawy, C. (2004). Avoidance of affect. In J. Bennett-Levy, G. Butler, M. Fennell, A Hackmann, M. Mueller, & D. Westbrook (Eds.), (2004, pp. 351–69). *Oxford guide to behavioural experiments in cognitive therapy.* Oxford: Oxford University Press.

Butler, G., Wells, A., and Dewick, H. (1995). Differential effect of worry and imagery after exposure to stressful stimulus. *Behavioural and Cognitive Psychotherapy*, 25, 45–56. https://doi.org/10.1017/S1352465800017628

Cisler, J. M., & Koster, E. H. (2010). Mechanisms of attentional biases towards threat in anxiety disorders: An integrative review. *Clinical psychology review*, 30(2), 203–216. https://doi.org/10.1016/j.cpr.2009.11.003

Clark, D. A., & Beck, A. T. (2011). *Cognitive therapy of anxiety disorders: Science and practice.* New York: Guilford Press.

Cusack, K., Jonas, D. E., Forneris, C. A., Wines, C., Sonis, J., Middleton, J. C., Feltner, C., Brownley, K. A., Olmsted, K. R., Greenblatt, A., Weil, A., & Gaynes, B. N. (2016). Psychological treatments for adults with posttraumatic stress disorder: A systematic review and meta-analysis. *Clinical Psychology Review*, 43, 128–141. https://doi.org/10.1016/j.cpr.2015.10.003

Dugas, M. J., Gagnon, F., Ladouceur, R., & Freeston, M. H. (1998). Generalized anxiety disorder: A preliminary test of a conceptual model. *Behaviour Research and Therapy*, 36, 215–226. https://doi.org/10.1016/S0005-7967(97)00070-3

Farrell, N. R., Deacon, B. J., Kemp, J. J., Dixon, L. J., & Sy, J. T. (2013). Do negative beliefs about exposure therapy cause its suboptimal delivery? An experimental investigation. *Journal of Anxiety Disorders*, 27, 763–771. https://doi.org/10.1016/j.janxdis.2013.03.007

Foa, E. B., & Rothbaum, B. O. (1998). *Treating the trauma of rape: Cognitive behavioral therapy for PTSD.* New York: Guilford Press.

Foa,, E. B., Hembree, E. A., & Rothbaum, B. O. (2007). *Prolonged exposure therapy for PTSD: Emotional processing of traumatic experiences: Therapist guide.* New York: Oxford University Press.

Grey, N. (Ed.). (2009). *A casebook of cognitive therapy for traumatic stress reactions.* New York: Routledge.

Harvey, A., Watkins, E., Mansell, W., & Shafran, R. (2004). *Cognitive behavioural processes across psychological disorders: A transdiagnostic approach to research and treatment.* Oxford: Oxford University Press.

Hebert, E. A., & Dugas, M. J. (2019). Behavioral experiments for intolerance of uncertainty: Challenging the unknown in the treatment of generalized anxiety disorder. *Cognitive and Behavioral Practice*, 26(2), 421–436. https://doi.org/10.1016/j.cbpra.2018.07.007

Hirsch, C., & Mathews, A. (2000). Impaired positive inferential bias in social phobia. *Journal of Abnormal Psychology*, 109, 705–712. https://doi.org/10.1037/0021-843X.109.4.705

Huppert, J. D., Moser, J. S., Gershuny, B. S., Riggs, D. S., Spokas, M., Filip, J., Hajcak, G., Parker, H. A., & Baer, L. (2005). The relationship between obsessive-compulsive and post-traumatic stress symptoms in clinical and non-clinical samples. *Journal of Anxiety Disorders*, 19, 127–136. https://doi.org/10.1016/j.janxdis.2004.01.001

Kennerley, H., Kirk, J., & Westbrook, D. (2017). *An introduction to cognitive therapy: Skills and applications* (3rd ed.). London: Sage.

Leahy, R. L., Holland, S. J. F., & McGinn, L. K. (2012). *Treatment plans and interventions for depression and anxiety disorders* (2nd ed.). New York: Guilford Press.

McManus, F., Clark, D. M., Grey, N., Wild, J., Hirsch, C., Fennell, M., Hackman, A., Waddington, L., Liness, S., & Manley, J. (2009). A demonstration of the efficacy of two of the components of cognitive therapy for social phobia. *Journal of Anxiety Disorders, 23*, 496–503. https://doi.org/10.1016/j.janxdis.2008.10.010

McManus, F., Sacadura, C., & Clark, D. M. (2008). Why social anxiety persists: An experimental manipulation of the role of safety behaviors as a possible maintaining factor. *Journal of Behavior Therapy and Experimental Psychiatry, 39*, 147–61. https://doi.org/10.1016/j.jbtep.2006.12.002

Mahoney, A., Hobbs, M., Newby, J., Williams, A., & Andrews, G. (2018). Maladaptive behaviours associated with generalized anxiety disorder: An item response theory analysis. *Behavioural and Cognitive Psychotherapy, 46*(4), 479–496. https://doi.org/10.1017/S1352465818000127

Mansell, W., Harvey, A., Watkins, E., & Shafran, R. (2009). Conceptual foundations of a transdiagnostic approach to CBT. *Journal of Cognitive Psychotherapy, 23*, 6–19. https://doi.org/10.1891/0889-8391.23.1.6

Nordahl, H. M., Borkovec, T. D., Hagen, R., Kennair, L. E. O., Hjemdal, O., Solem, S., Hansen, B., Haseth, S., & Wells, A. (2018). Metacognitive therapy versus cognitive-behavioural therapy in adults with generalised anxiety disorder, *British Journal of Psychiatry, 4*(5), 393–400. https://doi.org/10.1192/bjo.2018.54

Padesky, C. A. (2020). *The clinician's guide to CBT using Mind Over Mood, 2nd ed.* New York: Guilford Press.

Padesky, C. A. & Beck, J. S. (2014). Avoidant personality disorder. In A. T. Beck, D. D. Davis, & A. Freeman (Eds.), *Cognitive therapy of personality disorders* (3rd ed., pp. 174–202). New York: Guilford Press.

Rachman, S., Radomsky, A. S., & Sahfran, R. (2008). Safety behaviours: A reconsideration. *Behaviour, Research and Therapy, 46*, 163–173. https://doi.org/10.1016/j.brat.2007.11.008

Salkovskis, P. M. (1991). The importance of behaviour in the maintenance of anxiety and panic: A cognitive account. *Behavioural Psychotherapy, 19*, 6–19. https://doi.org/10.1017/S0141347300011472

Salkovskis, P. M., Clark, D. M., & Gelder, M. (1996). Cognition behaviour links in the persistence of panic, *Behaviour Research and Therapy, 34*, 453–458. https://doi.org/10.1016/0005-7967(95)00083-6

Salkovskis, P. M., Clark, D. M., Hackmann, A., Wells, A., & Gelder, M. (1999). An experimental investigation of the role of safety-seeking behaviors in the maintenance of panic disorder with agoraphobia. *Behavior Research and Therapy, 37*, 559–574. https://doi.org/10.1016/S0005-7967(98)00153-3

Simos, G., & Hofmann, S. G. (2013). *CBT for anxiety disorders: A practitioner book.* Chichester: Wiley-Blackwell.

Torres, A. R., Dedomenico, A. M., Crepaldi, A. L., & Miguel, E. C. (2004). Obsessive-compulsive symptoms in patients with panic disorder. *Comprehensive Psychiatry, 45*, 219–224. https://doi.org/10.1016/j.comppsych.2004.02.011

Waller, G. (2009). Evidence-based treatment and therapist drift. *Behaviour Research and Therapy, 47*, 119–127. https://doi.org/10.1016/j.brat.2008.10.018

Watkins, L. E., Sprang, K. R., & Rothbaum, B. O. (2018). Treating PTSD: A review of evidence-based psychotherapy interventions. *Frontiers of Behavioral Neuroscience, 12*, 1–9. https://doi.org/10.3389/fnbeh.2018.00258

Williams, J. M. G., Watts, F. N., MacLeod, C. & Mathews, A. (1997). *Cognitive psychology and emotional disorders* (2nd ed.). Chichester: Wiley.

Yiend, J. (2004). *Cognition, emotion and psychopathology: Theoretical, empirical and clinical directions.* Cambridge, UK: Cambridge University Press.

5

Imagery: The Language of Emotion

Christine A. Padesky and Emily A. Holmes

Imagine a recent very pleasant event in your life. Allow yourself a few minutes to focus on this imagery before you continue reading this paragraph. What did you see? Hear? Feel in your body? Taste? Is your memory of this event the same as the experience of the event itself? How is it similar or different? Was your recollection accompanied by any physical or emotional reactions? Take a moment and fully experience your memory in as many dimensions as possible.

Now imagine a future positive event that has not yet occurred but which you hope will happen. You might envision a celebration, a holiday, a promotion, completion of a task which is challenging, a new friend or baby. Take a few moments to fully develop vivid imagery of this future event before you continue reading this paragraph. What do you see? Hear? Feel in your body? Taste? Do you think your imagination of this event is similar or different to what the event itself will be like? How? Did you experience emotional reactions to what you imagined? Did these emotions feel real even though the event that evoked them has not occurred?

Whether we are consciously aware of it or not, imagery plays a major role in our thoughts about the past and future. Imagery can direct and change our memories, our aspirations or goals, and our emotional reactions to everything we experience in life. Just as in dreams, when we are awake, imagery makes up a significant proportion of our thought processes compared to words or abstract reasoning thoughts. And yet many therapists neglect to actively assess and work with imagery in therapy. When therapists do access client imagery, they sometimes feel hesitant or uncertain how to work with it. This chapter summarizes research relevant to imagery in psychotherapy and also demonstrates how guided discovery can be especially important in exploring and learning from imagery.

What Is Mental Imagery?

Mental imagery refers to sensory processing in the absence of sensory stimuli. Mental imagery is different from perception which is a response to sensory stimuli. For example, you can directly look at an apple or experience a family dinner (perception). Similar to the exercise at the beginning of this chapter, you can also bring to mind an image of that apple or a vivid sensory memory of that family dinner when the apple or family are not actually present (mental image). We can have mental images of single objects (like the apple), general events (a typical family dinner), or very specific events (e.g., that family dinner when the candle set the tablecloth on fire).

The word "image" conjures up the idea of a picture—but it is important to remember that images are not only visual pictures. Mental imagery can occur in any sensory modality: one can see with the "mind's eye," hear with the "mind's ear," and so forth (Kosslyn et al., 2001). In a mental image of a family dinner one might simultaneously visualize the faces of people sitting round the table, have auditory imagery of the click of knives and forks, have olfactory imagery of the smell of a steaming curry, and imagine tasting it. Mental images can be multimodal—that is incorporate several sensory modalities at once as in real life, or they can be predominantly in just one modality. For example, one can imagine the tune of the song "happy birthday" and only imagine the melody without any visual imagery. When using guided discovery regarding client imagery, it is therefore important to avoid a bias toward seeking visual imagery.

Keep in Mind

Imagery can involve any or all the senses: visual, taste, smell, hearing, or body sensations. Be sure to ask clients about multiple modalities.

We are also adept at combining images in novel ways to construct things we have never directly perceived together. For example, if you have at some point seen an apple tree and at another point seen a clock, you can imagine clock faces hanging like apples from the branches of an apple tree despite having never seen such a surreal object in real life. Thus, mental images can capture real and accurate memories or create combinations of things that have never been perceived before. In fact, one of the advantages of the brain's ability to generate mental imagery is that we can use it for "mental time travel" and, in doing so, use our imagination to anticipate and simulate what might happen in future events (Schacter et al., 2007). Imagining the future can be useful for planning an upcoming event. Imagining future bad outcomes either can be unhelpful and increase feelings of anxiety and depression or can be used as motivation to prepare for and mitigate future problems (Norem, 2001).

Importance of Imagery in Psychotherapy

There is a long history of research in experimental psychology on the topic of mental imagery. Indeed, mental imagery has been a topic of interest from the very earliest days of psychology as a discipline, and has generated lively debate over the decades (Baddeley & Andrade, 2000). Aaron T. Beck emphasized the importance of mental imagery at the inception of cognitive behavior therapy (CBT) (Beck et al., 1974). However, it is only in the past two decades that experimental psychology research on mental imagery has been linked directly to CBT. One of the first books to fully address the topic was the *Oxford Guide to Imagery in Cognitive Therapy* (Hackmann et al., 2011). More recently, this topic has been explored in rich detail by Stopa (2021) and various imagery techniques are more fully described in Holmes et al. (2019).

Mental imagery is important for the treatment of emotional disorders for a variety of reasons (Holmes & Mathews, 2010) and psychotherapists may be limiting treatment effectiveness if they do not incorporate imagery into their work (Blackwell, 2019, 2021; Pearson et al., 2015). The next sections highlight empirical findings about mental imagery relevant to therapy and illustrate the important role Socratic Dialogue can play in unpacking their therapeutic utility.

Imagery has stronger emotional impact than verbal processing

The conscious contents of our cognition can take the form of either verbal thoughts or mental images. For example, one can have the verbal thought "I am trapped" using language of the sort we use when we write or speak. Alternatively, one can imagine the experience of being trapped, such as being stuck in an elevator without the lights on, getting hotter and hotter, and starting to feel panicky. Research supports the hypothesis that compared to verbal thoughts, mental imagery about the same topic has a more powerful impact on emotion (Holmes & Mathews, 2010). Perhaps one reason for these findings is that imagery feels more "real" than verbal thoughts (Mathews et al., 2013). A myriad of cognitive meanings and emotional reactions can be attached to imagery no matter which sensory modes are involved. Because strong emotions may be attached to images, therapists should be alert to the possibility that some clients can feel overwhelmed by the emotional impact of images.

Keep in Mind

It is good practice to assess client capacity to manage intense emotions when working with traumatic images or other potentially overwhelming images. When clients don't have internal resources for emotion management, teach them methods for grounding and managing strong emotion before working with the most distressing images.

In a series of experiments, participants were asked to listen to a number of descriptions about events. For each description they heard, participants were asked to either focus on the words and meaning (verbal condition) or imagine it (imagery condition). In one experiment, all the descriptions had negative outcomes, e.g., "you hear footsteps behind you and realize it is a mugger." Those participants who had been assigned to the imagery condition had significantly greater levels of anxiety than those in the verbal condition (Holmes & Mathews, 2005). In another experiment, all the descriptions resolved positively, e.g., "you hear a sudden noise at night and realize with relief it is your partner coming home" or "You have been looking forward to your holiday. When you arrive at your destination you realize it is even better than you expected." Compared to those who were given verbal thoughts instructions, those participants who had imagined the positive events experienced significantly greater increases in positive affect (Holmes, Mathews et al., 2006). Strikingly, thinking about the same positive events in a verbal condition was not only less effective than using mental imagery, but even made people feel worse (Holmes et al., 2009). This general pattern of results has been replicated using a different type of experimental paradigm (Holmes, Mathews et al., 2008).

Overall, these results suggest that compared to verbal thought, mental imagery has a more powerful impact on emotion. The impact applies to both negative and positive events and moods. This is helpful for therapists to know as it underscores that it is important to work with imagery (not only verbal thoughts). During assessment, it is important to check for the presence of unhelpful imagery because unhelpful imagery can have a more toxic impact on emotions than verbal thoughts. In order to encourage positive emotions throughout treatment it is important to use mental imagery of positive events and gains instead of simple word descriptions. The experiments above demonstrate both that imagery is more powerful as an induction for positive mood and that, when thoughts about positive events are solely verbal, then mood may worsen.

Intrusive negative mental imagery occurs in a wide range of disorders

Many of the key negative thoughts that a CBT therapist will want to target take the form of images. For example, clients with post-traumatic stress disorder (PTSD) often have flashback imagery to trauma (Holmes et al., 2005), clients with social anxiety report images of themselves performing badly in social situations (Hackmann et al., 2000), and images of entrapment and humiliation occur in agoraphobia (Day et al., 2004). Images are also found in health anxiety (Wells & Hackmann, 1993), generalized anxiety disorder (Tallon et al., 2020), depression (Patel et al., 2007), suicidal thoughts (Holmes, Crane et al., 2007), bipolar disorder (Holmes, Geddes et al., 2008), schizophrenia (Malcolm et al., 2015; Morrison et al., 2002), and so forth. This has led researchers to suggest that imagery is widespread across psychological disorders and should be routinely asked for in assessment (Blackwell, 2021; Brewin et al., 2010; Di Simplicio et al., 2012; Hackmann & Holmes, 2004; Holmes, Arntz et al., 2007; Holmes & Mathews, 2010; Ji et al., 2019).

Imagery can boost client confidence in alternative beliefs

It is common in therapy for clients to test a belief and then say, "I *know* logically it's not true, but it still *feels* true." Given the special impact of imagery on emotion, for a client to also "feel" something is true they may need to use imagery to envision an alternative perspective and the emotions that accompany it. For this reason, many successful CBT approaches prompt clients to use vivid imagination during treatment procedures. For example, Ehlers and Clark's (2000) PTSD protocol introduces restructured, updated meanings into a traumatic image during reliving exercises. CBT interventions for suicide include active constructive imagery of coping with life post-suicide crisis as well as a relapse management program that relies on imagery exercises to assess the person's ability to deal with past and future suicidal crises using skills learned in therapy (Wenzel et al., 2009). Exposure using imagery modification has been shown to be as effective as in vivo exposure in treatment of snake phobias and led to a better response in highly fearful subjects (Hunt et al., 2006). Josefowitz (2017) suggests therapists can enhance the benefits of using thought records with depression and other moods if imagery is incorporated into them. For example, she suggests therapists can increase client engagement and confidence in alternative or balanced thoughts by vividly imagining situations consistent with them.

Keep in Mind

- Imagery makes up a significant portion of our thought processes and can include all sensory modalities (sight, sound, smell, taste, touch).
- Therapists who don't include imagery in their work are most likely limiting their therapy effectiveness.
- Imagery has a stronger emotional impact than thoughts stated in words.
- Imagery is present in most psychological disorders and should be routinely asked about in assessment.
- Therapists can increase client engagement and confidence in alternative beliefs by vividly imagining situations consistent with them.

Therapist Neglect of Imagery in Therapy: Common Traps

Why don't all therapists ask about mental imagery if it is so common? Often therapists don't even think to ask about imagery because their training did not include information about its importance. Even therapists who know imagery is important may not ask about it because they feel uncertain or less skilled in assessing and processing mental imagery than in discussing other types of thoughts. The first step to addressing these traps is to recognize that the same guided discovery methods used with other types of thoughts work well with imagery.

Imagery in Psychotherapy: Common Traps

Trap 1
When asked, a client denies having images and the therapist does not enquire further.

Trap 2
The therapist is anxious or uncertain how to work with imagery and so asks about images very lightly or refrains from asking at all.

Use of Socratic Dialogue to identify imagery

Trap 1

When asked, a client denies having images and the therapist does not enquire further.

It is not uncommon for clients to say they do not have any images if the therapist simply asks, "Do you have images?" This client response sometimes is the result of client uncertainty about what the therapist means by "imagery." Denial of imagery also reflects the quick and fleeting nature of some images. Just as clients are often not aware of verbal automatic thoughts at the beginning of therapy, they may not be aware of their automatic images. Some clients worry that having imagery might be a sign they are "crazy" and so they are reluctant to report images to the therapist. Some images may prompt uncomfortable feelings in the client such as embarrassment or shame and clients may be reluctant to tell these to a therapist, particularly in early sessions. Since nearly all clients have imagery, it is important that therapists actively enquire and help clients identify the imagery connected to moods and behaviors linked to therapy goals.

Trap 2

The therapist asks about images very lightly or refrains from asking at all.

Just as clients are often unaware of their own imagery or reluctant to reveal details about it, therapists also sometimes avoid pursuing the identification of images. Once therapists know the importance of imagery, imagery avoidance often is a result of therapist uncertainty about how to work with it. Therapists wonder:

- How do I talk to my client about imagery?
- How do I help my client identify images?
- What if my client doesn't report or experience imagery?
- What do I do when a client does report imagery?
- What if it opens a can of worms or my client thinks I'm flakey to ask about images?

The following sections address these questions and demonstrate how to use Socratic Dialogue to work effectively with client imagery.

How to talk with clients about imagery

Imagery is such a common part of human experience that there are many ways to introduce it into therapy discussions. In early sessions, imagery can be included in educational information about identifying thoughts:

Therapist: I notice you seem a bit sad right now. What went through your mind?

Rob: I thought you were probably disappointed with me.

Therapist: Did you have any images or memories related to that?

Rob: (Pause.) When you asked me about my homework, I felt a bit like I used to when my dad would ask me about my chores. I always felt like a disappointment to him.

Therapist: That fits with your facial expression. I wonder, did an image of your dad actually flash through your mind? Or the sound of his voice? Or his smell or any other strong sensation?

Rob: Now that I think about it, I could smell his aftershave. And hear the tone of his voice ... "Now, Robbie!"

Therapist: Did you see him?

Rob: I don't think so. I was looking at you but hearing him.

Therapist: Thank you for this information. It seems your sadness is linked to your thought you might be disappointing me and also to some powerful imagery connected to memories of your father asking about your chores.

Rob: I think so.

Therapist: Do you think these images ... his smell and the sound of your father's voice were an important trigger for your feelings of sadness?

Rob: Yes, definitely.

Therapist: Often, when we have strong feelings, there are images attached to these feelings. I don't just mean mental pictures. Like you experienced today, images can be in the form of smells, sounds, or even body sensations ... like a creepy feeling that crawls up your neck just before you get scared in a movie. It is really important that you try to notice these images and the other thoughts that go through your mind because these can help us figure out why your moods shift as they do.

Rob: Uh-huh.

Therapist: With your permission, I will ask you about thoughts and images to help remind you.

Rob: OK.

Therapist: Let's look now at this thought you had that you probably disappointed me and your image of your dad's smell and disappointed tone of voice. How do you think this connects with what I was asking about your homework?

In the Therapist's Mind

His therapist asks Rob about images or memories, recognizing that images can be linked to memories, and memories take the form of images. The client does not initially report imagery but when he offers a memory the therapist enquires about visual, auditory, olfactory and other sensations linked to this memory. In this way, the therapist Socratically guides the client to become aware of mental imagery processes. Before processing the meanings connected to the imagery, the therapist gives a rationale for its importance and invites Rob to collaborate in future searches for imagery.

How to help clients identify images

Clients typically will not mention images unless explicitly asked by their therapist (Hales et al., 2014). Questions enquiring about imagery can be preceded by educational information to normalize the presence of images that the client might find disturbing or be hesitant to report. This can be especially important in treatment of anxiety, psychosis, and suicide, for example. Consider the following interchange with a woman experiencing severe post-partum obsessive-compulsive disorder:

Therapist: Did you have any images?

Marta: No.

Therapist: That is interesting. Most people who are anxious have images that go along with their other thoughts. In fact, it is quite common to have images that are quite weird or even disturbing.

Marta: Like what?

Therapist: Well, some women have images of hurting her baby in some way. Others might imagine themselves screaming terrible things at the baby. These images can be quite frightening; especially if you worry you might really do it. And it can be scary to report these images to a therapist because you might worry you will be seen as a danger to your child, especially if you don't know these types of thoughts are common with anxiety.

Marta: I might sometimes have thoughts like that.

Therapist: Would you be willing to tell me about those images so we can see how they might link to your anxiety?

Notice that this therapist is very direct in giving examples of imagery that are common for new mothers. Giving a few examples of "weird" or socially unacceptable imagery can pave the way for a client to reveal her own imagery, especially if the therapist is matter of fact about their common frequency and link to anxiety.[1]

With psychosis, it can be important to acknowledge the client's convictions about whether an experience is imagined or real, especially when the imagery is a vivid hallucination or delusion. It is also important to sensitively judge when the timing is right to discuss these issues.

Therapist: You said sometimes voices tell you to do hurtful things.

Gomez: Yes.

Therapist: Do you think these voices are in the room outside of you or are they happening in your mind?

---

[1] Notice that Marta's therapist gives a variety of general and common examples of "weird images" and then asks an open question which invites Marta to report her own images. This is quite different from a therapist who repeatedly asks a client to report images related to a particular event in the absence of client reports of such events (e.g., "Did someone molest you? What images or memories do you have of being molested?"). Questions that guide clients to repeatedly imagine things they have not experienced can lead to false memories and are to be avoided (Hyman & Pentland, 1996; Loftus, 1997a; Otgaar et al., 2019).

Gomez: They are really there.
Therapist: What convinces you of that?
Gomez: I can hear them so clearly. I'm not making this up.
Therapist: I don't think you are making it up. I just know I have sometimes heard voices that seem like they are right there in the room with me and I later realized they were in my mind.
Gomez: These are really there.
Therapist: OK. We will need to learn more about these voices so we can understand where they come from. Do you have any ideas?
Gomez: I know they are evil.
Therapist: What gives you that idea?

In the Therapist's Mind

This therapist decides it is premature to ask her client to consider the voices may be a form of mental imagery we call hallucination. This idea can be introduced more slowly over time using guided discovery methods, such as a series of guided observations and experiments regarding the voices Gomez hears.

When people are convinced hallucinations are real, it is generally advantageous for a therapist to take the stance of a curious investigator rather than try to convince someone their beliefs are inaccurate. A Socratic approach reduces the risk of an alliance rupture that easily can occur if the therapist directly challenges a client's tightly held beliefs. In time, the therapist can elicit a client's cooperation to consider two hypotheses: (1) the voices are from real entities or (2) the voices come from the client's mind. Experiments can be devised to evaluate which of these is most consistent with the client's experiences. For example, if the voices are really in the room, is there evidence other people hear them? Would the client expect them to show up on a voice recorder? If the client ignores the voices' instructions, do bad things happen as the voices predict/threaten? Use of guided discovery methods for testing hallucinations and delusions are covered in more detail by Beck et al. (2020), Morrison (2001), and Wright et al. (2009).

What if clients don't report or experience imagery?
Brain trauma or neurological damage can interfere with the ability to experience or report mental imagery. Recently a condition called anphantasia has

been identified in less than 1% of the population whereby people lack the ability to voluntarily visualize though they typically can dream (Wicken et al., 2021). Therapists, of course, do not need to access imagery with the rare cases of clients who truly do not experience them. However, unless there are these types of brain deficits, nearly all people experience mental imagery—although people may claim they don't until they understand what the therapist means. Thus, when a client doesn't report imagery, the first approach is to educate them about what is meant by the words "mental imagery" or "images."

Assuming therapists have already followed the methods described previously in this chapter, they can use guided discovery to help clients examine their own experiences in the hope this leads to a better understanding of images. One approach is to ask someone to imagine and describe somewhere safe that is not connected to therapy issues, such as a favorite place. Alternatively, clients can be asked to silently sing a song or remember what it feels like to stand in a cold wind. If the client is able to do any of these tasks, the client is capable of experiencing imagery in at least one modality but is not aware enough to report it. In this instance, the therapist can give a rationale for why it is so important to notice imagery (e.g., "imagery often provides important clues as to why we behave and feel the ways we do"). Then the therapist can continue to demonstrate an interest in imagery and allow the client silent time in session to access it.

Therapists are advised to be alert to their own biases in the search for imagery. Many therapists predominantly enquire about visual imagery. Some client experiences such as childhood trauma may be linked to images coded in other sensory modalities more than visual ones. The following dialogue illustrates this:

Maija: (With eyes closed) I'm getting really scared. I don't want to talk about this anymore.

Therapist: That's OK. You can tell me to stop anytime you like. (Pause.) Would it be OK if I ask just a few more questions to help me understand why this is difficult for you?

Maija: (Silently nods.)

Therapist: What is going through your mind?

Maiji: (Silently shakes head "No.")

Therapist: Do you feel something in your body?

Maija: (Client nods slightly.)

Therapist: What do you feel?

Maija: (Pause.) Cold.

Therapist: Does the cold have a color or shape?

Maija: Hard. Red.
Therapist: Is the cold everywhere or in a certain spot?
Maija: My arms and legs.
Therapist: Is the rest of your body warm?
Maija: (Shakes head "No.") Can't feel it.
Therapist: So your arms and legs feel this hard, red, cold feeling but you don't feel anything in the rest of your body. Is that right?
Maija: (Nods.)
Therapist: Let's do an experiment to see if we can get rid of the cold feeling. Would that be alright?
Maija: (Nods.)

In this session, the therapist recognizes that Maija begins to dissociate when the therapy discussion approaches a topic likely to trigger memories of the abuse she experienced as a child. Her therapist has learned this abuse began before the age of eight, her abuser remained silent, and it occurred in the dark. As such it may be more likely to have kinesthetic/non-visual sensory associations than verbal ones. Also it is common for trauma experiences at any age to be encoded in kinesthetic sensations, body or tactile sensory experiences including temperature, weight, or equilibrium. Thus, her therapist shifts to asking questions about body sensations when Maija reports "nothing" is going through her mind. Her therapist could also inquire about other sensory experiences such as sounds, smells, tastes, or visual experiences, keeping in mind that each of these dimensions can evoke strong emotions when associated with trauma.

Keep in Mind

- Clients are often unaware of their imagery or are reluctant to reveal it. Therefore, therapists need to directly ask.

- Memories are encoded in imagery. Asking clients for memories and prompting them to describe sights, smells, sounds, and other sensory experiences linked to those memories can be a good introduction to what is meant by imagery.

- Even though someone has a vivid imaginal memory, this does not necessarily mean their memory is an exact representation of the event. People are capable of building memories post-hoc that may or may not reflect what actually happened.

- Normalizing the common occurrence of disturbing images is helpful for people experiencing anxiety, trauma, obsessive-compulsive disorder, psychosis, and suicidal ideation who are likely to have disturbing images themselves.
- Therapists can be aware of their own biases (e.g., to mainly enquire about visual imagery) and counter these habits showing awareness that trauma and other clinical issues are often encoded in other sensory modalities.

How to know if an image is important

Just as with other types of thoughts, therapists look for imagery most closely linked to the emotions or behaviors that are the focus of therapeutic discussions. Thus, an image of tonight's dinner is less likely to be relevant for a client who is highly perfectionistic than the image of making a mistake. Beck's theory of cognitive specificity (Beck, 1976) guides therapists to the types of content most likely to be associated with particular emotions. Themes of loss and failure accompanied by negative thoughts about the self, others, and future characterize depression (Beck et al., 1979); themes of threat, danger, and an inability to cope are associated with anxiety (Beck et al., 1985); anger often reflects fears or hurt feelings related to perceived violations of rules or trust with accompanying negative thoughts about other people and their motives (Beck, 1988; 1999).

Research on imagery related to particular disorders provides additional guidance for therapists. For example, research on imagery people have while suicidal or planning non-suicidal self-injury reveals that there are nearly always detailed images of future suicide or self-injury attempts (Hasking et al., 2018). These images in people contemplating suicide have been called "flash forwards" (Holmes & Butler, 2009; Holmes et al., 2007). Of concern is that these images are often accompanied by positive affect, which can serve to reinforce the imagery and increase the amount of time the person spends thinking about suicide. Therefore, it can be therapeutic to identify such suicidal images and transform their positive meanings into more negative ones. One strategy is to extend the image past the point of death and to consider aspects of death besides relief from distress. For example, the therapist can ask the client to imagine the impact on friends and family when they discover the body or learn about the suicide, and the lifelong emotional struggles those people might experience in order to come to terms with the meaning of this death.

Some of the most extensive research on imagery has been conducted in relation to traumatic events. While therapists have recognized for decades the therapeutic importance of flashbacks for trauma disorders, more recent studies reveal that people who have experienced trauma frequently have three or four different images that form these flashbacks. These key images are often linked to traumatic moments and meanings that carry the greatest emotional intensity for the person. For this reason, these particular images have been called "hotspots" (Holmes et al., 2005). Therapists help clients link emotions (e.g., anger) and cognitions (e.g., "they can't defend themselves") to identified imagery (e.g., soldiers are surrounded and being methodically shot).

What to do after a client reports imagery

The same interventions used to test out and evaluate verbal thoughts can be used with imagery. For example, in the treatment of PTSD, trauma experts recommend therapists prioritize hotspots over less emotionally charged memories of the trauma in order to help clients recover more quickly. Key therapy tasks are to use Socratic Dialogue to test for distortions in hotspot imagery and to transform the meanings associated with these hotspots (Grey & Holmes, 2008; Grey et al., 2001; Grey et al., 2002; Holmes et al., 2005).

The following dialogue illustrates these two processes. The discussion begins as the therapist is about to test out one hotspot image a soldier recalls from a traumatic day when his entire platoon was surrounded and killed by the opposing forces.

Therapist: Let's examine this event more closely. If I understand correctly, you are blaming yourself for their deaths because you saw them being surrounded and you did not move forward quickly enough to shoot the enemy.

Rich: Yes. The scene plays over and over in my mind. It was my fault. I didn't move fast enough.

Therapist: Please help me understand the situation better. (Therapist gathers great detail about the soldier's location, the location of the other soldiers, time of day, weather, etc. Hand drawings are made to make sure the therapist and Rich are talking about the same relative locations and distances.) So, given these locations, how would you have moved forward to kill your men's attackers?

Rich: (Pointing to drawings.) I would have followed this line of cover here. Because of the snipers, I would have crawled on my hands and knees through this section (pointing).

Therapist: How many meters do you think you would have needed to crawl?

Rich: About 10.

Therapist:	How much time do you think it would take to do that?
Rich:	Maybe 10 seconds.
Therapist:	Would you be willing to test that out here?
Rich:	What do you mean?
Therapist:	My office is about 4 meters. Maybe you could show me how you would have needed to crawl, carrying all your gear. Let me see if you can get from one side to the other in about 4 seconds.
Rich:	It would not have been a straight shot like in here. I would have had to navigate around quite a bit of rubble.
Therapist:	And keep your head down and carry all your gear?
Rich:	(Nods thoughtfully.)

Further discussion and a timed experiment of crawling with simulated gear and rubble reveals that it probably would have taken Rich at least 1 minute to get into position with his weapons to fire on the soldiers who had captured his men.

Rich:	Whenever I've imagined this, I thought I could have saved them so quickly.
Therapist:	You could move and position yourself much more quickly in imagination.
Rich:	Yes.
Therapist:	How much time do you think elapsed between when you saw your men were surrounded and when they were shot?
Rich:	It happened in such slow motion. It seemed like a long time. But I think it was only a few seconds.
Therapist:	And could you have fired on the attacking soldiers from your position when you saw them?
Rich:	No. Not without killing my own men because they were in between us.
Therapist:	What does this new information about the distance and timings mean to you? How much responsibility do you hold for their deaths?
Rich:	(Slowly.) There was not enough time. Even though I could see them and knew what was going to happen ... it was a nightmare I couldn't stop.
Therapist:	Yes, a nightmare. A tragedy. (Long silence.) One you couldn't prevent.
Rich:	(Tears in his eyes.) I'm so sorry. (Pause.) But maybe it was not my fault.

In this session, his therapist carefully unpacks the image of a war event that has plagued Rich for many years. As it happens, the details of the image contain distortions (e.g., Rich's image allows him to move to a new location much more quickly than would have been possible; his image neglects to include rubble he needs to crawl over and around). Once these distortions are identified and corrected, Rich comes to a new conclusion about his responsibility, which transforms the meaning of this event for him. Had his image not been distorted, the therapist would have focused on the meaning of Rich's inaction. Did he freeze? How can he understand this? Did this help save his own life? Was saving his own life the sole cause of the other men's deaths? How can he reach some acceptance of the consequences of his behavior? Does he feel the need to make reparations of some sort to his dead platoon mates? As described in Chapter 2, Socratic explorations do not have a fixed end in mind.

Therapist fears it will open a can of worms or clients will think it is flakey to ask about images

As shown in the previous dialogue with Rich, there are many directions of discovery the therapist can take depending upon what a client reveals about the content and meaning of imagery reported. If client reactions are mixed and complex, the proverbial "can of worms," the therapist is often fortunate to be working with imagery because simple changes in imagery can lead to multilevel changes in emotions and beliefs. This is because imagery is more multidimensional than word thoughts are. Consider the difference between shifting a core belief, "I am inadequate," and altering a related image of oneself as lying inanimate on a couch. It can be much easier to help someone imagine sitting up and gradually taking action than to change a word thought to "I can be effective."

If a client thinks identifying and talking about imagery is "flakey," the therapist can backtrack and do more education with the client about the role and importance of imagery in understanding emotional reactions. Even getting an image of what the therapist will look like or do if she is flakey and comparing this to the reality of the imagery explorations that have been done so far can help. A guided discovery exercise working with a simple image can also help the client understand the utility of image exploration and test out whether this feels flakey. For example, the client can be asked to imagine an upcoming event in both positive and negative ways. The therapist can draw out and write down the moods, motivation, and behaviors engendered by each image. Then the therapist can ask the client an analytical question such as "When you look at these observations we've summarized here, how do you think imagery might prove helpful to us in therapy?"

The remainder of this chapter highlights a variety of useful imagery interventions. And you will learn how research can be very helpful in guiding therapist choices as to when and how to intervene with imagery.

Imagery and Socratic Dialogue

As stated in the previous section, just about any therapy intervention that can be done with word thoughts can be done with images. Thus, imagery can play an important role in case conceptualization, examination of key beliefs, behavior change interventions, homework development, and every other treatment process familiar to therapists. Throughout this work, Socratic Dialogue can be used to help make sure the links discovered between imagery and emotions, beliefs, behaviors, and physiological responses reflect and explore meanings that come from the client rather than the therapist. As we explore uses of Socratic Dialogue with imagery, we will address the following common traps:

Socratic Dialogue and Imagery: Common Traps

Trap 3
The client reports an image, which evokes a variety of meanings and associations in the therapist's mind; these intrude on the therapist's processing of client reactions.

Trap 4
Imagery evokes strong reactions and the client and/or therapist feel overwhelmed with emotion.

Trap 5
The client reports several images and the therapist is not sure which of the images are important to explore.

Trap 6
The imagery involves smells, kinesthetic sensations, or other nonverbal content and the therapist is uncertain how to proceed.

Trap 7
The therapist is pretty certain the imagery described did not really occur and yet the client has strong emotional reactions to it and cannot easily dismiss the image out of mind.

Collaborative case conceptualization

It can be very useful to include imagery during case conceptualization because imagery often incorporates the cognitive, affective, behavioral, and physical client experiences of central importance to understanding a particular issue. Therapists are encouraged to use Socratic Dialogue during case conceptualization in order to develop a shared understanding of the origins and maintaining factors for client issues. Forming the conceptualization collaboratively helps therapists guard against the clinical bias which is introduced when the therapist relies on their own ideas about the client's issues more strongly than the client's perspective (Kuyken et al., 2009; Padesky, 2020).

Conceptualization often relies on a person's memories of life events. Memory about the self is called "autobiographical memory." There is a vast experimental psychology and neuroscience literature on this topic. An aspect particularly relevant to mental imagery and case conceptualization is that our memory for past events takes the form of mental images rather than just verbal thoughts. This type of memory has been referred to as sensory-perceptual episodic memory (Conway, 2001). For example, if you are asked to remember the last visit you paid to the dentist you are likely to remember this in the form of a sensory mental image of the sight of the treatment room, the smell of the mouthwash, and perhaps the sound of a drill. Our memories of the past inform our sense of self, who we think we are, who we think we will become. Such memories help shape the goals we set and strive for (Conway et al., 2004; Stopa, 2009).

Clinicians are well aware of the power of memory, its effect on a client's sense of self, and their hopes for the future. Since research tells us episodic memories take the form of images, when our clients give us factual, logical statements during assessment it is unlikely they are tapping into memories of a specific event. Asking for more concrete details can help gather the information important for a conceptualization. Observe how Ali's therapist uses imagery to gather information that can help them understand some of the factors contributing to his struggling marriage:

Ali:	Adilah and I were happy in the early years of our marriage. After five years, things started to fall apart. (*Factual, logical statement.*)
Therapist:	Can you describe to me one event early in your marriage that captures how happy you were?
Ali:	Yes. We started a small restaurant and we were so excited on opening night.
Therapist:	Imagine that night. Describe to me what you see, smell, hear, and feel. Especially the parts that capture your happiness with Adilah. (Ali describes opening night in some detail, describing the intimate moments he and Adilah shared.)
Therapist:	It sounds like you were both very happy together. And you both were attentive to each other, even in the midst of a busy night.
Ali:	Yes. But then it all fell apart.
Therapist:	Did it fall apart all at once or over time?
Ali:	Slowly, over time.
Therapist:	Is there some event or interaction that symbolizes to you what things were like when they began to "fall apart"?

In the Therapist's Mind

By asking Ali to choose memories to represent different stages in his marriage, his therapist hopes to learn more about the meanings and themes regarding their relationship that are most important to Ali. These themes are elaborated through his vivid imagery of these events. His imagery captures emotional moments and meanings likely to be missing from a purely verbal discussion of their marital history.

Sometimes client images closely match the therapist's own images. This can result in the therapist making an error of assuming that image details or meanings are the same for the client as they would be for the therapist. Consider a client who reports an image of sailing in a boat to a therapist who is an avid sailor. This therapist will need to actively guard against merging his or her own associations to sailing with those of the client. Maintaining a Socratic stance and asking the client to unpack his or her own image will help do this.

Trap 3

The client reports an image that evokes a variety of meanings and associations in the therapist's mind; these intrude on the therapist's processing of client reactions.

When images evoke strong emotional reactions in the therapist

The potential for clinical bias can increase when images are identified as part of a conceptualization process. This is because images also evoke stronger emotional reactions in the therapist than words alone do.

Trap 4

Imagery evokes strong reactions and the client and/or therapist feel over-whelmed with emotion.

In the following dialogue, this therapist initially does a good job of using Socratic Dialogue to help Akiko identify images. However, when the images reported by Akiko evoke strong emotional reactions in the therapist, the therapist's use of Socratic Dialogue is derailed.

Therapist: So far Akiko we have listed three things that you know increase your sadness: lying in bed for longer than 10 minutes, staring at the stacks of paper on your desk, and when your boyfriend tells you he is disappointed in you. Are you aware of any images that increase your sadness? Images can be mental pictures, sounds, smells, or body sensations.

Akiko: Sometimes I just hear a tone in my boyfriend's voice and I know he is unhappy with me. Is that what you mean?

Therapist: It could be, especially if you hear that tone even when your boyfriend is not there. Or, if when you hear that tone in his voice when he is there, it brings some thoughts and memories to mind that go beyond the situation you are in.

Akiko: Yes. I think I understand. Sometime when I hear that tone in his voice it reminds me of the wind in the trees that I heard from my room as a child. I was so lonely after my mother died and felt so sad.

Therapist: When you hear that tone in his voice, does a vivid memory come to mind of yourself as a child listening to the wind in the trees and feeling so lonely and sad that your mother was gone?

Akiko: Yes. Not always. But when it does, I feel really sad in a deep way in my chest.

Therapist: **Losing a parent is very hard. I wonder if you worry that you will lose your boyfriend if he is disappointed in you.**

Akiko: Hmmm ... I'm not sure.

Therapist: **When we are close to our parents, it can be such a loss when they die. This can make it even harder to face the possibility of loss of other important people in our life.**

This therapist did a good job of asking Akiko for images connected to her feelings of sadness. However, in the last two therapist comments (in bold type) we observe the therapist has a theory connecting Akiko's loss of her mother in childhood to her sadness in reaction to her boyfriend's disappointment. Rather than pursue a Socratic line of questioning to find out Akiko's associations between childhood and her current situation, the therapist offers her own interpretation. Even when Akiko indicates that this may not be right, "Hmmm ... I'm not sure," the therapist proceeds putting this hypothesis forward.

How did this occur, given that this therapist generally tries to be Socratic? This therapist's mother was aging and the therapist realized her mother would probably die within the next few years. Akiko's image of the wind in the trees was so vivid it triggered the therapist to imagine her own mother's death and she felt a deep sadness in response to that image. When the therapist turned her mind back to the issue of Akiko's sadness related to her boyfriend's disappointment, the therapist looked for links with her mother's death because this was the most salient part of Akiko's imagery in the therapist's mind. With her own associations and meanings activated, the therapist imagined how hard it would be to contemplate losing a love relationship at the same time her mother was dying, even though this was not Akiko's situation.

When we experience strong emotions and reactions to client images, it is very helpful to enlist supervision or consultation to help us manage and separate our own reactions from our client's. If these reactions are frequent or particularly strong, we may even decide to find a therapist for ourselves to process our reactions. Let's observe the differences that occur when Akiko's therapist shakes off immersion in her own imagery, meanings, and associations to Akiko's image and instead maintains a Socratic stance. The therapist's new questions and responses are in bold type as she probes for Akiko's meanings attached to her imagery. The dialogue begins two-thirds of the way through the previous example:

Therapist: When you hear that tone in his voice, does a vivid memory come to mind of yourself as a child listening to the wind in the trees and feeling so lonely and sad?

Akiko: Yes. Not always. But when it does, I feel really sad in a deep way in my chest.

Therapist: How do you think this image and memory from childhood relates to what you are experiencing now?

Akiko: (Pauses.) When I listened to the wind in the trees as a child, the sadness was so deep because I loved my mother and it was hard to understand she was gone forever. There was nothing I could do. The "nothing to do" made me especially sad. When my boyfriend is disappointed, sometimes when I am depressed it seems I am incapable of doing what I want to do to make things better. It is like I can see the path but I can't take the first step, my legs are too heavy.

Therapist: **So your sadness is linked to feeling incapable of doing what you can think of to make your relationship better? Your legs are too heavy?**

Akiko: Yes. I want to be more connected to him and have fun like we used to but my sadness makes it almost impossible for me to do this, even when I can see it would help us both.

Therapist: **What parts of that image are most important to write down on our conceptualization here?**

Akiko: I think we should write: "Like when I was a child, I feel incapable of changing things. My legs feel too heavy."

When her therapist holds back on expressing her personally generated hypotheses linking Akiko's mother's death with fears of losing her boyfriend, Akiko is more engaged in the conceptualization. Akiko makes a link that was not obvious to the therapist. Her childhood image is linked by virtue of a similarity in the difficulty to do something to change the situation. She also offers an additional contemporary image: "I can't take the first step, my legs are too heavy." This image can be used metaphorically in therapy to help Akiko begin to take small positive steps, even when her "legs feel too heavy."

When images evoke strong emotional reactions in the client

Sometimes it is the client who is overwhelmed by the emotionality of an image. When a client becomes tearful or frightened in response to an image, these emotional reactions can be explored compassionately just as is done with word thoughts. The therapist can ask what the image means to the client and what parts of the image or its meaning evoke the emotions experienced. Some clients who experience particularly intense emotional reactions may dissociate in response to images. As shown in the example with Maija earlier in this chapter, this response can occur in clients who have experienced severe trauma.

As Maija's therapist demonstrated, using Socratic Dialogue can help therapists stay engaged with a client who is dissociating. In this instance, the therapist will combine Socratic Dialogue with more direct methods designed to help the client become grounded and leave the dissociated state. Kennerley's chapter on "Impulsive and Compulsive Behaviors" (Chapter 7) describes these methods and their rationale in more detail.

> **Trap 5**
> ___
> The client reports several images and the therapist is not sure how to know which of the images are important to explore.

What to do when there are several images

As happened with Akiko, sometimes one image leads to another. At times, therapists face a cornucopia of images. How does one decide which of the images are important to include in a conceptualization or explore in therapy? Generally, the client is the best guide to making these choices. Akiko's therapist asks, "What parts of that image are most important to write down on our conceptualization here?" When there are multiple images, it is helpful to ask, "Which of these images do you think are most important for us to write down and explore?"

An additional guideline is that imagery most strongly connected to the client's presenting issues is often most important. Thus, for clients who are anxious, images that connect to hotspots, the most intense anxiety, are probably most important to examine in therapy (Holmes et al., 2005). Similarly, "hot" images connected to depression, anger, or other moods which are the focus of therapy should be prioritized. If the goal of therapy is behavior change, images that connect most strongly with target behaviors may be the most important to examine. For example, images that trigger substance misuse or eating problems are important to identify and explore if these behaviors are treatment foci. In addition, images that promote desired behaviors can boost the effectiveness of therapy as described later in this chapter.

Exploring and testing imagery

How do we test central beliefs when they take the form of imagery? The same methods discussed elsewhere in this book apply. One can use Socratic Dialogue, behavioral experiments, thought records, role play, and other methods to test out and examine imagery. This is true whether the imagery pertains to actual or imagined experiences. In order to put these statements in context, it is helpful to realize that imagery is just like real perception and uses the same neural processes.

We know this from brain neuroimaging research that investigates which neural systems are activated when participants conduct particular tasks. Many experiments have been conducted which contrast direct perception with the corresponding mental imagery. For example, if you scan the brain of someone directly seeing the letter A, or forming a visual image of the letter A, results show that the same or similar parts of the brain are used in direct perception as in mental imagery (Ganis et al., 2004; Kosslyn et al., 2001; Pearson et al., 2015). This overlap in brain regions used applies not only for different aspects of visual mental imagery (e.g., color, size), but to other sensory modalities. For example, the mental practice of movement produces similar cortical activation patterns to actual movement. The power of imagery is such that imaginal practice of movement can impact the physical recovery of movement in stroke patients (Carrasco & Cantalapiedra, 2016). Though more complex stimuli have been less well researched, a similar pattern of results is emerging. For example, looking at a frightening face activates a brain region associated with fear—the amygdala. Simply imagining such faces also activates this region (Kim et al., 2007).

Overall, these types of studies tell us that mental imagery and direct perception are similar in terms of brain response. This is helpful for therapists to know as it suggests that imagining an event can have the same impact as actually seeing/hearing that event happen. It can be helpful to normalize for a client that their negative imagery is understandably upsetting as it can have a similar impact to experiencing a real event. Child therapists can be aware that children can have traumatic reactions to witnessing events either in real life or on television. This may account for why children who watch more television coverage of a disaster are more likely to experience traumatic-stress symptoms, especially if they have pre-existing PTSD symptoms (Weems et al., 2012). Similarly, positive imagery can lead to the same degree of joy and happiness as real world experiences.

Trap 6

The imagery involves smells, kinesthetic sensations, or other nonverbal content and the therapist is uncertain how to proceed.

How to explore imagery that involves smells, kinesthetic sensations, or other nonverbal content

In terms of Socratic Dialogue, research suggests that when target cognitions are images, the therapist should respond to these similarly as one would verbal thoughts. This is true even when imagery involves smells, body sensations, or other nonverbal content. When using Socratic Dialogue, the evidence gathered to test a belief can be solely derived from information gathered within the image itself as demonstrated in the following excerpt of a therapy session with Saul who experiences chronic rheumatoid arthritis:

Saul: The pain has been so bad lately. I don't think I can manage it.

Therapist: Can you describe your pain to me? (*Informational question*)

Saul: Like I told my wife this morning, it feels like there are hot coals in my joints.

Therapist: Oh! That sounds really painful. (*Empathic listening*)

Saul: Yes, I can't stand it.

Therapist: (After she gathers more information about which joints are affected, pain ratings, and other relevant information to the pain treatment.) Let's return to this image you have of a hot coal in your joints.

Saul: (Rolling his eyes.) Do we have to?

Therapist: (Smiling.) Well, it's up to you but we've discussed how important your images are.

Saul: Yes, actually I'm just joking. I know that coal image makes my pain worse.

Therapist: What about the pain is like a hot coal?

Saul: It feels like my joints are burning. And the pain is really intense. I see the pain as an orange and red color. And my joint feels about the same size as a coal.

Therapist: Is there anything in your experience that is not like a hot coal?

Saul: Well, if it were a hot coal, I could pour water on it and cool it down.

Therapist: Good point. (Writes it down.) Anything else?

Saul: I guess a hot coal gradually gets cooler over time. It burns out on its own. My joints have not been settling down all week.

Therapist: That's an interesting observation. What can you think of that is hot like your pain and can stay hot without cooling down?

Saul: Well, a radiator would do that if you keep the heat on.

Therapist: Good. I've written down your three ideas here: (1) If it is a hot coal, I could pour water over it and cool it down, (2) if it is a hot coal, it will burn out on its own, and (3) if it doesn't cool down, then it is more like a radiator which has to be turned off. (*Written summary*)

Saul: OK. What am I supposed to do with that?

Therapist: I'm not sure. Why don't you look at these three ideas here and see what comes into your mind. You might need to be a bit creative. (*Analytical prompt instead of a question*)

Saul: (After a minute of silence.) I suppose I could use imagery to pour some cool water over my joints. (Still staring at the written list.) It would help to know the pain won't be this intense forever; it will cool down. And if it doesn't cool down, then that means I need to find a way to go to the source and turn it off.

Therapist: How would you do that?

Saul: Well, the nurse at my doctor's office showed me how to apply pressure in certain spots to help ease the pain. And you've taught me how imagery can help relieve the pain. Maybe I could start with imagery of pouring cold water over the joint and allow a bit of time for this cooling image to work. If this doesn't help, then I could imagine those pressure points are the turn off valve for the radiator. I could press the turn off switch and wait for the radiator to cool down.

Therapist: How does that plan sound to you?

Saul: It's worth a try. I could stand the pain better if I knew it wouldn't last all day and there was something I could do about it.

Saul's therapist used Socratic Dialogue to help Saul test out whether his arthritic pain really was like a hot coal and to generate ideas to help evaluate whether he could manage or cope with it. She stayed within his image and asked him for ideas, listened empathically, and made a written summary of his observations. Then she encouraged Saul to be creative and use the ideas from the summary to see how they could help him. Note that the plan Saul suggested involved a series of images. Clients often are quite creative in using images in metaphorical ways to solve a problem. Working directly with Saul's image of the hot coal led to a resolution that could be easier for him to remember and implement than ideas derived from a dialogue about pain management that did not incorporate his imagery. Despite the imaginary nature of his metaphors, they might seem more "real" to Saul than verbal dialogue.

Auditory hallucinations as imagery

Auditory hallucinations are a type of imagery quite common in psychosis. Guided discovery methods can be used to test out beliefs and interpretations made about the voices heard during auditory hallucinations (Beck et al., 2020; Beck et al., 2009; Morrison, 2001, 2009). As with most imagery, voices heard in hallucinations sound very real, as real as voices in any other conversation. Thus, trying to "convince" the client that these voices are in their mind and not in the room is not usually the best strategy. Instead, therapists can use guided discovery methods such as behavioral experiments to test out relevant beliefs about the voices and allow people to come to their own conclusions about where the voices come from.

For example, Jamal and his therapist devised a series of behavioral experiments regarding the voice he heard. Initially these experiments tested out whether the voice was in the room. Jamal agreed that if the voice was in the room, then other people would react, at least nonverbally, when it began to shout at Jamal. Also, he predicted it could be recorded on the voice recorder on his phone so his therapist could hear it as well. As with all behavioral experiments, Jamal wrote down his predictions ahead of time and recorded his observations when each experiment finished (Bennett-Levy et al., 2004). He was genuinely surprised when other people did not react to the voice. When he asked two of his friends, "Did you just hear someone shouting?" they said no. His attempts to record the voice on his audio recorder also failed. This series of experiments led Jamal to shift his belief that the voice could be heard by anyone.

However, even if only he heard the voice, Jamal believed it had great power over him. Thus, Jamal's therapist worked with him to construct a hierarchy of experiments to test out this belief. Figure 5.1 shows some of Jamal's behavioral experiments and their outcomes.

The types of experiments that Jamal and his therapist conducted can have a powerful therapeutic effect on people who hear voices. When voices are perceived as omnipotent or dangerous, both frequency and distress regarding voices increase (Chadwick & Birchwood, 1994; Gaudiano & Herbert, 2006).

Experiment	Prediction	What Happened	What did I learn?
Delay responding for 5 seconds	Voice will get angry and hurt me	Nothing	The voice is not as dangerous as I thought. If I don't do what it says or if I ignore it or play music, I'm still OK. It doesn't hurt me. I can decide whether to listen to it or not.
Delay responding for 15 seconds	Voice will get angry and hurt me	I was scared but nothing happened	
Turn on some music and make it loud	Voice will get louder. He might turn off the music.	Music played on and on. I couldn't hear voice and when I turned the music off, the voice was gone.	
Say, "You are just a voice and have no power over me."	Something bad. The voice won't like this.	I missed my bus home but I'm not sure the voice caused this. It wasn't too bad.	

Figure 5.1 Jamal's behavioral experiments to test the power of the voice he hears.

Behavioral experiments provide the type of real-world experience that has much higher credibility to the person who hears voices than is provided by verbal educational information. Thus, behavioral experiments are an important form of guided discovery with auditory hallucinations. As shown in Figure 5.1, Jamal's therapist guided him to debrief these experiments using the guided discovery methods of prediction, observation, written summaries, and analytical/synthesizing questions (i.e., the fourth column of the chart, "What did I learn?").

Distortions in imagery

Our perceptions of events are often distorted, so it is not surprising that imagery also often includes distortions. Helping people recognize and correct distortions in imagery can be a fruitful pathway for changing the meanings about them and emotional reactions to them. Consider Charlene who has been depressed and suicidal. She sees herself as "useless" and therefore proclaims there is no reason she should live. As one small part of a concerted suicide intervention plan, her therapist explored images related to her belief she is useless.

Therapist: When you say the word "useless" you sound disgusted with yourself.

Charlene: I am. That's a good word for it.

Therapist: Do any images come to mind when you say, "I'm useless?"

Charlene: I suppose so. I see myself as I am.

Therapist: What is that like? Tell me exactly what you see.

Charlene: Well, I'm ugly and dirty, wearing ragged clothes. I'm smelly like a homeless person. But I don't have dignity like a homeless person who is homeless because of bad luck. I'm disgusting because it's my own fault I'm so useless.

Therapist: This image that you have of yourself being ugly, dirty, ragged, smelly—can you describe more about your clothes, your hair, anything else that seems important? (Charlene offers more details and the therapist writes them all down.)

Therapist: We experience lots of emotion in reaction to our images. That's why it can be helpful to make sure our images are fair and balanced.

Charlene: I am useless.

Therapist: Let's put "useless" on the side for the moment. I've written down your description of your image. Let's take each part and see if it is a fair description of you. For example, in your image, your hair is

> matted and dirty. Your hair doesn't look like that to me. How would
> you describe your hair today?

Charlene: I'm not sure.

Therapist: Would it be OK to take your picture with your phone's camera?
Then we can look at your photo and compare it to your image of
yourself.

Charlene: Yeah, that would be alright.

When clients report negative or disturbing images, it is important to get
as many details as possible. If the images relate to real people or events, then
the details of the images can be compared with direct observation, just as
Charlene's therapist is beginning to do with her. Once distortions are revealed, the client can be asked to see how their reactions are different when
the image is aligned more closely with their observations of the live event
or people. For example, one woman who was intimidated by a man yelling at her realized he towered over her in her image but in reality he was
shorter than she was. When she adjusted the image to him looking up at her
while he yelled, she felt more in control of her emotions. Toward the end of
their meeting, Charlene's therapist asked her to reflect on the impact of her
adjusted image:

Therapist: When you see yourself more like you look in this photo, does that
have any effect on your feelings toward yourself?

Charlene: Yes. It really made a difference when we talked about my eyes.
I look so tired. In my mind my eyes are nasty and saying to the
world, "I don't give a f—." My eyes here (pointing to her photo) are
just tired. No wonder I don't do things. I'm worn out by feeling so
down and having so many problems for so long. A worn-out couch
is not useless, it is just used up.

Therapist: Yes. And a worn-out couch can be recovered and filled with new
stuffing and made fresh and useful again.

Charlene: I'm not sure I'm up to it but that's a nice thought.

Once again, notice that her therapist is attuned to notice slight changes in
imagery that offer hope to Charlene. When Charlene refers to herself metaphorically as a worn-out couch, her therapist extends that metaphor and talks
about how a couch can be rebuilt and made useful again. Imagery provides a
fertile ground for metaphors that offer possibilities for change, growth, and
recovery.

Keep in Mind

- Case conceptualization and empirical research are good guides to the imaginal themes that are most likely to be important for a particular issue.
- The same interventions used to test verbal thoughts can be used with imagery.
- Get as many details as you can about images. Details help reveal distortions and aspects of the image that can be tested.
- Evidence relevant to evaluating and learning from an image can often be found within the image itself.
- Imagery can often prompt clients to generate creative ideas to help themselves.
- Just as for verbal thoughts, imagery often includes distortions. Identifying and providing corrective information for these distortions often relieves the distress of disturbing images.

How can images of events that didn't really occur be tested?

Sometimes people have images of things that have never really occurred and yet they have strong emotional reactions to them and cannot easily dismiss these images out of their mind. In fact, imagery increases the likelihood the person will believe something will or did occur. A wealth of studies shows that when people are asked to imagine an event they are more likely to believe later that the imagined event actually occurred. For example, someone who is told to imagine knocking over a punchbowl at a wedding when they were young is likely to later believe that this really did occur (Loftus, 1997a and 1997b). People vary in how well they are able to distinguish between real and imagined events—a process known as reality monitoring (Johnson & Raye, 1981). Also, imagining events in the future inflates the likelihood someone believes that the event will occur. For example, the ease of imagining symptoms of a disease increases people's ratings of how likely they think it is that they will contract that disease (Sherman et al., 1985). People who imagine winning a lottery are more likely to inflate the odds that they will win.

Trap 7

The therapist is pretty certain the imagery described did not really occur and yet the client has strong emotional reactions to it and cannot easily dismiss the image out of mind.

One implication of these findings that imagery strengthens beliefs something actually happened or will happen is found in the "false memory" literature (Andrews et al., 1995). Therapists who ask repeatedly about childhood trauma when clients have not reported such experiences are likely to induce clients to believe they were victims of childhood trauma. Therapists should never ask clients to deliberately imagine traumatic events that have not been reported by the client because this increases the likelihood they will believe such imagined events really occurred (Otgaar et al., 2019). Of course, suggesting what clients imagine is not consistent with Socratic Dialogue in any case.

When images are troublesome for clients and yet do not relate to real people or events, therapists can intervene just as they would with images that relate to actual experiences. Brief case examples illustrate each of these four prime strategies:

- Probe for distortions in the image.
- Transform the image in helpful ways.
- Help the client construct an alternative image.
- Collaboratively evaluate the meanings and implications of the image.

Probe for distortions

Lee felt very guilty that three of his friends were killed in a fatal auto accident that occurred when they drove home from an evening class. An image kept coming into his head in which he said to them, "Let me drive you home." In this image his friends all got into his car and were driven home without incident. Lee could not shake his guilt because he thought he could have intervened to prevent their deaths. His therapist used Socratic Dialogue with Lee to test out the reality of this image and see whether it might be distorted in any way. By the end of the session, Lee acknowledged that it was very unlikely he would have made such an offer or his friends would have accepted it because: (1) they lived in a different part of town than he did, (2) one of his friends had driven his own car to class; to accept a ride, this friend would have had to leave his car at the university overnight, and (3) Lee had musical instruments in his car and it would have been impossible for all three friends to fit in the remaining space. Once he realized the distortions in his image, Lee was able to set aside his guilt and grieve the loss of his friends.

Transform the image

Maria had recurrent nightmares. These were often dreams that she and her therapist believed related to the sexual abuse she endured in her childhood. One recurrent nightmare included a man with many heads walking slowly toward her. Each head had many eyes which all leered at her in a threatening manner. In her dream, she was backed up against a wall next to a bed and could see nowhere to hide or run. Her therapist decided to help Maria transform the imagery in this dream using methods from Imagery Rehearsal Therapy (IRT), which has been demonstrated to be an effective treatment for recurrent nightmares (Krakow, 2004). Once she and Maria documented the various elements of the nightmare, her therapist gave Maria the following instructions:

Therapist: I want you to think of your nightmare as a movie.

Maria: A very scary movie!

Therapist: That's right. Imagine you are the director of a new movie. This new movie starts the same way as your nightmare. But in this new movie, you have all the special effects that you want and need. You can make anything happen. I want you to figure out something that changes your dream in some way where you are taking actions that help you feel safe and protected.

Maria: What kind of changes should I make in it?

Therapist: Whatever you like. Take a few minutes now and see what comes to your mind.

Maria: (After a few minutes of silence, a big smile comes over Maria's face.) I got it!

Therapist: Do you want to tell me?

Maria: The man is coming at me. When he gets close, I pull the blanket off the bed and throw it over him!

Therapist: What happens then?

Maria: He disappears!

While the initial nightmare implied Maria was powerless in protecting herself from threatened abuse, her transformed dream incorporated an action that led Maria to feel she could protect herself. Maria was instructed by her therapist to rehearse this new dream while she was awake several times a day over the next week. This rehearsal was meant to increase the likelihood that she would be able to transform her dream before it became a nightmare if it occurred again. As happens in about 90% of cases in research studies on IRT (Krakow, 2004), Maria's nightmare of the man with many heads never recurred. After she went through these same steps of transforming the imagery of one other recurrent nightmare, her nightmares stopped entirely for the first time in her life.

Notice that imagery transformation does not need to follow the rules of the real world. Maria's nightmares began when she was 4 years old and her transformation of this dream was a 4-year-old's solution. Throwing a blanket over the monstrous man made him disappear. This case example underscores the importance of the therapist maintaining a Socratic stance during imagery transformation. Therapist suggestions are never as likely to be as effective as client ideas for how to alter personal imagery.

Sometimes therapists will want to encourage clients to edit the initial imagery transformations they propose. For example, some abuse survivors will initially propose imagery that involves hurting their abuser. This type of transformed image can leave survivors of abuse viewing themselves as bad/abusive/ "no better than my abuser." When violent images are proposed, ask clients to think about developing an image that enables them to feel safe, free of blame and stigma, and importantly, fundamentally different from their abuser in ways congruent with their personal values.

Construct an alternative image

Research demonstrates that distressing imagery strengthens a person's conviction that the event is real or will happen. This effect can occur even when a person realizes that the imagery is unlikely to be true. Logic can be ineffective in tackling such beliefs. Recruiting alternative imagery can be more effective than disputing the veracity of existing imagery. Consider Viola who was still acutely grieving 3 years after her husband Victor's death. When she began therapy she was nearly housebound; she believed it would be disloyal to Victor's memory to participate in and enjoy social activities.

Her therapist inquired whether Viola believed Victor would want her to stay home grieving. Viola did not think so but reported an image of Victor on his death bed and how weak and sad he looked. She could not shake this image even though she knew he was no longer in his ill state. It did not seem acceptable for Viola to laugh and have fun when he was still lying in bed in her mind. Her therapist decided it might help Viola if she could construct an alternative image. She began by finding out if Viola could replace his dying image with a happier image such as people are able to imagine when they believe in life after death:

Therapist: Do you believe in an afterlife, Viola?

Viola: Yes ... I'm not sure. But I hope there is one.

Therapist: If there is one, what do you think Victor looks like now?

Viola: I don't know. I can't picture it. I'm not sure.

Therapist: Sometimes after people die, family members sense their presence. Do you ever feel like Victor is in the room or that he has come back to communicate with you?

Viola: No. Sometimes I have wished for that. But it never happened.

In the Therapist's Mind

Viola does not seem to have any clear images of life after death and so she does not have any preformed images to draw upon. It might be better to suggest a more creative process for generating an alternative image. Sometimes dreams can be used for this purpose.

Therapist: I wonder if you would be willing to try to have a dream that would send you a message to help you know how to handle this dilemma?

Viola: What do you mean?

Therapist: I've heard some people say how their loved one appeared in a dream long after death and gave them a message. Perhaps you could ask Victor to come to you in a dream and give you a message about what he wants for you now. Or you could hope for some other kind of dream that would give you a message that would help you.

Viola: That's an odd idea. I've not thought of doing that.

Therapist: It's not something I usually think to do in therapy. But since some people find it helpful, you could try and see what happens. What do you think?

Viola: Do I just hope for a message?

Therapist: I'm not sure how or if this will work. Maybe just before you go to sleep you could hope for a message from Victor. Do this for several nights and see what happens.

Viola returned to the next therapy appointment and reported that Victor had appeared in an interesting dream. Instead of looking ill, he looked as healthy as he had before his illness and was playing a guitar as he had done in his youth. When Viola tried to approach him, he shook his head with a smile and walked away. When she woke up, Viola felt sad to see him go and yet she experienced a sense of calm.

Therapist: What do you think this dream means?

Viola: I think Victor wants me to know that he is happy and has moved on. He was giving me permission to move on as well.

Therapist: What parts of the dream stand out for you and give you this message?

Viola: The fact that he was playing his guitar again. He always liked music and now he can play to his heart's content. When he walked away

Therapist: from me he smiled which told me he is happy. I could see in his eyes he wanted me to be happy too and this can't happen if he is the center of my life now. (Pause.) He walked away not because he was rejecting me but because he wants me to find new happiness.

Therapist: What difference does this message make for you?

Viola: I feel more at peace now. I think I can start doing things and keep this new image of Victor in my mind to make that feel alright.

The alternative image that came to Viola in a dream helped her move beyond daily grieving more effectively than hours of therapy discussion. This case example illustrates once again that alternative imagery that the client constructs, even in a dream, is much more potent than any imagery a therapist might suggest.

Evaluate the meanings and implications of an image

People with health anxiety have frequent imagery about disease (Wells & Hackmann, 1993). The research from experimental psychology cited earlier suggests that these images will increase client belief that they will really contract diseases. This type of belief lends itself readily to Socratic Dialogue, at the level of both (1) meta-cognitive beliefs about imagery (e.g., "because I can see this happen to me, it must real") and (2) the content of the imagery (e.g., an image of contracting HIV AIDS and dying). In addition, exploring the meanings and implications of imagery can sometimes lead to useful interventions.

Roberto's health anxiety centered on fears that he would contract HIV and then become extremely ill with AIDS. One recurring theme in his imagery was that his parents and people in his workplace would deduce from his illness that he was gay and reject him. Rather than simply test out his fears about illness, Roberto's therapist explored the implications of this particular illness:

Therapist: Which is worse for you when you imagine this? Developing AIDS or having people discover you are gay?

Roberto: Having no control over people finding out I am gay. I've been so careful to only tell people I know will support me. I don't want to live with the judgment and rejection I will have to go through.

For Roberto, the most frightening meanings and implications of his image were that his identity as a gay man would be discovered by his parents and others and lead to disastrous consequences. His therapist used Socratic Dialogue to help Roberto examine the likelihood of his feared consequences and his ability to handle these in a way that would preserve his positive self-esteem as a gay man. As described by Padesky (1989), these interventions included discussions of how to constructively manage his parent's homophobic beliefs to increase the likelihood that they would accept Roberto over time. In addition, they explored strategies for managing social pressures he could face in his workplace and elsewhere. These discussions greatly eased Roberto's fears of the interpersonal consequences that might result if he did contract AIDS and if people subsequently became aware he was gay. Roberto was then able to benefit more readily from standard health anxiety treatment protocols (Axelsson et al., 2020; Clark et al., 1998; Furer et al., 2007; Taylor & Asmundson, 2004).

Imagery, behavior change, and learning assignment adherence

In addition to powerfully affecting people's beliefs and emotions, imagery also increases the chances that they will take action. In a seminal study about elections in the United States, one group of participants was asked to imagine (just once!) voting and one group was not. Those who had engaged in voting-related mental imagery, compared to those who had not, were significantly more likely to actually cast their vote in the ballot box in the forthcoming (real) election (Libby et al., 2007). Other experiments show that the power of imagery to increase the likelihood of taking action applies to a range of events—from signing up for cable TV (Gregory et al., 1982), to exam revision (Pham & Taylor, 1999) to blood donation (Carroll, 1978). Thus, when we want clients to take positive action, it may be helpful to first ask them to imagine doing this action.

Imagining desired behaviors or even upcoming learning assignment efforts has the added benefit of identifying both helpful resources which can support change and roadblocks that might block it. The following example illustrates these possibilities:

Therapist: Before you leave today, let's take a few minutes so you can imagine starting that conversation with Kim at work.

Sean: Just do it in my head?

Therapist: Yes, but try to imagine it as vividly as possible. See if you can smell the coffee in the break room. Pay attention to the sounds you hear and the "feel" of the room. Does it feel warm and stuffy or cool and open? Once you are vividly "there" then put you and Kim in the room and start the conversation. Take as much time as you need and then you can tell me about it.

Sean: (Quiet for about 90 seconds.) That was something else!

Therapist: What do you mean?

Sean: Well, I got myself in the room ... Smelled the coffee and could see Kim pouring herself a cup. Then I asked her if she had a minute. She said OK and we started to talk like you and I practiced but then Jim came into the room and just started talking about his weekend and it was hard to get him to stop talking. So Kim and I didn't get to finish our conversation.

Therapist: That's so funny. Do you think that might happen?

Sean: It really could. Jim follows Kim into the break room all the time.

Therapist: So how does this affect your plan?

Sean: I think I should ask Kim to talk somewhere other than the break room.

Therapist: You thought the break room would be the most natural place. What other ideas do you have?

Sean: Well, when I was imagining talking to her just now, I noticed how she was really happy to talk to me. I guess when I think about it, she is easier to talk to than I usually imagine when I'm anxious. So maybe I could just ask her to take a break with me and walk outside for some fresh air so I could talk to her about something.

Therapist: See if you can vividly imagine that right now and let's see how it goes.

One could argue that nearly all at-home learning assignments can benefit from imagery rehearsal before leaving the session. Imagery rehearsal can also be inserted into other CBT interventions such as Thought Records. For example, clients can be asked to develop vivid images related to an alternative or more balanced thought in column 6 of a 7-Column Thought Record (Greenberger & Padesky, 2016) and to focus on these images prior to rating how strongly they believe these thoughts (Josefowitz, 2017).

Use of Socratic Dialogue to develop positive images that promote change

Many people imagine themselves doing various behaviors in advance of an event (e.g., job interviews, making a speech, disciplining a child, presenting a gift). Imaginal rehearsal helps us refine our approach and also gives us opportunities to develop experience so we can act with greater confidence and improve the likelihood we will behave in the ways we want. Including imaginal rehearsals in therapy and also as part of homework assignments helps clients gain both experience and confidence in new behaviors they want to develop. Recall that when envisioning positive events, compared to thinking about them in words, imagery is linked to more positive mood (Holmes et al., 2009).

While images can be of objects and events they can also represent much broader domains such as a person's sense of self. The generation of positive imagery about oneself in the past and future is an important part of CBT treatment approaches for personality disorder (Arntz & Weertman, 1999; Padesky & Mooney, 2007). To develop a more positive sense of self that is believable, it is important for the client to generate their own mental imagery. More recently, Hallford and colleagues (Hallford, Barry et al., 2020; Hallford, Sharma et al., 2020) empirically demonstrate the benefits of increasing positive future images in the treatment of major depression. For a review of imagery interventions and their role in treating mood, anxiety, and stress-related disorders see Hitchcock et al. (2017).

Positive imagery is also central to Padesky and Mooney's (2012) Strengths-Based CBT approach for building resilience. As described in Chapter 2, they highlight a number of nonverbal and verbal differences that are important for therapists to incorporate when using Socratic Dialogue to help clients generate new, more positive beliefs and imagery. First, clients often require positive encouragement to develop positive imagery and new belief systems. In fact, therapist neutrality can be considered a negative intervention in the context of imagining something new. Consider the differences in these two therapist responses to Gina, a client with borderline personality disorder who says, "I would like to be more connected to other people."

Neutral Therapist: What would that look like to be more connected to others?

Positive Therapist: I can see how that would be good for you. What would it look like to be more connected to others?

Although the neutral response is acceptable, this client might feel uneasy not knowing if the therapist endorses her positive goal or is skeptical. The positive, encouraging therapist response openly endorses the client's aspirations before inquiring further. This supports the client's positive goal.

Of course, as emphasized throughout this chapter, words are not as powerful as imagery. In fact, the positive therapist's response is strengthened further when accompanied by a big smile and when strong interest is conveyed in the vocal tone of the question:

Positive Therapist: (Big genuine smile.) I can see how that would be good for you. (With enthusiastic interest in voice.) What would it look like to be more connected to others?

In addition to expressed positive support and therapeutic smiling, Padesky and Mooney (2012) recommend therapists who are working with clients toward the development of new positive qualities or sense of self allow periods of therapeutic silence to allow for client creativity in the construction of something new. Use of positive imagery and metaphors are also emphasized. Finally, they suggest that questions in Socratic Dialogue should be constructive rather than deconstructive when developing positive beliefs and imagery (Mooney & Padesky, 2000). Compare the differences between these two types of questions in the following Socratic Dialogue:

Therapist:	(With an encouraging smile.) Gina, take a minute and imagine how it would look and feel if you were connected to other people.
Gina:	I wouldn't be so tight around them.
Therapist—Deconstructive:	What happens when you are tight?
Therapist—Constructive:	How would you like to be instead?

The deconstructive question requires Gina to think about her old interaction style. The constructive question encourages Gina to imagine something new, to create a more positive image of her interactions. This is how Gina responds to the constructive question:

Gina:	Hmmm. I'm not sure. (Silence.) I guess I'd be more relaxed. (Silence.) If I was relaxed I could be myself, maybe even be funny and trust that they wouldn't judge me.
Therapist—Deconstructive:	Have you had experiences like that?
Therapist—Constructive:	(Smiling.) That would be so nice. If they weren't judging you, how would they be thinking about you? What would you like them to be thinking about you?
Gina:	(Quietly.) I'd like them to like me. (Pause.) I'd like them to be glad they are with me.

Again, the deconstructive question leads Gina away from her positive imagery while the constructive responses support and enhance the development of her positive imagery.

When using Socratic Dialogue to develop positive imagery, it is important that therapists incorporate these positive and constructive elements into the four stages of Socratic Dialogue:

- Stage 1—Informational questions: ask constructive questions, smile and actively encourage client's positive imagery;
- Stage 2—Empathic listening: listen with encouragement (head nods, smile as appropriate);
- Stage 3—Written summaries: make summaries that sift out negative elements and retain positive elements; and
- Stage 4—Analytical/synthesizing questions: ask the client analytical/synthesizing questions such as "What would that be like for you?", "How do you feel when you imagine that?", "Is that the best you can imagine or is there something even more positive?", and "What does this image allow you to do/feel/experience?"

Positive imagery such as Gina is beginning to develop can be used in therapy to help people imagine a different future as well as new behaviors, emotions, and beliefs. In turn, this imagery can be used to guide and encourage Gina as she tries out new behaviors and attitudes in her interpersonal interactions. Behavioral experiments can be used in a somewhat novel way to test the viability of her positive imagery (Padesky & Mooney, 2012). These behavioral experiments can be debriefed using the constructive aspects of Socratic Dialogue summarized here so that Gina has opportunities to move toward enacting her positive imagery with or without modifications, based on her experiences.

Keep in Mind

- Imagining action increases the likelihood someone will take that action.
- Adherence to at-home learning tasks is likely to be improved by imaginal rehearsal before the end of a therapy session.
- Imagery of future positive events can increase positive mood, even in clients experiencing depression.
- When helping clients develop positive imagery, therapists are advised to employ positive encouragement, constructive language, a genuine smile, to reflect client-generated metaphors, and to allow greater periods of silence to make room for client creativity.

Summary

As research on key aspects of mental imagery demonstrates, imagery is central to our mental processes and has a profound influence on the ways our minds work. Therapists are encouraged to identify and work with client imagery because imagery has a stronger emotional impact on clients than verbal summaries of cognitions and events. As illustrated in this chapter, imagery has a role to play in all the methods of guided discovery commonly used in CBT (e.g., Socratic Dialogue, behavioral experiments, thought records, role plays, exposure).

Intrusive negative mental imagery occurs in a wide range of disorders. Socratic Dialogue can be used to explore the details and meanings of imagery so therapist and client can make sense of why people do things they do not want to do. For example, repeated checking of a stove as part of one client's obsessive-compulsive disorder might be fueled by a recurrent image of the house on fire. This chapter illustrates a variety of ways guided discovery methods are used to identify mental imagery even when clients initially may not be aware of what mental imagery is compared to verbal thought. Many case examples and therapist–client dialogues are presented to demonstrate methods to explore, examine, test, and transform a variety of types of imagery—visual, auditory, kinesthetic, and olfactory—whether these images link to real-life experiences, dreams, hallucinations, or false memories.

In addition, guided discovery methods can be used to employ imagery as a pathway to positive transformation. A focus on imagery can boost client confidence in alternative beliefs, whether on a thought record, in a Socratic Dialogue, or during debriefing of a behavioral experiment. Imagery can be used to increase the likelihood of behavior change or to imagine and evaluate the usefulness of new behaviors and behavioral experiments. Verbal and nonverbal modifications to the four stages of Socratic Dialogue were presented that can enhance its effectiveness in the development of positive imagery.

Throughout every stage of therapy from case conceptualization to relapse management planning, imagery can be woven into the fabric of therapeutic interventions. Fortunately, the same guided discovery methods that work effectively in the identification and exploration of verbal cognitions work equally well with imagery. In fact, for all the reasons outlined in this chapter, embedding imagery into every aspect of guided discovery is likely to enhance its therapeutic impact.

Reader Learning Activities

- What percentage of your therapy sessions incorporated imagery prior to reading this chapter? What percentage of your therapy sessions do you think would benefit from incorporating imagery in light of the information in this chapter?

- Identify two ways you could increase the intentional use of imagery in your sessions (e.g., asking about imagery and their details during case conceptualization, allowing time for imaginal rehearsal of learning assignments).

- Identify any images you have that inhibit you from greater use of imagery in therapy.

- What guided discovery methods could you use to deal with unhelpful imagery that you or your clients experience (e.g., Socratic Dialogue, behavioral experiments, imaginal rehearsal, role plays)?

- What guided discovery methods can be used with you or your clients to promote more constructive and rewarding imagery?

- Choose one Socratic method illustrated in this chapter that you think would be helpful to try out with appropriate clients in the coming weeks. Predict what you think will happen when you use it. Try it at least five times and see how the outcomes compare with your predictions.

- If you struggle in eliciting and working with imagery even after experimenting with methods described in this chapter, read more about imagery and consider getting supervision or consultation from someone with experience using imagery in therapy.

References

Andrews, B., Morton, J., Bekerian, D. A., Brewin, C. R., Davies, G. M., & Mollon, P. (1995). The recovery of memories in clinical-practice—experiences and beliefs of British-Psychological-Society practitioners. *The Psychologist, 8*(5), 209–214.

Arntz, A., & Weertman, A. (1999). Treatment of childhood memories: Theory and practice. *Behaviour Research and Therapy, 37*(8), 715–740. https://doi.org/10.1016/S0005-7967(98)00173-9

Axelsson E., Andersson E., Ljótsson B., Björkander D., Hedman-Lagerlöf, M., & Hedman-Lagerlöf, E. (2020). Effect of internet vs face-to-face cognitive behavior therapy for health anxiety: A randomized noninferiority clinical trial. *JAMA Psychiatry, 77*(9), 915–924. https://doi.org/10.1001/jamapsychiatry.2020.0940

Baddeley, A. D., & Andrade, J. (2000). Working memory and the vividness of imagery. *Journal of Experimental Psychology-General, 129*(1), 126–145. https://doi.org/10.1037/0096-3445.129.1.126

Beck, A. T. (1976). *Cognitive therapy and the emotional disorders*. New York: New American Library.

Beck, A. T. (1988). *Love is never enough*. New York: Harper & Row.

Beck, A. T., (1999). *Prisoners of hate: The cognitive basis of anger, hostility and violence*. New York: HarperCollins.

Beck, A. T., & Emery, G. (with Greenberg, R. L.). (1985). *Anxiety disorders and phobias: A cognitive perspective*. New York: Basic Books.

Beck, A. T., Grant, P., Inverson, E., Brinen, A. P., & Perivoliotis, D. (2020). *Recovery-oriented cognitive therapy for serious mental health conditions*. New York: Guilford Press.

Beck, A. T., Laude, R., & Bohnert, M. (1974). Ideational components of anxiety neurosis. *Archives of General Psychiatry, 31*, 319–325. https://doi.org/10.1001/archpsyc.1974.01760150035005

Beck, A. T., Rector, N.A., Stolar, N., & Grant, P. (2009). *Schizophrenia: Cognitive theory, research, and therapy*. New York: Guilford Press.

Beck, A. T., Rush, A. J., Shaw, B. F., & Emery, G. (1979). *Cognitive therapy of depression*. New York: Guilford Press.

Bennett-Levy, J., Butler, G., Fennell, M., Hackmann, A., Mueller, M., & Westbrook, D. (2004). *Oxford guide to behavioural experiments in cognitive therapy*. Oxford: Oxford University Press.

Blackwell, S. E. (2019). Mental imagery: From basic research to clinical practice. *Journal of Psychotherapy Integration, 29*, 235–247. https://doi.org/10.1037/int0000108

Blackwell, S. E. (2021). Mental imagery in the science and practice of cognitive behaviour therapy: Past, present, and future perspectives. *International Journal of Cognitive Therapy, 14*(2), 160–181. https://doi.org/10.1007/s41811-021-00102-0

Brewin, C. R., Gregory, J. D., Lipton, M., & Burgess, N. (2010). Intrusive images in psychological disorders: Characteristics, neural mechanisms, and treatment implications, *Psychological Review, 117*(1), 210–232. https://doi.org/10.1037/a0018113

Carrasco, D. G., & Cantalapiedra, J. A. (2016). Effectiveness of motor imagery or mental practice in functional recovery after stroke: a systematic review. *Neurología* (English Edition), *31*(1), 43–52. https://doi.org/10.1016/j.nrleng.2013.02.008

Carroll, J. S. (1978). The effect of imagining an event on expectations for the event: An interpretation in terms of the availability heuristic. *Journal of Experimental Social Psychology, 14*, 88–96. https://doi.org/10.1016/0022-1031(78)90062-8

Chadwick, P., & Birchwood, M. (1994). The omnipotence of voices: A cognitive approach to auditory hallucinations. *British Journal of Psychiatry, 164*, 190–201. https://doi.org/10.1192/bjp.164.2.190

Clark, D. M., Salkovskis, P. M., Hackmann, A., Wells, A., Fennell, M., Ludgate, J., Ahmad, S., Richards, H. C., & Gelder, M. (1998). Two psychological treatments for hypochondriasis. A randomised controlled trial. *British Journal of Psychiatry, 173*, 218–225. https://doi.org/10.1192/bjp.173.3.218

Conway, M. A. (2001). Sensory-perceptual episodic memory and its context: Autobiographical memory. *Philosophical Transactions of the Royal Society of London Series B-Biological Sciences, 356*(1413), 1375–1384. https://doi.org/10.1098/rstb.2001.0940

Conway, M. A., Meares, K., & Standart, S. (2004). Images and goals. *Memory, 12*(4), 525–531. https://doi.org/10.1080/09658210444000151

Day, S. J., Holmes, E. A., & Hackmann, A. (2004). Occurrence of imagery and its link with early memories in agoraphobia. *Memory, 12*(4), 416–427. https://doi.org/10.1080/09658210444000034

Di Simplicio, M, McInerney, J. E., Goodwin, G. M., Attenburrow, M. J., & Holmes, E. A. (2012). Revealing the mind's eye: bringing (mental) images into psychiatry. *American Journal of Psychiatry, 169*(12), 1245–1246. https://doi.org/10.1176/appi.ajp.2012.12040499

Ehlers, A., & Clark, D. M. (2000). A cognitive model of posttraumatic stress disorder. *Behaviour Research and Therapy, 38*(4), 319–345. https://doi.org/10.1016/s0005-7967(99)00123-0

Furer, P., Walker, J. R., & Stein, M. B. (2007). *Treating health anxiety and fear of death: A practitioner's guide.* New York: Springer.

Ganis, G., Thompson, W. L., & Kosslyn, S. M. (2004). Brain areas underlying visual mental imagery and visual perception: An fMRI study. *Cognitive Brain Research, 20*(2), 226–241. https://doi.org/10.1016/j.cogbrainres.2004.02.012

Gaudiano, B. A., & Herbert, J. D. (2006). Believability of hallucinations as a potential mediator of their frequency and associated distress in psychotic inpatients. *Behavioural and Cognitive Psychotherapy, 34*(4), 497–502. https://doi.org/10.1017/S1352465806003080

Greenberger, D., & Padesky, C. A. (2016). *Mind over mood: Change how you feel by changing the way you think* (2nd ed.). New York: Guilford Press.

Gregory, W. L., Cialdini, R. B., & Carpenter, K. M. (1982). Self-relevant scenarios as mediators of likelihood estimates and compliance—does imagining make it so. *Journal of Personality and Social Psychology, 43*(1), 89–99. https://doi.org/10.1037/0022-3514.43.1.89

Grey, N., & Holmes, E. A. (2008). "Hotspots" in trauma memories in the treatment of post-traumatic stress disorder: a replication. *Memory, 16*(7), 788–796. https://doi.org/10.1080/09658210802266446

Grey, N., Holmes, E. A., & Brewin, C. R. (2001). Peritraumatic emotional "hot spots" in memory. *Behavioural and Cognitive Psychotherapy, 29*(3), 357–362. https://doi.org/10.1017/S1352465801003095

Grey, N., Young, K., & Holmes, E. A. (2002). Cognitive restructuring within reliving: a treatment for peritraumatic emotional hotspots in PTSD. *Behavioural and Cognitive Psychotherapy, 30*(1), 37–56. https://doi.org/10.1017/S1352465802001054

Hackmann, A., Bennett-Levy, J. & Holmes, E. A. (2011). *Oxford guide to imagery in cognitive therapy.* Oxford: Oxford University Press.

Hackmann, A., Clark, D. M., & McManus, F. (2000). Recurrent images and early memories in social phobia. *Behaviour Research and Therapy, 38*(6), 601–610. https://doi.org/10.1016/S0005-7967(99)00161-8

Hackmann, A., & Holmes, E. A. (2004). Reflecting on imagery: A clinical perspective and overview of the special edition on mental imagery and memory in psychopathology. *Memory, 12*(4), 389–402. https://doi.org/10.1080/09658210444000133

Hales, S. A., Blackwell, S. E., Di Simplicio, M., Iyadurai, L., Young, K., & Holmes, E. A. (2014). Imagery based cognitive-behavioral assessment. In G. P. Brown & D. A. Clark (Eds.), *Assessment in Cognitive Therapy.* New York: Guilford Press.

Hallford, D. J., Barry, T. J., Austin, D. W., Raes, F., Takano, K., & Klein, B. (2020). Impairments in episodic future thinking for positive events and anticipatory pleasure in major depression. *Journal of Affective Disorders, 260*, 536–543. https://doi.org/10.1016/j.jad.2019.09.039

Hallford, D. J., Sharma, M. K., & Austin, D. W. (2020). Increasing anticipatory pleasure in major depression through enhancing episodic future thinking: A randomized single-case series trial. *Journal of Psychopathology and Behavioral Assessment, 42*, 751–764. https://doi.org/10.1007/s10862-020-09820-9

Hasking, P. A., Di Simplicio, M., McEvoy, P. M., & Rees, C. S. (2018). Emotional cascade theory and non-suicidal self-injury: The importance of imagery and positive affect. *Cognition and Emotion, 32*(5), 941–952. https://doi.org/10.1080/02699931.2017.1368456

Hitchcock, C., Werner-Seidler, A., Blackwell, S. E., & Dalgleish, T. (2017). Autobiographical episodic memory-based training for the treatment of mood, anxiety and stress-related disorders: A systematic review and meta-analysis. *Clinical Psychology Review, 52*, 92–107. https://doi.org/10.1016/j.cpr.2016.12.003

Holmes, E. A., Arntz, A., & Smucker, M. R. (2007). Imagery rescripting in cognitive behaviour therapy: Images, treatment techniques and outcomes. *Journal of Behavior Therapy and Experimental Psychiatry*, *38*(4), 297–305. https://doi.org/10.1016/j.jbtep.2007.10.007

Holmes, E. A., & Butler, G. (2009). Cognitive therapy and suicidality in PTSD: And recent thoughts on flashbacks to trauma versus 'flashforwards to suicide'. In N. Grey (Ed.), *A case book of cognitive therapy for traumatic stress reactions* (pp. 178–194). Hove: Routledge.

Holmes, E. A., Crane, C., Fennell, M. J. V., & Williams, J. M. G. (2007). Imagery about suicide in depression—"Flash-forwards"? *Journal of Behavior Therapy and Experimental Psychiatry*, *38*(4), 423–434. https://doi.org/10.1016/j.jbtep.2007.10.004

Holmes, E. A., Geddes, J. R., Colom, F., & Goodwin, G. M. (2008). Mental imagery as an emotional amplifier: Application to bipolar disorder. *Behaviour Research and Therapy*, *46*(12), 1251–1258. https://doi.org/10.1016/j.brat.2008.09.005

Holmes, E. A., Grey, N., & Young, K. A. D. (2005). Intrusive images and "hotspots" of trauma memories in posttraumatic stress disorder: An exploratory investigation of emotions and cognitive themes. *Journal of Behavior Therapy and Experimental Psychiatry*, *36*(1), 3–17. https://doi.org/10.1016/j.jbtep.2004.11.002

Holmes, E. A., Hales, S. A., Young, K., & Di Simplicio, M. (2019). *Imagery-based cognitive therapy for bipolar disorder and mood instability*. New York: Guilford Press.

Holmes, E. A., Lang, T. J., & Shah, D. M. (2009). Developing interpretation bias modification as a 'cognitive vaccine' for depressed mood—Imagining positive events makes you feel better than thinking about them verbally. *Journal of Abnormal Psychology*, *118*(1), 76–88. https://doi.org/10.1037/a0012590

Holmes, E. A., & Mathews, A. (2005). Mental imagery and emotion: A special relationship? *Emotion*, *5*(4), 489–497. https://doi.org/10.1037/1528-3542.5.4.489

Holmes, E. A., & Mathews, A. (2010). Mental imagery in emotion and emotional disorders. *Clinical Psychology Review*, *30*(3), 349–362. https://doi.org/10.1016/j.cpr.2010.01.001

Holmes, E. A., Mathews, A., Dalgleish, T., & Mackintosh, B. (2006). Positive interpretation training: Effects of mental imagery versus verbal training on positive mood. *Behavior Therapy*, *37*(3), 237–247. https://doi.org/10.1016/j.beth.2006.02.002

Holmes, E. A., Mathews, A., Mackintosh, B., & Dalgleish, T. (2008). The causal effect of mental imagery on emotion assessed using picture-word cues. *Emotion*, *8*(3), 395–409. https://doi.org/10.1037/1528-3542.8.3.395

Hunt, M., Bylsma, L., Brock, J., Fenton, M., Goldberg, A., Miller, R., Tran, T., & Urgelles, J. (2006). The role of imagery in the maintenance and treatment of snake fear. *Journal of Behavior Therapy and Experimental Psychiatry*, *37*, 283–298. https://doi.org/10.1016/j.jbtep.2005.12.002

Hyman, I. E., & Pentland, J. (1996). The role of mental imagery in the creation of false childhood memories. *Journal of Memory and Language*, *35*, 101–117. https://doi.org/10.1006/jmla.1996.0006

Ji, J. L., Kavanagh, D. J., Holmes, E. A., MacLeod, C., & Di Simplicio, M. (2019). Mental imagery in psychiatry: Conceptual and clinical implications. *CNS Spectrums*, *24*(1), 114–126. https://doi.org/10.1017/S1092852918001487

Johnson, M. K., & Raye, C. L. (1981). Reality monitoring. *Psychological Review*, *88*(1), 67–85. https://doi.org/10.1037/0033-295X.88.1.67

Josefowitz, N. (2017). Incorporating imagery into thought records: Increasing engagement in balanced thoughts. *Cognitive and Behavioral Practice*, *24*(1), 90–100. https://doi.org/10.1016/j.cbpra.2016.03.005

Kim, S. E., Kim, J. W., Kim, J. J., Jeong, B. S., Choi, E. A., Jeong, Y. G., Kim, J. H., Ku, J., & Ki, S. W. (2007). The neural mechanism of imagining facial affective expression. *Brain Research*, *1145*, 128–137. https://doi.org/10.1016/j.brainres.2006.12.048

Kosslyn, S. M., Ganis, G., & Thompson, W. L. (2001). Neural foundations of imagery. *Nature Reviews: Neuroscience, 2*(9), 635–642. https://doi.org/10.1038/35090055

Krakow, B. (2004). Imagery rehearsal therapy for chronic posttraumatic nightmares: A mind's eye view. In R. I., Rosner, W. J., Lyddon, & A. Freeman (Eds.), *Cognitive therapy and dreams* pp. 89–109. New York: Springer Publishing.

Kuyken, W., Padesky, C.A., & Dudley, R. (2009). *Collaborative case conceptualization: Working effectively with clients in cognitive-behavioral therapy*. New York: Guilford Press.

Libby, L. K., Shaeffer, E. M., Eibach, R. P., & Slemmer, J. A. (2007). Picture yourself at the polls: Visual perspective in mental imagery affects self-perception and behavior. *Psychological Science, 18*(3), 199–203. https://doi.org/10.1111/j.1467-9280.2007.01872.x

Loftus, E. F. (1997a). Creating false memories. *Scientific American, 277*, 70–75. https://doi.org/10.1038/scientificamerican0997-70

Loftus, E. F. (1997b). Memory for a past that never was. *Current Directions in Psychological Science, 6*(3), 60–65. https://doi.org/10.1111/1467-8721.ep11512654

Malcolm, C. P., Picchioni, M. M., & Ellett, L. (2015). Intrusive prospective imagery, post-traumatic intrusions and anxiety in schizophrenia. *Psychiatry Research, 230*(3), 899–904. https://doi.org/10.1016/j.psychres.2015.11.029

Mathews, A., Ridgeway, V., & Holmes, E. A. (2013). Feels like the real thing: Imagery is both more realistic and emotional than verbal thought, *Cognitive and Emotion, 27*(2), 217–229. https://doi.org/10.1080/02699931.2012.698252

Mooney, K.A., & Padesky, C.A. (2000) Applying client creativity to recurrent problems: Constructing possibilities and tolerating doubt. *Journal of Cognitive Psychotherapy: An International Quarterly, 14*(2), 149–161. https://doi.org/10.1891/0889-8391.14.2.149

Morrison, A. P. (2001), Cognitive therapy for auditory hallucinations as an alternative to anti-psychotic medication: A case series. *Clinical Psychology & Psychotherapy, 8*, 136–147. https://doi.org/10.1002/cpp.269

Morrison, A. P. (2009). Cognitive behaviour therapy for first episode psychosis: Good for nothing or fit for purpose? *Psychosis: Psychological, Social and Integrative Approaches, 1* (2), 103–112. https://doi.org/10.1080/17522430903026393

Morrison, A. P., Beck, A. T., Glentworth, D., Dunn, H., Reid, G. S., Larkin, W., & Williams, S. (2002). Imagery and psychotic symptoms: A preliminary investigation. *Behaviour Research and Therapy, 40*(9), 1053–1062. https://doi.org/10.1016/S0005-7967(01)00128-0

Norem, J. K. (2001). *The positive power of negative thinking: Using defensive pessimism to harness anxiety and perform at your peak*. Cambridge, MA: Basic Books.

Otgaar, H., Howe, M. L., Patihis, L., Merckelbach, H., Lynn, S. J., Lilienfeld, S. O., & Loftus, E. F. (2019). The return of the repressed: The persistent and problematic claims of long-forgotten trauma. *Perspectives on Psychological Science, 14*(6), 1072–1095. https://doi.org/10.1177/1745691619862306

Padesky, C. A. (1989). Attaining and maintaining positive lesbian self-identity: A cognitive therapy approach. *Women & Therapy, 8* (1, 2), 145–156. https://doi.org/10.1300/J015v08n01_12 [available from: http://padesky.com/clinical-corner/publications].

Padesky, C.A., (2020). Collaborative case conceptualization: Client knows best. *Cognitive and Behavioral Practice, 27*, 392–404. https://doi.org/10.1016/j.cbpra.2020.06.003

Padesky, C. A., & Mooney, K. A. (2007). *The NEW Paradigm CBT approach to personality disorders*. Unpublished manuscript.

Padesky, C. A., & Mooney, K. A. (2012). Strengths-based cognitive-behavioural therapy: A four-step model to build resilience. *Clinical Psychology and Psychotherapy, 19* (4), 283–290. https://doi.org/10.1002/cpp.1795

Patel, T., Brewin, C. R., Wheatley, J., Wells, A., Fisher, P., & Myers, S. (2007). Intrusive images and memories in major depression. *Behaviour Research and Therapy, 45*(11), 2573–2580. https://doi.org/10.1016/j.brat.2007.06.004

Pearson, J., Naselaris, T., Holmes, E. A., & Kosslyn, S. M. (2015). Mental imagery: Functional mechanisms and clinical applications, *Trends in Cognitive Sciences, 19*(10), 590–602. https://doi.org/10.1016/j.tics.2015.08.003

Pham, L. B., & Taylor, S. E. (1999). From thought to action: Effects of process- versus outcome-based mental simulations on performance. *Personality and Social Psychology Bulletin, 25*(2), 250–260. https://doi.org/10.1177/0146167299025002010

Schacter, D. L., Addis, D. R., & Buckner, R. L. (2007). Remembering the past to imagine the future: The prospective brain. *Nature Reviews: Neuroscience, 8*(Sept), 657–661. https://doi.org/10.1038/nrn2213

Sherman, S. J., Cialdini, R. B., Schwartzman, D. F., & Reynolds, K. D. (1985). Imagining can heighten or lower the perceived likelihood of contracting a disease: The mediating effect of ease of imagery. *Personality and Social Psychology Bulletin, 11*(1), 118–127. https://doi.org/10.1177/0146167285111011

Stopa, L. (Ed.). (2009). *Imagery and the threatened self: Perspectives on mental imagery and the self in cognitive therapy.* Hove: Routledge.

Stopa, L. (2021) *Imagery in cognitive-behavioral therapy.* New York: Guilford Press.

Tallon, K., Ovanessian, M. M., Koerner, N., & Dugas, M. J. (2020). Mental imagery in generalized anxiety disorder: A comparison with healthy control participants. *Behaviour Research and Therapy, 127,* 103571. https://doi.org/10.1016/j.brat.2020.103571

Taylor, S., & Asmundson, G. J. G. (2004) *Treating health anxiety: A cognitive–behavioral approach.* New York: Guilford Press.

Weems, C. F., Scott, B. G., Banks, D. M., & Graham, R. A. (2012). Is TV traumatic for all youths? The role of preexisting posttraumatic-stress symptoms in the link between disaster coverage and stress. *Psychological Science, 23*(11). 1293–1297. https://doi.org/10.1177/0956797612446952

Wells, A., & Hackmann, A. (1993). Imagery and core beliefs in health anxiety: Content and origins. *Behavioural & Cognitive Psychotherapy, 21,* 265–273. https://doi.org/10.1017/S1352465800010511

Wenzel, A., Brown, G. K., Beck, A. T. (2009). *Cognitive therapy for suicidal patients: Scientific and clinical applications.* Washington, DC: American Psychological Association.

Wicken, M., Keogh, R., & Pearson, J. (2021). The critical role of mental imagery in human emotion: Insights from fear-based imagery and aphantasia. *Proceedings of the Royal Society B, 288*(1946), 20210267. https://doi.org/10.1098/rspb.2021.0267

Wright J. H., Turkington D., Kingdon D., & Basco M. (2009). *Cognitive therapy for severe mental illness: An illustrated guide.* Arlington, VA: American Psychiatric Publishing.

6
Inflexible Beliefs

Helen Kennerley and Christine A. Padesky

> One man was so convinced he was dead that his family finally took
> him to a therapist. His therapist tried many different interventions to
> help him see that he was alive. Nothing budged the man's belief that
> he was dead.
>
> Finally his therapist showed him textbooks and websites that pro-
> vided lots of evidence that dead men don't bleed. After hours spent
> reviewing all this information, the man finally seemed convinced that
> dead men don't bleed.
>
> **Therapist:** Do you now agree that dead men don't bleed?
> **Man:**   Yes.
> **Therapist:** OK. I'm going to prick your finger with this pin.
>   (As she pricks his finger, it begins to bleed.)
> **Man:**   What do you know? . . . Dead men do bleed!
>
> —Joke of unknown origin

The man in the above joke is caught in the trap of inflexible beliefs—because
he believes that he is dead, he interprets his experiences in that light and because he interprets his experiences in that light, he "confirms" that he is dead.
How often do you find yourself and other people caught in similar traps?

> I'm unattractive so I don't believe compliments. I don't get believable com-
> pliments; therefore I must be unattractive.
>
> I'm stupid and only achieve by luck, not because of my ability; because
> I don't make real achievements, I must be stupid.

It can be very frustrating for therapists when client beliefs remain inflexible even in the face of clear contradictory evidence or multiple attempts

244 Dialogues for Discovery

to loosen these beliefs via guided discovery. At the same time, clients can also become frustrated or experience therapists as unsupportive when they are continually questioned about the ideas that they believe are absolutely "true." Unfortunately, prolonged frustration can lead to hopelessness and disengagement—for both parties. Warning signs of hopelessness might include clients not engaging in homework or missing sessions, or therapists feeling discouraged when seeing a client's name in their schedule, for example.

This chapter describes methods for using guided discovery with people with inflexible beliefs in ways that are not alienating and that minimize the risk of creating a therapeutic impasse. To begin, we offer a number of guiding principles that are illustrated throughout this chapter to help therapists navigate common challenges:

Keep in Mind

- **Understand what lies behind inflexible beliefs**—clients always have "good reasons" for their beliefs (Mooney & Padesky, 2004).

- **Adopt a genuinely curious rather than a challenging stance** and maintain an open, investigative approach.

- **Generate alternative beliefs** so that your client's experiences can be weighed in terms of whether they fit better with the inflexible belief or the alternative belief. When no alternative is identified, it can be more difficult to reconsider an inflexible belief.

- **Attend to the relationship**—test inflexible beliefs only when the alliance is relatively strong.

- **Match intervention to the level of cognition** (Mooney & Padesky, 2000, 160; Padesky, 2020a):
  - Automatic thoughts—gather evidence from the specific event(s).
  - Underlying assumptions—use behavioral experiments.
  - Core beliefs—continuum work, positive data logs, role-plays.

- **Keep the work fresh** even when it takes a long time:
  - Use humor (sensitively).
  - Co-develop new ideas language with your client.
  - Be patient and also stay active.

Understanding Inflexible Beliefs

It is interesting how the same simple gesture can trigger very different responses:

> A stranger offers a bus seat to a woman—she thanks him for his offer and enjoys the opportunity to sit down.
>
> A stranger offers a bus seat to a woman—she rejects his offer and keeps a close eye on him for the rest of the journey.
>
> A stranger offers a bus seat to a woman—she accepts his offer but sits uncomfortably imagining that others pity her, too.

In order to understand these different reactions, we need to know the beliefs of each woman. Beliefs come in all shapes and sizes—some are emotionally charged, some not at all; some beliefs are flexible and easily modified and others are hard to shift. Yet all beliefs have a foundation in personal reality. They are understandable in the context of someone's personal life experiences and our first task is to appreciate this. Guided discovery methods help us learn why beliefs make sense to particular individuals.

Over a lifetime we build beliefs about ourselves, the world around us, and the future. We develop a notion of who we are, what we can do, and what we can expect. This begins even before we have the capacity to use language or even form enduring images. Our beliefs and the meanings that we make of our world make personal sense in the light of our experiences and these meanings can be held as words, images, or simply a "felt sense." Our beliefs framework then gives rise to our "rules for living," our outlook in life, and shapes our expectations and the conclusions we draw from situations.

Thus, someone who is indulged as a child might grow to believe that they are unusually special and assume that others should meet their needs, while a neglected or abused youngster might develop beliefs that they are not worthy, that others are harmful, and they might predict that others will hurt them. These beliefs will make sense to the child, will feel "true," and can become very well established. Beliefs that are sufficiently "fixed" or rigid continue into adulthood and continue to influence interpretations and behaviors even when the environment and relationships have changed.

Looking back at the bus scenarios, the stranger might have offered the bus seat to a woman who had a childhood of reasonable indulgence and she would assume that the gesture fitted with the notion that others do things for her, that her needs matter, and she would probably take the seat and feel better because of it. No problem for her. The very same act might trigger suspicious thoughts for a woman who had endured hurt or neglect ("Why is he doing this? He's probably up to something. What's his ulterior motive? It's probably hurtful.") or for a woman who had experienced a lifetime of denigration ("I must look desperate—what a sad creature I am."). These latter two women might well reject his offer or accept it and then feel suspicious, worried, or embarrassed. Their beliefs would stop them from being able to even consider that his was a friendly or polite gesture. They are unlikely to experience pleasure or feelings of acceptance or to view others as benign—responses that might otherwise help consolidate a positive experience.

It is common for long-held unhelpful beliefs to be rigid as well as extreme. This combination of unhelpful content and inflexibility is powerful. Some clients' beliefs are so tightly held that therapists struggle to make any progress and this can trigger our own inflexible beliefs:

> I am a terrible therapist
> Other therapists would know what to do—they are all better than I am.

You probably know your own Achilles' heel. This reminds us how important it is to monitor therapy closely, to consider our own reactions and our own contributions to stuck points. It can be helpful to test our own beliefs using guided discovery methods in self-supervision (Padesky, 2006), with a supervisor, or another therapist. This is a recurring theme in this chapter because it is crucial that we reflect on our practice and gain supervision when struggling in therapy, and therapy challenges are common when working with inflexible belief systems.

Therapy Approaches for Working with Inflexible Beliefs

In cognitive behavioral therapy (CBT) we tend to address the *emotionally charged beliefs* that cause or maintain distress. These take different forms. Some are underlying assumptions that reflect "if ... then" conditional predictions and rules for living ("if I do not check, then the house will burn down" or "if something goes well, then something is soon bound to go wrong" or "if thin is attractive, then fat is gross and intolerable") or they can be core beliefs that are absolute ("I am unlovable" or "the world is a very dangerous place"). Underlying assumptions can often be effectively tested within several weeks using behavioral experiments, while core beliefs can be more difficult to shift as they are unconditional and considered completely "true." For this reason, clinical progress can often be made more quickly if therapist and client work at the underlying assumption level.

Underlying assumptions are linked to core beliefs. Thus, a client who holds the core belief "I'm worthless" most likely also holds related underlying assumptions such as "If I make a mistake, then my efforts are worthless." Behavioral experiments in which people rate the value of imperfect efforts can begin to shift the underlying assumption and indirectly begin to weaken the strength of the related core belief. Thus, it is often advisable to work at the underlying assumption level of belief for an extensive period of time before deciding whether it is necessary to work directly with core beliefs (Padesky, 2020a).

Core beliefs are the most inflexible level of beliefs, and if left unaddressed they sometimes perpetuate problems. Therefore, much of this chapter explores how to work with core beliefs. Since the 1990s, therapists have described strategies for modifying core beliefs. Classic CBT interventions have been adapted and elaborated to be more effective with these absolute and rigidly held beliefs. Succinct descriptions can be found in Beck et al. (2015), Padesky (1994; 2020a), and Young et al. (2006). The most commonly used interventions are summarized in this chapter's Appendix. To be effective, a therapist must also develop a positive alliance and engage the heart and mind of the client holding fixed beliefs while using these strategies. Without the full participation of the client, these strategies are likely to prove fruitless.

The first step toward engagement is to help clients appreciate a rationale for using strategies that might otherwise seem potentially threatening or futile. A good starting point, structured as a Socratic Dialogue, is Padesky's prejudice analogy (Padesky, 1991; 2003). It reveals the nature of core beliefs and how these are maintained over time, provides a rationale for interventions, and instills hope.

Padesky's prejudice metaphor

As illustrated in Padesky's (2003) video demonstration on constructing new core beliefs, a client is asked to name someone she knows who holds a prejudice but one that the client does not share. This sets up a discussion in which the client has more flexible thinking about the topic than the person they are imagining. For example, the client might choose a neighbor who thinks people of a certain ethnicity are "lazy."

Next, Padesky asks the client to describe how their neighbor is likely to interpret a person of that ethnicity who appears lazy (e.g., "Just as I thought!")

or does not appear lazy. In response to the second instance (which contradicts the neighbor's belief) the client can be asked a number of questions to elicit four common schema maintenance processes (Padesky, 1994):

- not noticing contradictory information,
- discounting contradictory information,
- distorting experiences, and
- claiming an observation is an "exception to the rule."

Each of these client predictions of their neighbor's response is written down by the therapist who exhibits great curiosity about these processes the client anticipates from her neighbor.

The following brief dialogue illustrates how this can be done. Notice how the therapist proposes various circumstances in order to elicit the four common schema maintenance processes (highlighted parenthetically).

Therapist: So how do you think your neighbor would react to someone who is a new immigrant and yet they are not lazy?

Client: I think he might say, "Well, that is just one person. They don't fit the mold." (*Exception to the rule*)

Therapist: OK, let's write that down. (Writing.) "They don't fit the mold." It's like he's saying that there are exceptions to every rule but that doesn't mean the rule is not true.

Client: Exactly. That is how he would think.

Therapist: How would you think about this?

Client: I would think, "Everyone is different. You can't make one rule to cover all people—even people of a single immigrant group."

Therapist: Let's capture these two ways of thinking on this paper here. So your neighbor would think . . .

Client: Everyone in this group is the same, even if one person doesn't fit the mold.

Therapist: And you would think . . .

Client: One rule can't cover everyone in a group. People are different.

Therapist: Let's consider another circumstance. Suppose the first immigrant your neighbor saw who appeared to be lazy happens to mention that they are feeling much better now. They were sick the previous week when the neighbor saw them. What might your prejudiced neighbor think?

Client: He might think, "That's just an excuse. I can see that they are lazy." (*Distorting experiences*)

Therapist: And you would think?

Client: This is new information. I would think differently about what I saw.

Therapist: Let's write those two ideas down in our columns labeled, "My neighbor thinks" and "I think." (Prompts client to begin writing.)

Therapist: What if that immigrant who your neighbor thinks is lazy is outside one afternoon doing lots of strenuous yardwork. Do you think your neighbor would pay attention to this and reconsider his beliefs?

Client: No, he might not even pay attention to this. (*Not noticing contradictory information*)

Therapist: Do you think it is kind of easy to ignore information that doesn't fit our beliefs?

Client: Yes, I think it is.

Therapist: Why don't you write that in the neighbor column, "Ignores information that doesn't fit his beliefs." (Pauses while client writes.) And if you pointed out to your neighbor that the immigrant he thought was lazy was working very hard in the yard, what might he say?

Client: He would probably say, "Oh, he's not working so hard. I work harder." (*Discounting contradictory information*)

Therapist: Write that down. (Pauses while client writes.) What might you think when he says that?

Client: You think you are right but different information is right in front of you.

Therapist: That's really interesting. Write that idea down in the "I think" column.

The client is then asked how she would go about changing her neighbor's prejudice. Here the therapist asks questions to prompt consideration of how difficult it is to change a firmly held point of view. Questions can be asked to cue the client to consider the necessity for generating multiple contradictory pieces of evidence, writing these down for the neighbor, and pointing out experiences that do not fit with prejudicial beliefs.

Finally, the client is asked why she thinks the therapist is going into such detail with her about changing her neighbor's prejudicial beliefs. At this point, clients often have an "aha" moment; perhaps their own strongly held negative beliefs, like a prejudice, are maintained by confirmatory experiences as well as contradictory experiences that are discounted, distorted, not noticed, or seen as an exception to the rule. This insight is used by the therapist as a rationale for core belief change methods used in CBT: the importance of noticing many different experiences (especially those which contradict the firmly held beliefs), writing these down, and allowing the therapist to notice and point out relevant information the client may have not noticed. Therapists are wise to set up this plan as an experiment rather than asserting the client's rigidly held beliefs are prejudices. A therapist might say, "We don't know if your belief is true or really a prejudice. Let's look carefully at the information we gather over the next number of weeks to find out. Would you be willing to do that with me?"

Once our clients understand the nature of fixed beliefs and the challenges in countering them, we can continue to use guided discovery methods as we:

- "unpack" and understand key beliefs (both those of the client and therapist);
- collect information to develop a shared formulation;
- provide rationales for interventions; and
- instill hope in the face of relapse and pessimism.

The rest of this chapter demonstrates how to achieve these aims and illustrates common traps to avoid when working with clients with inflexible beliefs. Readers are also referred to the section in Chapter 7 that reviews in depth the principles of relapse management. Clients with inflexible beliefs are particularly vulnerable to lapses and it is crucial that they learn how to manage them effectively.

Keep in Mind

- Tightly held beliefs are understandable once personal meanings are unpacked.
- Rapid change in beliefs only happens at the level of automatic thoughts or underlying assumptions. Core beliefs and other tightly held beliefs can be expected to change slowly.
- Relapse is common. Be prepared for this.
- Therapists also need to attend to their own unhelpful beliefs. Ensure that you have sufficient supervision or consultation with experienced colleagues.

Common Therapy Traps: Inflexible Beliefs

Holding these preceding principles in mind will no doubt help both you and your client. In addition, keep in mind that the work can still be fraught and challenging, particularly as there are some common therapist traps into which we can fall. We will now systematically address each of the five common traps working with inflexible beliefs listed in Box 6.1.

Box 6.1 Common Traps Working with Inflexible Beliefs

Trap 1
Therapist continues therapy without a sound working alliance—often just hoping for the best.

Trap 2
Therapist doesn't grasp the reasons for the client's belief(s) or misses difficult-to- access beliefs, and persists in ineffectual therapy.

Trap 3
Therapist and client go over the same issues, session after session, in repetitive ways.

Trap 4
Therapist becomes hopeless (this can "trap" our clients, too).

Trap 5
Client inflexible beliefs trigger therapist (unhelpful) inflexible beliefs.

Trap 1

Therapist continues therapy without a sound working alliance

The quality of a therapy alliance is not constant. With some clients, it is difficult to establish and maintain a collaborative, working alliance. With other clients, an established therapy alliance is fragile or frequently ruptured. It can be tempting to settle for less than a sound therapeutic relationship and just try to move forward in a given session. However, alliance difficulties can compound if we do this. Alliance difficulties arise for many reasons, including:

- Tensions develop because a client's beliefs are very different from our own. As a result, we fail to "get it," our summaries frustrate our client because they miss the mark, or we even lose curiosity and begin to challenge rather than test their beliefs.
- Our client mistrusts us, which prevents proper engagement and investment in the relationship.
- Client beliefs (often unexpressed) contribute to difficulties maintaining a truly "working" alliance.

These problems can be frustrating, but are not insurmountable.

Client beliefs are very different from therapist beliefs

It is not uncommon that client and therapist beliefs differ but the discrepancy can be particularly marked when clients present with problems that, at least superficially, their therapist can't grasp. For example, some therapists find it difficult to relate to anorexic beliefs, clients who experience profound worthlessness and hopelessness, or obsessive-compulsive disorder (OCD)-related thinking. It can also occur when clients with personality disorder traits exhibit extreme and erratic perspectives and behaviors that violate their therapist's values or tolerance.

Clients are often aware that their therapist holds *very* different beliefs than they do. When this happens, it is easy for them to conclude that you don't understand them. A sense of being misunderstood by someone who is meant to be helpful can certainly strain the relationship. Other times they hold such store by their beliefs that they really do not want to give them up and fear that you will try to make them do so. Clients might be convinced that they are doing something worthwhile in starving, exercising, obsessively checking, or even killing themselves and they fear that you will try to stop them. If you pose a threat to what they believe is their "best path" they are not going to be motivated to work *with* you.

It is understandable that clients might lack confidence in our ability to be empathic and appreciate how their inner world works. As we have already suggested, you might actually find yourself struggling to grasp what drives them from time to time. When this happens, it is very important that you explore, with genuine curiosity, why certain client beliefs and behaviors are so compelling. Keep asking yourself: "Just why do these beliefs/behaviors make sense to this person?" Stay curious and you'll get there. Preface questions with goodwill. For example, "I know you must have good reasons for XYZ, can you help me understand what those are?"

Therapy texts always say that therapists should adopt a nonjudgmental stance. It really is crucial to do so as clients can feel embarrassed about, or even shameful of, their beliefs and behaviors. You need to create the right milieu for them to feel confident in sharing information with you.

The therapist's challenge here is twofold:

1. to communicate that you do understand their fears and goals even though you might not share them, and
2. to help them see that it is worthwhile to take a chance on engaging in the therapy with you.

Let's see how the following therapist works to meet these two challenges simultaneously. She is working with Alan, a 45-year-old man who had difficulty controlling anger outbursts:

Therapist: (Looking at Alan's written notes from the previous week.) Here you write that you got angry and verbally assaulted a man—yet you rated it a very good evening. I'm not sure that I understand. Could you run through that episode last night?

Alan: Yeah, but I don't really expect you to get it—to understand why I need my anger, why I like it. I was having a drink with mates. Relaxing a bit, you know? We were having a laugh and I felt quite good. This bloke in a suit—don't know what he was doing in our part of the city—pushed his way past me to the bar. I saw red and laid into him.

Therapist: You saw red? Can you say a bit more about what that was like?

Alan: It's just "whoosh" and I'm furious and I just want to let someone have it.

Therapist: Can you say more about the feelings you have—the "whoosh"?

Alan: I feel electric, charged, ready for anything: I feel like a lion.

Therapist: So this is a good feeling? (Alan nods.) And what's going through your mind at that point?

Alan: I want respect and I want people to see that no one gets one over on me.

Therapist: I can understand that. So what happened next—when you "laid into him"?

Alan: I shouted at him—told him never to touch me. Never. I said he'd better say sorry or he'd be sorry.

Therapist:	What did you mean?
Alan:	I don't know really—it just felt like the right thing to say and it really scared him. I would have punched him if he'd pushed me to it but he apologized and left soon after.
Therapist:	And how were things with you then?
Alan:	Great—I felt that I'd made my point and people would realize that you don't mess with Alan.
Therapist:	What so good about that?
Alan:	I feel safe. I spent my childhood feeling scared of everyone and I can feel safe because people are scared of me.
Therapist:	So being angry seems to feel like a good thing for you—the sensation makes you feel powerful and it achieves two really good goals—feeling safe and feeling respected. (Alan nods.) I can see why it's such an important and powerful reaction for you. (Pause.) Is there ever any down side?
Alan:	Sometimes I feel that people don't respect me, they are just scared of me—but that's OK 'cos I still feel safe.
Therapist:	Anything else?
Alan:	I do get into trouble from time to time: the police have pulled me in, I've been banned from a couple of places and it's ended some relationships pretty quickly. I'm here because the police pulled me in.
Therapist:	What happens when you are pulled in by the police?
Alan:	It's a pain—it's a waste of time, I get a bad reputation at work and it's expensive: the fines I've paid! And actually I find it embarrassing. My girlfriend gives me grief as she has to come and collect me and she resents the cost.
Therapist:	So if you do get in trouble with the police—how do you end up feeling?
Alan:	Not good—I get angry with myself and I feel ashamed that I've let down my boss and my girlfriend—then I feel insecure.
Therapist:	And how do you feel about being banned from places?
Alan:	Initially I don't care but later I get annoyed with myself and embarrassed when I have to tell friends that I'm not allowed into certain places.
Therapist:	What about the relationships that end because of your angry outbursts—how does that leave you feeling?
Alan:	That's a really big problem. I feel weak rather than strong. Sometimes I get even angrier and that gives me an even worse

reputation as a worker and as a boyfriend. Word gets around. I often end up feeling really worthless because I've brought this on myself.

Therapist: Let me see if I've understood this: there are times when being angry seems great—you feel safe, powerful, and respected; then there are times when the consequences of your anger outbursts bring you a lot of grief and you end up feeling worthless and insecure. Quite a dilemma.

Alan: Yes it is. I don't know what to do really. There's no way I want to feel or be seen as weak but I don't want the downside of my anger. Having said that—It feels so good, I don't know if I want to give that up either.

Therapist: So you want to feel safe, respected, and you want that great feeling from time to time?

Alan: Yes—that's about it.

Therapist: These are all good goals. Would you be willing to see if we could we try to think of ways of achieving them that don't have such a big downside? Then you could feel safe and respected and occasionally get that high feeling, but in ways that are not so disruptive to your life?

In the Therapist's Mind

In this dialogue, the therapist creates a safe environment for Alan to tell her about his anger by simply being curious and non-confrontive. She doesn't focus on his saying that he's prepared to punch a man, for example, although this has not escaped her notice and she will be paying attention to the risk that Alan poses to others. Through curious questions, she first encourages him to explain why anger is something he feels good about. Only when she understands the attraction of anger (and he has expressed that) does she raise the possibility of there being a downside to it. She decides to help him express the dilemma posed by his anger. At this stage in therapy she feels it is important that they both appreciate this conflict as this might give him the motivation to work with her and give her the compassion to understand what drives his angry behavior. Finally she offers hope in suggesting that they work together to achieve his goals in a more adaptive way.

Client mistrusts the therapist

Some clients with inflexible beliefs will struggle to engage with you at all. Memories of being hurt, betrayed, and rejected may be revived in the therapeutic relationship. These will activate fixed beliefs about the dangers of trusting and they will try to protect themselves by overtly or covertly failing to engage with you.

Your challenge as a therapist in this instance is to demonstrate that it is safe to trust you as a therapist while being realistic about what you can offer. In the following dialogue, Caroline, a 35-year-old single woman experiencing post-traumatic stress disorder (PTSD), expresses a variety of concerns about how safe and trustworthy therapy and this therapist will be.

Therapist:	It can be helpful if we set the scene for our sessions so that you feel as comfortable as possible in them.
Caroline:	You mean that I won't have to feel bad?
Therapist:	Well, there will be times when we need to explore things that could be distressing but we can think how to do this so you feel as strong and as in control as possible.
Caroline:	How are you going to do that, then?
Therapist:	Not "me" so much as "us." I need your help in appreciating what will be helpful for you at times when you are feeling upset or scared. How does that sound to you?
Caroline:	Sensible I suppose.
Therapist:	Given what you are expecting in these sessions, could I ask what worries you most?
Caroline:	I don't want to get flashbacks: I can't cope with them. That's what scares me most.
Therapist:	Well that's understandable—so in the early sessions we could focus on helping you develop some flashback management strategies so that you might be able to manage them, making them less overwhelming. What do you think?
Caroline:	Sounds good in theory—I can't imagine being able to do it though.
Therapist:	Is there anything that you already do that helps you cope with them?
Caroline:	Well I have a drink and that can take the edge off things. I don't go to certain places or watch certain TV programs in case they trigger them. If I think that I'm going to have one I try to keep myself busy.
Therapist:	It sounds as if you are already doing things we can build on. Very importantly, you have learnt to recognize when you are vulnerable.

	We can now work on developing more ways of taking the edge off the flashbacks and ways of distracting yourself from them. If we did that, how do you think you would feel about the sessions?
Caroline:	Safer, I suppose.
Therapist:	Can you think of anything else that would help you feel safer?
Caroline:	Knowing that what I say here is confidential—I need to know what happens to the notes you make and I need to know who you'll be talking to.
Therapist	Everything you say here is confidential—your written notes stay here in my filing cabinet and it is locked when I'm not in the room. Any other notes stored on the computer are only accessible using my password. As I told you in our first appointment, there are some legal limits to that confidentiality. Do you remember what we discussed then?
Caroline:	Not really.
Therapist:	Let's go through them again. For example, if I learn that you are a threat to yourself or other people ... (Therapist reviews various legal limits to confidentiality.) In addition, my secretary sees correspondence concerning you, but she is bound by confidentiality laws and the only person I would discuss your progress with is my supervisor—who does not know your real name. It is a professional requirement for me to have a supervisor as it protects you from getting substandard treatment, and I find it helpful to get advice and ideas from an experienced practitioner. How do you feel about my talking with my supervisor?
Caroline:	I hadn't thought about it before but I feel glad that you get some advice. But what if I want to kill myself?
Therapist:	That is what I mean by a "threat to yourself." What is your understanding of my professional duty if you become suicidal?
Caroline:	You have to let people know—my family doctor, a psychiatrist. You can get me put away. You might as well know that I just won't tell you.
Therapist:	You are quite right that there are other professionals who would need to be informed and I would have to do that if I believed that your life was at risk. I can understand that you would be reluctant to put yourself in that position. However, I want you to know that I would not take the decision to break confidentiality lightly and would do my very best to first discuss it with you and I would continue to be your therapist and support you through the consequences.

Caroline: Big deal your help would be if they lock me up in a hospital.

Therapist: The hospital is not my first choice either. I would hope that we could talk to see if we could address your feelings in the session. If we could, we might be able to organize more support, and we might be able to ease the suicidal feelings enough so that it was not necessary for the information to leave the room. No one else would be involved in that case. But that would rest on you being able to tell me how you felt. Hearing this, what do you think?

Caroline: I can see your point—I hadn't thought of it like that before—that there might be something in it for me if I told you how suicidal I felt.

Therapist: Is there anything that I could do to make you feel more able to tell me?

Caroline: Being open like this helps me feel that you have my interests at heart and that you are not hiding anything—I have to know that you are not hiding anything.

Therapist: How can I help you feel confident about that?

Caroline: I'd like to see the notes you write.

Therapist: I can photocopy them for you—we can also audio-record the sessions so that you can review the meetings and come back with anything about my practice that seems unclear or worries you.

Caroline: OK—I didn't know that was possible. I thought therapy was more "cloak and dagger" than this. (Smiles.)

Therapist: Anything else that might help you feel more at ease?

Caroline: Can't think of anything right now.

Therapist: OK, so why don't I pose a couple of questions—how do you want me to respond if you get distressed in sessions or if you have a flashback in the session? Different people have different preferences.

Caroline: Good questions. If I start to cry then I'd just as soon you don't make a big issue of it. Don't ignore it but just pass me some tissues and never, never try to hug me.

Therapist: I wouldn't normally touch clients at all. Would that be an acceptable ground rule—no touching?

Caroline: Certainly would—and if I have a flashback could you try to get me out of it as soon as possible—I'm not sure how but I'd want you to help me end it.

Therapist: That's something we'd already planned to work on, so yes. Now is there anything else?

Caroline: This might sound silly but could I sit over there? I just feel better with my back against a wall.

Therapist: That's easily done. Why don't you move there right now? (Client moves.) Anything else?

Caroline: No, I think that's it.

Therapist: Good, but how about we keep things under review in case something else comes up? Our "ground rules" aren't set in stone.

Caroline: I like that; it helps me feel safer.

Therapist: Excellent. So, in summary: I'll be as open as I can and you can see my therapy notes and review recordings of our sessions if you like. You will sit over there as you feel more comfortable with that. If you get upset in sessions, I'll acknowledge it but I won't make a big thing of it; if you have a flashback I'll try to help you come out of it and we'll work on strategies aimed to do just that; if you are feeling suicidal, you will let me know so that we can talk and try to ease those feelings first in here, just the two of us. And if you are at risk of killing yourself I will let your doctor and the psychiatrist know. I will discuss this with you and offer continued support. And you can be confident that I won't touch you. How does that sound?

In the Therapist's Mind

In this dialogue, Caroline's therapist begins by taking the lead in stating that he wants to establish as comfortable an alliance as possible. Here (and elsewhere in the session) he knows he could have been more Socratic and first encouraged Caroline to realize the advantages of doing this—but with a wary and ambivalent client it is often easier to be more Socratic after an alliance is developed. Mistrustful clients can interpret Socratic questioning in early sessions as the therapist trying to "trick" or influence them. He is hoping direct information sharing will build trust more quickly. Later, Caroline stated that she wanted her therapist to be open. This confirmed his hypothesis that overusing the Socratic approach could have resulted in her feeling that he was being opaque. Sometimes it is better to "put your cards on the table" and give information. In this instance, he hoped information-giving offered her immediate assurance of his concern and openness.

Even when you opt for information-giving you can begin to introduce a Socratic style by asking, "What do you make of that?" or "How does that fit with your experiences?" and so on, just as this therapist does. Doing so will prompt reflection and consideration of the implications of the information. As therapists, we always need to ask ourselves—"What do I want to achieve here?" and "Is using Socratic Dialogue the best way of doing this?" The use of Socratic Dialogue was appropriate in clarifying just what Caroline feared in therapy and it would have been remiss to have assumed her fears.

The therapist also used Socratic Dialogue in drawing out her coping strategies and helping her realize that she had strengths they could build on—that he was not going to take away her ways of dealing with her fears but rather improve them. Thus, even though she mentioned some suboptimal methods of coping with her flashbacks (taking a drink and avoidance), her therapist credits her with doing her best to cope. The aim of this was to help her feel safer in therapy and to instill hope. The therapist also used direct questions, such as "How do you want me to respond if you get distressed in sessions ... ?", as he did not want certain issues to be overlooked because they had not been raised by Caroline.

An important and simple Socratic question that was used to good effect here was the " ... and is there anything else?" question. This maximizes the chances of uncovering Caroline's major fears and identifying her range of coping strategies.

Client beliefs interfere with the alliance

Many beliefs can interfere with establishing and maintaining a good therapy alliance. For example, some clients will feel compelled to develop a dependent relationship rather than a collaborative one. They will have "good reasons" for doing this: it can be fueled by inflexible beliefs such as "incompetency" core beliefs, or powerful beliefs and fears about being weak or stupid, or convictions that you, the therapist, are omniscient. Other clients might form a superficial relationship and do or say whatever they believe will please us rather than genuinely participate in therapy because they fear criticism and rejection. Clients can sometimes have a strong sense of entitlement and believe that their needs should be met by others, so they may sit back in therapy, thinking the therapist should always be there for them and do all the work.

When inflexible client beliefs interfere with the therapy alliance, you need to unpack the idiosyncratic meanings of these beliefs and help the client find good reasons to collaborate with you.

Here, the therapist's challenge is to communicate realistic parameters of working together and your own limitations without dashing hope that you can help. You want to form a constructive working alliance in which the client collaborates with you. Siobhan is a 43-year-old, single woman experiencing major depression and reporting a family history of gross parental neglect. Observe how her therapist works with her to achieve some level of collaboration:

Therapist: Let's think about our agenda for this session. Let's make a list of . . . .

Siobhan: (Jumping in before the therapist has finished her sentence.) Well it's all been bad really, a terrible week. I feel worse than ever—I've been so looking forward to seeing you. I find it such a long time to wait between sessions. I thought today would never arrive. Christopher was ever so rude to me at work and nobody there actually cares about my feelings, so no one stood up for me and I just sat on my own at lunch time and felt like crying. I just feel so unimportant, so alone, not worth bothering about. But, you know me, I just got on with my job in the afternoon—soldiered on. Typical Siobhan. But I'm crying on the inside. My boss, Bethany, says that I am the most reliable of her staff. She says she can rely on me to put the job first and not to think about myself. I suppose that's what I've always done—put myself last. But it's never really done me any good—there's never really been any thanks for this, I'm just exploited. Good old Siobhan, you can rely on her, you can put on her, you can be really rude to her.

Therapist: Could we just pause there? It does sound as though the week was difficult and some upsetting things happened for you that we may want to talk about. I am wondering just what we need to put on the agenda to make sure we address the issues you feel are most important? We can begin with the review of the assignment from last session—you were going to try to keep a log of your activities and note how pleasurable and how difficult each was—then what else do we need on the agenda?

Siobhan: Erm, the issue—you always ask me this. I'm not sure, I suppose I want to talk it through—why people are so horrid to me and I want to feel better.

Therapist: There's a good goal—wanting to feel better. "Talking it through" might be a good way to achieve that or perhaps there are other ways of getting there.

Siobhan: I always feel better when I talk with you, so I think that's what I need to do.

Therapist: Now that's interesting because you said that you were feeling worse than ever this week. Does that mean that the feeling better after the session wears off?

Siobhan; Yes—that's why I'm so worried about them coming to an end—how many more sessions have we left?

Therapist: This is our third session, so there are twelve left.

Siobhan: Don't say that—that scares me. Only twelve. What am I going to do when I can't see you anymore?

Therapist: It sounds as though we have an important item for the agenda: something around how you might best use the remaining twelve sessions. So you can make good use of what you've learnt even when you aren't coming here anymore. What do you think?

In the Therapist's Mind

Her therapist decides to consciously avoid unpacking Siobhan's emotions, and even her thoughts, at this point. In previous sessions they identified her "poor me— competent other" and her "poor me—cruel other" core beliefs. Her therapist knows that focusing on core beliefs in brief depression treatment can actually lead to worsening depression (Hawley et al., 2017). Focusing in more detail on her experiences right now could be reassuring for Siobhan, but it does seem that this is not helpful in the longer term. Indeed, in-depth enquiry can become part of an unproductive reassurance-giving cycle with some people who tend towards dependency.

With all this in mind, her therapist instead acknowledges her distress and reflects that this might be an important item for the agenda and, at the same time, she maintains the structure of the session, creating an opportunity to collaborate within the framework of CBT. This is particularly important for Siobhan as she has difficulty in organizing her thinking and initiating problem solving. The therapist is modeling the rudimentary skills of problem solving by refining key issues.

You see Siobhan's therapist asking direct, if not leading questions—"Does this mean that feeling better after the session wears off?" and "It sounds as though we have an important item for the agenda: something around how you might best use the remaining twelve sessions." Although these are not Socratic questions, they invite Siobhan's collaboration for getting the session back on track. There is the danger that Siobhan will simply be agreeable to the therapist's suggestions, but this will soon be apparent as they explore these issues, and it is at least socializing Siobhan into a more focused way of working.

The therapist is conscientious in not engaging in reassurance and, despite Siobhan's worries, she keeps the end date clearly in view. This is particularly important with clients who have a tendency toward dependency as it is this endpoint that raises their most pertinent issue—fears around coping independently. However, the therapist continues to offer hope—suggesting that they work together to achieve good goals and to maximize the benefit of the CBT sessions.

Her therapist's plan, given what she already understands of Siobhan's inner world is to:

1. Review her Weekly Activity Schedule (WAS) homework (Greenberger & Padesky, 2016) and compare any positive ratings on this with Siobhan's negative feelings at beginning of session. Her hypothesis is that, in the longer term, the WAS will have been more effective in lifting Siobhan's mood than simply talking about her problems. The therapist may be wrong, but this is an opportunity to re-engage in Socratic exploration.

2. Explore Siobhan's inflexible beliefs with a view to helping her review them as possible "prejudices." However, if the therapist and Siobhan only talk about evidence of whether she needs help from others, her inflexible beliefs may be hard to budge. Concrete experiences in which Siobhan experiments with self-sufficiency are more likely to have an impact and be memorable for her once therapy ends. Therefore, Siobhan's therapist will help her test out these beliefs experientially by offering her opportunities to carry out experiments related to self-sufficiency in and outside the therapy session. This may take time and will only be productive if the therapist has successfully engaged Siobhan in CBT—hence the need to emphasize engagement and time frames for therapy at the outset.

Keep in Mind

- Use conceptualization to make sense of your client's difficulties. Devise conceptualizations collaboratively with clients to promote mutual understanding and also so you can predict barriers and setbacks (cf. Kuyken et al., 2009; Padesky, 2020b).

- Psycho-education and instilling hope are crucial. Padesky's (1991; 2003) prejudice metaphor is an effective way of helping clients understand how inflexible beliefs are maintained and the processes that can be employed to test them out.

- Pay attention to process issues. Client's inflexible beliefs will often have an impact on therapy processes. Use these opportunities to highlight beliefs and set up in-session experiments to test out their predictions.

Trap 2

Therapist doesn't grasp the reasons for client belief(s) or misses difficult-to-access beliefs and persists in ineffectual therapy

---

Not all exploration of automatic thoughts and beliefs goes smoothly. All therapists struggle at times to identify key cognitions. This perhaps happens more frequently with clients with longstanding, fixed, and distressing beliefs. Two particular challenges to understanding a client's inner world arise (1) when meanings are not formulated in words (or even pictures) and (2) when the client is highly avoidant of cognitive and emotional exploration because they fear they will become overwhelmed by emotions or traumatic memories.

When beliefs are not formulated as words or even pictures

On occasion clients report, "I just *feel* bad—I can't put it into words, there are no words or images in my mind." You might wonder how a therapist can proceed in that situation. First of all, we can keep in mind that meanings are constructed at different times in our development and some meanings developed at very young ages do not readily map onto language—they are held more like a "felt sense." This can also happen with beliefs that are so well established and entrenched that they have been transformed from something accessible to something more like an emotional "knee jerk reaction" and it can take time for your client to be able to figure out the cognitive content of a reaction.

The challenge here for therapists is twofold: (1) creating a means of exploring meanings that do not map onto language, and (2) enabling clients to explore cognitions linked with what seem like automatic emotional reactions. Ella is a 24-year-old student who struggles to control her weight. In the following dialogue, her therapist uses some of the imagery identification strategies described in Chapter 5 to help Ella identify memories and images that might help them both understand what evokes her "felt sense" desire to binge:

Therapist: You recorded all your episodes of binge-eating really well, but I notice you've not put anything in the thoughts and images column.

Ella: That's because I don't have any.

Therapist: That's interesting, that sometimes happens. Could we look at this most recent entry again, the one from last night, to see if we can find any explanations for that binge?

Ella: Yes, sure.

Therapist: Can you tell me a little bit more about what was happening around that time?

Ella: I had a pretty routine day of boring studies—stuff that I've got to get through for my exams. I had not eaten much during the day and was pleased about that. By seven o'clock I was really tired of studying and I simply felt "bingey." It was if I had to find something to eat—I just had to. I found myself in the kitchen looking through cupboards without having really thought about it.

Therapist: Can you say a little more about that feeling—"bingey"?

Ella: It's a feeling—perhaps an emotion—but I'm not sure it's even that—I'm just not sure.

Therapist: Maybe it is, maybe not—but can you recall how it felt physically? How it felt in your body? Where was it? Did it have a shape, a color, a temperature?

Ella: I feel physically agitated—sort of. There's a crawling sensation beneath my skin ... and there's a feeling in the pit of my stomach—it's hollow and silver and like jelly. That's funny I feel kind of tearful describing this: it isn't a nice feeling. When I think about it now I realize that I want to get rid of it and that I eat to stop the feeling.

Therapist: Would it be okay if I asked you to stay with that feeling so we could explore it a bit more?

Ella: Okay.

Therapist: See if you can close your eyes and get in touch with that hollow, silver, jelly-like feeling in the pit of your stomach. Have you captured it again?

Ella: Yes.

Therapist: Okay, can you tell me more about it? Anything that comes to mind.

Ella: I feel quite shaky and tearful. The hollow feeling gets stronger the more I focus on it. That's the worst part of it. I feel vulnerable, isolated—I feel unloved and unwanted, isn't that strange?

Therapist: How far back do these feelings go? Is there a time when you didn't have them?

Ella: I think that I've always had them and I've eaten or drunk to switch them off. That's probably why I was quite overweight as a child. My parents made it clear that I was a disappointment to them—I never felt wanted, I often felt criticized, and I had these feelings then.

Therapist: It sounds as though it is possible that you have felt unloved and unwanted since you were very small and that the hollow feeling is how you experienced it as a little child and that bodily sensation has stayed with you. You also said that it is a horrible feeling and so you try to manage it by comforting yourself with food or alcohol. What do you think about that?

Ella: That's probably right—but it's such a new idea that I'll need to think about it.

Therapist: Of course it's just an idea, a possibility. However, we could look at ways of replacing that hollow feeling with one which does not compel you to overeat or drink. What do you think about trying that?

Ella: Sounds like a good idea—what do I do?

In the Therapist's Mind

Ella's therapist seeks permission to explore her experiences, thus respecting their working alliance. Holding the hypothesis that Ella has a visceral reaction leading to binge-eating, the therapist asks her to recall the memory of a recent incident. Using informational questions, she begins to "unpack" the bodily sensations associated with the urge to overeat. She asks direct and evocative informational questions such as "Did it have a shape, a color, a temperature?" not to elicit a yes or no answer, but to encourage Ella to consider novel possibilities.

She asks about the origin of the sensations in order to get a better understanding of what is behind them—and offers a capsule summary to check out her understanding of Ella's experience and to help Ella better appreciate that there is a pattern here and it makes sense.

The pacing is gentle as Ella is reviewing "new territory" and will need time to assimilate this different perspective. Nonetheless, the therapist provides hope that they can begin the process of learning how to manage unhelpful sensations rather than staying with the distress for too long.

Client avoids therapy explorations because of fears of overwhelming emotion or traumatic memories

Some people experience intense emotions or flashbacks or nightmares when asked to reflect on their inner worlds. It is important to be sensitive to this and, at the same time, not err in the opposite direction by avoiding exploration of troubled thoughts. In these instances therapists can employ specific strategies to ground and stabilize clients while using Socratic Dialogue.

How can we create a sense of safety and be sensitive to clients' limitations while still exploring relevant cognitions and emotions? Jaochim is a 51-year-old man who is fearful of exploring his thoughts and feelings. His therapist discusses this with him to collaboratively find a way forward:

Therapist: Last session you said that you were nervous about trying to keep a diary that captured your feelings and thoughts—and from your feedback now, it looks as though it wasn't possible for you after all. That's okay—there are other ways for us to work together. I'm wondering though if we need to do some work on helping you feel more comfortable about exploring your feelings. What do you think?

Joachim: How do you mean? I can't imagine feeling comfortable.

Therapist: Maybe not, but perhaps we can make it less uncomfortable, a bit easier. Is there anything you found that made you feel a bit more comfortable when we met last time?

Joachim: The fact that you seemed to listen to me without passing judgment.

Therapist: That's helpful to know. Was there anything else?

Joachim: Maybe you telling me that I could ask you to stop and I could take a break at any time—I think that helped me open up more.

Therapist: Open up in what way?

Joachim: Well to say more about what I'd been through.

Therapist: Was there anything that helped you to open up more about your feelings and thoughts?

Joachim: Well I think that I did open up about that more than I ever have done because you weren't judging me and you gave me permission to stop things.

Therapist: Ok so how about we build on that? I'll try to continue to help you feel free from being judged here and you can always ask that we stop if that is what you need. Now, is there anything else that might help?

Joachim: I can't think of anything—I can always tell you if I think of something later.

Therapist: Please do—I would welcome regular feedback from you. Now can I ask what might sound like a strange question—if you were to get distressed, how would I know? I ask because, in my experience, everyone is a bit different in the way they show they feel upset.

Joachim: I get upset on the inside but I won't let you see that. I'll probably go quiet and after a while I'll start to get angry.

Therapist: If I notice you getting quiet, what's the best way for me to react so that you feel you can tell me what's going on for you?

Joachim:	Good question. I don't want you to ignore it—I'd rather you say straight out that you've noticed a change in me. If you say something about it early on I probably won't get angry because I won't feel that my feelings are being ignored. But the idea of talking about emotions still fills me with dread.
Therapist:	Why do you think that is?
Joachim:	No idea. (Joachim goes quiet and the therapist sits with this for a while and considers how to use the opportunity to respect what Joachim has just said.)

In the Therapist's Mind

His therapist thought it would be helpful for both of them if Joachim could explain his reluctance to explore his feelings. His terse response to her last question and the subsequent silence made her realize that she has probably overestimated his readiness to do so. She has mistaken his collaboration in looking at ways of making therapy feel safe for a willingness to explore thoughts and emotions.

His silence presents an opportunity to do what they had just agreed. So she acknowledges this and immediately offers him a way to deal with his difficulty. She hopes this will give Joachim the message that he can expect to get relief from his distress. Later in therapy, when he learns to tolerate distress better, she will encourage him to stay with his feelings at times like this.

Therapist:	Joachim, I'm wondering if you are quiet now because our discussion has triggered some difficult emotions. And, if so, what we can do to make things easier for you. I'll be guided by you, but I've some suggestions if you'd like to hear them.
Joachim:	No. I mean yes. I mean I have some bad feelings but I don't want to talk about it and I don't want you to do anything. Can we just go back to what we were talking about before?
Therapist:	OK, certainly. Let's make a written summary then so we both remember what we agreed. (Writing as she speaks.) In order for you to feel as comfortable as possible I'll try to listen carefully to you and be nonjudgmental. If I notice you becoming quiet I'll comment on it but I won't assume that you are ready to talk about your feelings as this is still difficult for you. How does that sound?

Joachim: About right. (Still rather reserved.)

Therapist: And when we just did this—acknowledged the silence and the possible distress underneath it—how was that?

Joachim: It worked actually. I could feel myself being pulled down by feelings and then your question and the comment about coping sort of broke the spell.

Therapist: And what does that tell you?

Joachim: You won't make me dwell on bad feelings and you might actually help me put a lid on them. So therapy might be bearable after all.

Therapist: Let's hope so! Now, has anything else come to mind that might be helpful that we should add to our summary? (Long pause.) For example, if you were to get angry or obviously distressed—how should we manage that?

Joachim: You should know that I wouldn't hurt you—I've never hurt anyone but myself—but I might walk out and I think you should let me be if that happens.

Therapist: OK—but what about coming back into the session—anything I could do that would make that easier for you?

Joachim: Well, you just saying that makes me feel as though I could come back in again.

Therapist: What should we write down here to help you remember that?

In the Therapist's Mind

His therapist immediately drew on Joachim's own experience, asking what had helped him in the previous session (and asking him to reflect on his experience within this session). This ensured that he had no difficulty in accessing relevant information and so he was able to engage in the dialogue. In turn, this offered an opportunity for the development of collaboration and shared responsibility.

The therapist kept her questions very transparent (for example giving a rationale for questions, "I ask because … "). This signaled to Joachim that her intentions were straightforward. She initially persevered with questions concerning his comfort to reinforce his sense of safety with her. It was wise of her to ask Joachim what "upset" looks like because people who fear emotions often camouflage their distress. It was good practice to ask how she should respond if he did get upset as this got them back on track and helped them develop a useful plan. This then put Joachim at ease.

It might seem that the therapist was laboring a point in focusing so heavily on creating a sense of safety but this is often necessary with fearful clients and it also introduces Socratic Dialogue processes in a non-threatening way. Later, when they had established a working relationship in which Joachim felt safe, he was able to answer his therapist's question concerning his fear of affect. He reported that "I could lose it—get overwhelmed—start crying. It feels as though a dam might break and I would cry myself crazy." These predictions paved the way for teaching affect management skills followed by behavioral experiments to help Joachim test his fearful images and build his confidence that he could tolerate both affect and crying.

Keep in Mind

- Meanings can be stored as words, pictures, or bodily sensations.
- It is important to form a sound therapeutic relationship and aim to make therapy feel "safe" by anticipating threatening obstacles and collaborating on making a plan to manage them.
- Stay curious. Don't jump to conclusions because of your expectations.

Trap 3

Therapist and client go over the same issues, session after session, in repetitive ways

---

Inflexible beliefs can take a long time to shift. A therapist and client can get into a rut and just keep saying the same things back and forth over and over again. It is our challenge as therapists to keep therapy fresh even when working with the same beliefs over a lengthy period of time. These three guidelines can help therapy stay fresh when working with inflexible beliefs:

1. Be patient and also stay active;
2. Use humor and a language the client can embrace; and
3. Develop imagery and case conceptualizations that bring ideas to life.

These recommendations are each illustrated in the following sections.

Be patient and also stay active

Inflexible beliefs are usually either underlying assumptions or core beliefs and so we can expect them to change more slowly than automatic thoughts. Therapists often feel better when they accept that some beliefs change slowly. However, sometimes when therapists expect slow change, they become passive or resign themselves to saying the same thing 100 times. Clients need to be actively engaged in examining inflexible beliefs. Therefore, therapists need to use active therapy methods and regularly vary these to maintain client curiosity.

Behavioral experiments are ideal for these purposes. To maximize learning from behavioral experiments, generate an alternative belief first so results of experiments can compare whether the client's inflexible belief or the alternative belief fit the data best. For example, instead of relying heavily on Socratic Dialogue in session to repeatedly look for evidence that supports and doesn't support an inflexible belief, use role-plays to help the client try on different perspectives.

Martine is a chef and believes "if something isn't perfect, it's worthless." She can be asked to role-play situations in which a dinner is flawed in some way that leads to a diner complaint. In a first role-play, the therapist can be the unhappy diner and Martine can experience and discuss her emotional and cognitive responses to the named imperfections in the food. Next, Martine can role-play a disgruntled diner. The therapist can role-play the chef in two ways—first, apologetic and convinced the meal is "worthless," and, second, accepting criticisms, asking for clarification, and assertively expressing appreciation for the diner's feedback. After these two role-plays, the client can be asked about the value of the experience for the customer and chef, depending upon the two different types of "chef" responses to imperfection. Learning from these and subsequent role-plays could help generate an alternative belief such as, "Even imperfect results can have value; at very least something can be learned from them."

To set up experiments outside of session, Martine and her therapist could create a written survey to give to real diners. This survey could ask them to rate that evening's food on a scale of perfection and another scale of its worth or value to the diner. Diners can be invited to make suggestions for improvement if the food was disappointing in some way. Martine's perfectionistic belief predicts that any diner who rates a meal less than perfect will also rate it as worthless. The alternative belief predicts diners will value even imperfect food and also that Martine can learn valuable things from the survey when the results are not rated as perfect.

As another experiment, Martine could interview friends and family about their most valuable experiences, accomplishments, or whatever category of experience links most closely to her perfectionistic standards. Once highest worth activities are identified, Martine could ask a series of questions (developed with the therapist) as a test of her inflexible perfectionism belief such as "Was this done perfectly? How perfectly on a 0–10 scale?", "How would you rate its worth to you on a 0–10 scale?", and "What made it worthwhile to you, if it wasn't perfect?"

Use humor and a language the client can embrace

Inflexible beliefs are usually held with great seriousness by clients. Early in their discussion, therapists demonstrate compassionate empathy regarding the origins of these beliefs and their impact on clients' lives. Once this has been done, the therapist can subtly shift the emphasis to compassionate empathy toward the client as someone who is trapped by this belief. This can be expressed in different ways with different clients, depending upon the metaphors and language that fits with the client's speaking style. Here are some sample therapist statements:

- There's that worthlessness belief again. I'm so sorry that every time you have a chance to make forward progress, that belief pops up and stops you in your tracks. It seems so unfair.
- Your belief that "people can't be trusted" surfaces every time we begin to talk more easily with each other. I think this belief wants to protect you from disappointment in case I let you down. It's trying to help you but also spoils your chance to feel good here.

Once your client is able to join you in seeing themselves as trapped by their inflexible beliefs, it is possible to invite the client to employ humor and more playful language to characterize these beliefs. Notice the emphasis on inviting the client to employ humor. Therapists should be cautious expressing their own humor about deeply held beliefs because this can fall flat and be experienced as insensitive by the client. The advantage of inviting a client to frame their inflexible beliefs in a humorous way is that seeing humor in a situation both requires and elicits thinking flexibility. The following dialogue illustrates this process with Jamal, a 22-year-old man plagued by self-critical thoughts:

Therapist: I imagine this little person on your shoulder, whispering in your ear this negative idea over and over again. Is that how you experience it?

Jamal: No, it's more like a finger-waving scold.

Therapist: I imagine that's rough to handle. Can you think of some way to make your belief lighter or more cartoon-like so it won't bother you so much?

Jamal: What do you mean?

Therapist: Well, sometimes in animated movies a scolding or scary character can actually be drawn in ways that look funny and therefore that character is less intimidating.

Jamal: Oh, you mean like the monsters in *Monsters, Inc.?*

Therapist: (Laughing.) Exactly. That's a perfect idea. Those monsters were acting scary to keep their jobs but they really weren't dangerous. Could you make your belief like that?

Jamal: I suppose so.

Therapist: What would your monster belief look like?

In this interchange, his therapist invites Jamal to develop a characterization for his belief that changes its emotional impact from intimidating to benign. Once this has been accomplished, Jamal's humorous image can be referenced whenever his belief is activated. Over time, this humorous characterization can help sap Jamal's conviction that his unhelpful belief is true.

Develop imagery and case conceptualizations that bring ideas to life

As demonstrated with Jamal in the previous dialogue, imagery can be employed to bring beliefs to life. Jamal is likely to be more engaged in thinking about and evaluating his belief when it becomes an animated monster of his own design rather than simply words that sting. Similarly, case conceptualizations can be collaboratively drawn to keep clients engaged in actively examining their inflexible beliefs. Initial conceptualizations can be descriptive and these can evolve over time to describe triggers and maintenance factors, or to capture the developmental history of inflexible beliefs (Kuyken et al., 2009; Padesky, 2020b). The key is to develop conceptualizations collaboratively with clients in ways that increase their awareness of and curiosity about inflexible beliefs.

The best conceptualizations of inflexible beliefs capture the flow of client experience. For example, one client found it interesting that she could hold onto good experiences for a while but eventually her inflexible belief, "No one can be trusted," spoiled all her relationships. She ended up drawing a conceptualization that looked like a bucket, "It's like I have a leaky bucket. When relationships begin, the bucket fills with water. Over time, the good experiences gradually leak away and when the bucket is empty I don't believe there was ever any real water there." This conceptualization and image of the impact of her negative core beliefs about trusting others led her to begin to consider how she could plug the holes in her bucket of experiences. This conceptualization and image captivated her and led to a number of useful interventions that she pursued with interest and curiosity.

Keep in Mind

- Aim to keep the work fresh even when the therapy takes a long time.
- Be patient and also stay active in session.
- Use humor sensitively! Ask your client to construct humorous ways to think about inflexible beliefs.
- Co-construct case conceptualizations and imagery that engages your clients and helps them gain fresh perspectives.

Trap 4

Therapist becomes hopeless

We have all been there: stuck, mystified by the lack of therapy progress, hoping our supervisor or colleague can show us the way out of a rut. Our client expresses a desire to change, yet all efforts are thwarted, all evidence contrary to existing beliefs is discounted, and little or nothing happens between sessions because beliefs aren't shifting enough. Sometime it is the opposite—progress is slow because so much happens between the sessions. We discover that clients' extreme beliefs are endorsed by unhelpful social, domestic, or professional networks. At other times we feel stuck because, despite what seems like best efforts, our client continues to relapse and we begin to share their pessimism. Therapist hopelessness is often accompanied by increasing ineffectiveness.

There are ways to navigate the hopelessness trap. As soon as you recognize the problem, formulate what is obstructing progress. There are many obstacles to consider, from a practical lack of resources to more complicated emotional, cognitive, and systemic "blocks" existing in either you or your client. If you realize your client is discounting evidence because their inflexible belief is a core belief, then switching to Socratic interventions such as continuum work can be more powerful than simple evidence gathering.

Another common obstacle is fear (fueled by inflexible beliefs). It can be useful to routinely ask clients how they view the prospect of change, using Socratic enquiry to explore this. In fact, exploring the consequences of change can be a fruitful part of any assessment and ongoing therapy. Sometimes it is not an individual client's fears that block change but a systemic fear such as a family's (or organization's) unwillingness to support change. Systems often operate to maintain the status quo—sometimes because of a lack of concern and sometimes because the "old way" has advantages for the social system. "Systems" can hold their own fixed beliefs. One of the authors can remember a distressed spouse turning up at a session pleading for the return of his "real" wife who had "disappeared" as a result of her therapy. He wanted the insecure woman who needed him to return to his life. He truly believed that the only way he could feel and appear to be a "real man" was if he was seen to be stronger than his wife. This prompted some very helpful couple therapy.

The following sections describe strategies well suited to managing three common obstacles that can fuel hopelessness:

- All evidence contrary to existing beliefs is discounted.
- Clients are so afraid of change that little or nothing happens between sessions.
- The client's inflexible beliefs are endorsed by unhelpful social, domestic, or professional networks.

All evidence contrary to existing beliefs is discounted

You are pleased with your work together: a well-executed behavioral experiment has led to a new intellectual conclusion. But how disappointing for both of you when it is swiftly dismissed with a "... yes but he was only saying that to be kind/... yes but they don't know the real me/... yes but I was just lucky that time."

Here the therapist's challenge is to resist feeling defeated *and* to stay engaged in constructing hopeful options. Fortunately, this "... yes but ..." situation need not be a cue for hopelessness (in client or therapist) as it can present an opportunity for taking a different "Socratic path."

Use of a continuum
When any and all evidence contradicting a belief is discounted, that belief is most likely an inflexible core belief. Using a continuum to evaluate a core belief will be more effective than simple evidence gathering because core beliefs are, by definition, absolute "all or nothing" beliefs. A continuum requires the client to consider the middle ground, the large area of experience that core

beliefs usually ignore. In reality, very few life experiences actually fit on the endpoints of a continuum. Thus, core beliefs are usually weakened when clients are asked to think in terms of a continuum. And, as you will see, a continuum offers alternative possibilities and this makes the process of easing inflexible beliefs all the more achievable.

Continuum work is generally more effective if the alternative belief is rated on the continuum rather than the unhelpful belief. This is because shifts in core beliefs are likely to happen slowly. Consider the impact of using a continuum if the belief shifts 1%. The client is already in new territory when they believe an alternative idea 1%; in contrast, they are still dwelling on familiar ground when confidence in a current belief drops to 99%. Thus, as shown in the following example, Caitlyn's therapist begins by simply asking her to define an alternative core belief before setting up the continuum. He does this in a straightforward manner by asking her, "How would you like to be?" Caitlyn is a 32-year-old woman who struggles with bulimia, social anxiety, and relationship conflicts.

Therapist: If you didn't see yourself as unlovable, how would you like to be?
Caitlyn: Loveable, I guess.
Therapist: OK. Let's draw a scale here that rates lovability from 0 to 100%. (Draws this continuum scale.) How would you define 100% lovable?

Notice that her therapist begins by asking Caitlyn to define the endpoints of the scale. These are easier to define because they match up well with the nature of core beliefs and Caitlyn's established perspective. He works with her to make sure the qualities she chooses for the endpoints are extreme absolutes:

Caitlyn: If you are lovable, then people like you.
Therapist: So, I guess 100% lovable would mean everyone in the world likes you.
Caitlyn: I'm not sure that is possible.
Therapist: I don't think so either. But if being lovable means people like you, then 100% lovable would have to mean everyone in the world likes you.
Caitlyn: Oh, I guess that's right.

He does not question the criteria she sets up because this is her definition of lovability. However, he does make sure that the endpoints of her continuum are absolutes. After some discussion, she defines 100% lovable as everyone in the world likes you, you do everything well, and you are always in a good mood.

Therapist:	So, if that is 100% lovable, then we should write under the 0% point on the scale the opposite of those things. For example, if 100% lovable means everyone in the world like you, then 0% would mean?
Caitlyn:	Nobody likes you.
Therapist:	Write that under 0%.

In the Therapist's Mind

As Caitlyn writes her 0% definition ("nobody likes you, you do everything terribly, and you are always in a bad mood") on the continuum, her therapist considers how to begin to use this continuum. He decides to begin by asking Caitlyn about other people because she is so adamant about her own unlovability.

Therapist:	Let's see how we can use this scale. Where would you put your friend Paul on this scale?
Caitlyn:	He's lovable.
Therapist:	How lovable? Does everyone in the world like him? Is he always in a good mood?
Caitlyn:	A lot of people like him, but not everybody. And sometimes he is not in a good mood. I guess I'd put him at about 70%.
Therapist:	Who else can we put on this scale?
Caitlyn:	My father. I'd put him at 0%.
Therapist:	Nobody likes him, he does everything terribly, and he is always in a bad mood?
Caitlyn:	Well, not exactly. OK, maybe he would be at 10%.
Therapist:	That's interesting, when you begin to think about it, your father gets a 10% rating. OK. Who else?
Caitlyn:	Liza. She is between my father and Paul. Maybe 50%.
Therapist:	Where would you put yourself?
Caitlyn:	Oh, I'm at 0%.
Therapist:	Worse than your father, then? Nobody likes you, you do everything terribly, and you are always in a bad mood?
Caitlyn:	Maybe my father should be at 5% and I will put myself at 10%.
Therapist:	It's good to see how you really start to make this scale work for you as you think more deeply about personal qualities. This is the idea, so well done.

Notice that this therapist's use of the continuum with Caitlyn follows the 4-Stage Model of Socratic Dialogue (see Chapter 2). Her therapist begins by asking information questions (step 1) to define points on the continuum and to ask where various people would be rated on this scale. Her therapists listens (step 2) to Caitlyn's responses and makes sure her ratings are consistent with the criteria she defined at the beginning of the exercise. Her ratings that are marked on the continuum become the written summary (step 3) of their discussion as shown in Figure 6.1. Finally, these continuum ratings provide rich opportunities for the therapist to show curiosity through analytical and synthesizing questions such as:

- That's interesting. How is it that you care about Paul or Liza even though they are not 100% lovable?
- Can you think of a time when Paul seemed less than 70% lovable? If so, how did he become more lovable again after that time? I wonder what this says about being lovable? Does this give you any ideas about how you could become more than 10% lovable?
- Caitlyn can be encouraged to get even more curious and to rate herself on each of the criteria for lovability she set. She rates herself as 20% liked by others, 40% doing things well, and 15% of the time in a good mood. Her therapist then asks, "How might you understand why you are higher on these scores than the total lovability score you gave yourself (10%)?"

Use of 2 × 2 grid to test underlying assumptions

A single line continuum as used above to evaluate a core belief will not work as well if the client's inflexible belief is an underlying assumption. This is because underlying assumptions link two ideas in an "if.... then..." prediction. However, underlying assumptions can be tested in a similar way as illustrated above by creating both an *x*- and *y*-axis continuum (with the resulting two continua overlapping and looking like a plus sign) in order to examine the predictions of an underlying assumption. Even easier for most people to understand, the *x*- and *y*-axes can be drawn as a 2 × 2 grid as demonstrated in the following example.

Phil grew up in a chaotic family with parents who frequently fought physically and hit their children during alcoholic binges. As an adult, he avoided

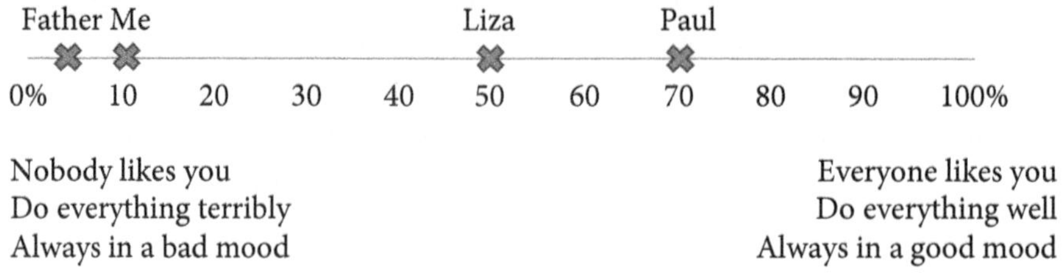
Father Me
Liza
Paul
0%
10
20
30
40
50
60
70
80
90
100%
Nobody likes you
Do everything terribly
Always in a bad mood
Everyone likes you
Do everything well
Always in a good mood

Figure 6.1 Caitlyn's continuum of lovability.

all conflict by withdrawing whenever he began to feel irritated with someone. This led to difficulties in his marriage because his spouse Erik wanted to actively discuss disagreements and the issues that led to conflict. Their couple's therapist helped Phil identify his belief that anger and conflict always lead to damage in a relationship. This belief was written on the white board as "Expressing anger is destructive."

Notice that Phil's belief has two interlinked concepts (expressing anger, destructive). It could be stated as an underlying assumption, "If I express anger, then it will have a destructive effect on our relationship". Stating it this way helps the therapist set up behavioral experiments so the couple can test whether Phil's belief reliably predicts outcomes in his relationship with Erik. Prior to doing these experiments, their therapist decided to draw out the implications of Phil's belief as shown in Figure 6.2.

Therapist: Phil, would you draw your belief this way? It shows that big expressions of anger are highly destructive, smaller expressions of anger are less destructive, small attempts to not express anger are a little bit constructive and big efforts to not express anger are very constructive.

Phil: Yes, that is exactly the way I see it.

Therapist: Erik, do you see it the same way?

Erik: No. I think you can express anger and have it be constructive and sometimes when you don't express anger, it can hurt your relationship.

Therapist: Can you give Phil and me some examples of what you mean?

Erik: OK. (Turning to Phil). Do you remember the time I told you I was angry that you kept texting while we were eating?

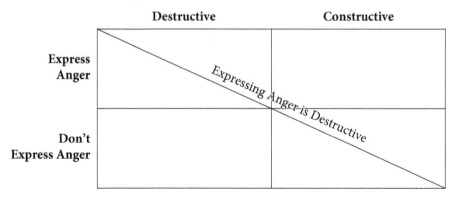

Figure 6.2 Phil's belief "Expressing anger is destructive" drawn on a 2 × 2 grid.

Phil: Of course. I don't do that anymore because I know it bothers you.

Erik: Yes, and that meant a lot to me that you stopped doing that. I think that has been better for our relationship.

Phil: Me, too.

Erik: So that would be an example of a time that expressing anger was constructive.

Therapist: Let me write that example in this upper right box (Writes as shown in Figure 6.3.) Phil, can you think of any examples of when you didn't express anger you felt and it had a destructive effect?

Phil: I suppose the time Erik was spending every Saturday morning with Boomer playing tennis. It made be jealous and angry but I didn't say anything for weeks. It started to drive us apart and Erik didn't even know it.

Therapist: What happened?

Phil: One day Erik came home early and I was crying. I told him how upset I was because I thought he might be having an affair with

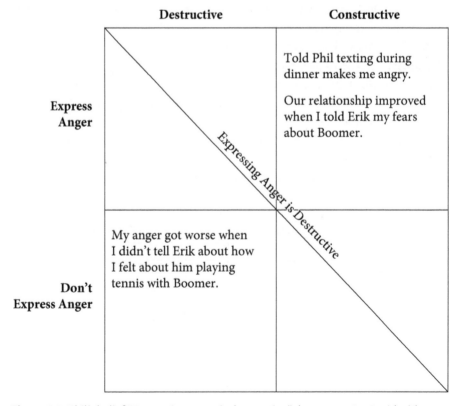

Figure 6.3 Phil's belief "Expressing anger is destructive" drawn on a 2 × 2 grid with contradictory evidence.

Boomer. He convinced me he was not and told me I was welcome to come with him to the tennis court whenever I wanted. I did go there a few times and once I got to know Boomer a bit better I realized they were just friends who liked to play tennis and I stopped being upset about it.

Therapist: So this was an example that shows when you did not express your anger it had a destructive effect on you and your relationship.

Phil: Yes.

Therapist: (Writing as shown on Figure 6.3). Let me put that in this lower left box. And, a few weeks later, when you did tell Erik you were jealous and angry, it had a constructive effect on you and your relationship. Is that right?

Phil: Yes, it did.

Therapist: Where should I write that, Phil?

Phil: I guess in that upper right box.

Figure 6.3 shows Phil's belief with contradictory examples summarized in the relevant boxes to record evidence that expressing anger can be constructive and not expressing anger can be destructive.

Therapist: We could get more information about exceptions to your belief, Phil. But it seems to me, the most important idea is that you want to be constructive, whether you express your anger or not.

Phil: That's right. I never thought about those other boxes ... how anger could actually help or how not saying you were angry could sometimes hurt.

Therapist: When you were growing up, it seems most of the time anger in your family was in the destructive box. So how were you to learn this? Would you be willing to do some experiments to see if you and Erik can learn to express anger and mostly stay constructive? And also learn how to tell if not expressing anger is constructive or destructive?

Phil: Absolutely. This is a very different way of looking at it.

Use of a continuum fits well with the four stages of Socratic Dialogue and is ideally suited to working with inflexible beliefs when the client discounts all evidence that contradicts their beliefs. As pointed out with Padesky's prejudice model described earlier in this chapter, core beliefs are also maintained because people don't notice or remember contradictory evidence. For this reason, core belief logs (also called positive data logs) are also used to strengthen alternative core beliefs (Padesky, 1994; 2020a). Core belief logs ask the client over a number of months to keep a daily record of evidence that is consistent with an alternative core belief. For example, Erik and Phil could be asked to keep a record of every time expressed anger leads to a constructive outcome. Other guided discovery methods can also be used to strengthen alternative core beliefs. For a more complete description of these methods see Padesky (2020a).

Clients are so afraid of change that little or nothing happens between sessions

When you suspect fear of change is leading to an impasse, you can use Socratic Dialogue to gain a better understanding of client fears and to help you co-create an atmosphere of safety and hope. Begin by asking questions to find out more about their beliefs. For example, 55-year-old Sharya had concluded that she would benefit from being more assertive and independent and yet she was quite nervous to take the first steps in doing so. Her therapist asked questions such as:

- I wonder, how might things change if you did express your views more?
- Let's imagine that you were now able to go shopping on your own. Can you see that in your mind's eye? How does it feel? Do you foresee any problems? How do you think your friends and family will react?
- When you can do these things, what will your view of yourself be? How will you see yourself?

As you and your client actively imagine and/or role-play what change might be like, you might discover additional inflexible beliefs that need to be tackled before your client can be confident that she can cope with the consequences of change.

Sharya realized that she was afraid that her behavioral changes would upset the family dynamics so much that she might lose the love and respect of her children and spouse. This reflected a core belief that "I am essentially unlovable" and an assumption that "If you displease someone, they will turn on you." She also had a nagging (but very longstanding) view (assumption) that "Assertive women are insensitive," and she did not want to view herself in that way. By far the most challenging realization, however, was that she was afraid of changing at this stage in her life as it left her with a profound sense of self-disappointment and grief: " ....why didn't I do something sooner?"

In the Therapist's Mind

Her therapist, quite understandably, now wants to help Sharya make a statement, rather than pose a question, because we cannot test and review questions. He aims to be cautious as he anticipated that (a) reflecting on this might activate painful, negative core beliefs (which it did) and (b) that she might experience enormous grief when she considered the magnitude of an (avoidable) loss.

Therapist: That question, "Why didn't I do something sooner?", seems to have brought up some really deep emotions. I wonder if you would be willing to explore with me why you think you did not make these changes earlier in your life? Would that be OK?

Sharya: Because I'm stupid, I'm weak, I'm worthless. I've thrown it all away. I've suffered all these years and I deserve to suffer for being so pathetic. It's my fault because I didn't do anything earlier. It's my fault that my children have not had a decent childhood. I've scarred them for life now. That's unforgivable. I am a worthless person and a worthless cause—better I'd never been born. Better if I weren't here now.

In the Therapist's Mind

Despite his forethought, the therapist had underestimated the cognitive and emotional impact of "scratching the surface." He immediately regretted opening a line of enquiry that propelled Sharya down an avenue of self-recrimination and possible suicidal intention. Fortunately, this was early on in their session and he could invest the remaining time to helping her gain control of the feelings and calm her self-recrimination.

He considered a Socratic approach of looking for "evidence against" her negative statements, but he knew her well enough to appreciate that she would not be able to generate counterbalancing statements and would probably feel all the worse because of it. Instead, he decided to gently encourage her to retreat to her "safe place in mind," a soothing and empowering image that they had been developing together. Over the next several minutes, this helped her regain some calm and self-compassion.

Once Sharya felt calmer, they reflected on what had just happened and discovered that she had been getting increasingly "wound up" behind a coping façade. She said that she rated her sense of being "wound up" 7/10 before he asked his question and 10/10 the moment she heard it. They agreed that in future she would tell her therapist when she reached a rating of 7/10 so they could jointly make some decisions about whether and how to ease up. In this instance, the Socratic enquiry about her level of stress was appropriate; enquiry about the content of her distress would have risked triggering too much emotion.

Once through this impasse, they continued their task of formulating "obstacles to change" together, using Socratic questions but keeping the exercise as "intellectual" as possible and purposely avoiding "hot" cognitions for the remainder of this session. In order to maintain a sense of safety, Sharya's therapist took time to address these fears before resuming her graded behavioral experiments in acting more assertive and independent.

The client's inflexible beliefs are endorsed by social, domestic, or professional networks

Sometimes social, family, or professional networks actually help maintain inflexible beliefs. Consider and ask questions to understand any systemic factors that might make change difficult for your client. When these are identified, devise a systemic strategy for change with your client.

As occurred in the following illustration, systemic factors sometimes are tangentially mentioned during the process of debriefing between session learning assignments. Mikey was a 20-year-old man in therapy for treatment of PTSD following a road traffic accident. He had been trying to return to the site of his accident in order to test his old prediction that he could not tolerate the emotions this would evoke. His beliefs had, once again remained fixed, so his therapist asked more about his support network asking questions such as:

- Let's review last Thursday when you tried to revisit the site of the accident. You said your mother went with you. Can you tell me more about that? For example, where was she? Did she stand with you or stay behind?
- How did she react ....?
- What did she say ....?
- ... and what did this mean to you?

It was helpful to review a recent and specific incident in detail because these questions revealed that Mikey's mother always walked and stood between him and the accident scene so that she could shield him if he became too distressed. Something else the therapist discovered was that Mikey's mother was herself distressed throughout this exercise and tried to leave the scene as quickly as possible. When the therapist asked the key question, "And what did this mean to you?", Mikey replied that, even though his mother had never said as much, her reactions confirmed that it was an emotionally overwhelming situation. They both felt compelled to leave the scene quite swiftly—that is, before the negative prediction was properly tested. In this case his mother had subtly supported Mikey's belief and undermined the potential value of his experiment.

In other instances support for a negative belief is not so subtle or well-intended. Many clients regularly hear statements such as "You are really stupid/ugly/worthless". These are often shameful and painful experiences to relate to a therapist and clients therefore may not report them without prompting. Be vigilant in identifying these experiences while making sure to ask about them in a sensitive manner.

Be mindful that attempts to change can put clients in danger if they are parts of systems that include domestic violence or other volatile interactions. Therefore, assessment of client environments and social contexts is highly relevant to planning change, especially changes that are interpersonal.

Cultural factors can also make changing inflexible beliefs easier or more difficult. Change is easier when cultural values are congruent with change efforts. When change requires experimenting with countercultural beliefs or behaviors, we can predict people will experience headwinds to their efforts, both internally and socially. Whenever possible, take cultural values into account and try to co-create change plans that are compatible with a client's closely held cultural values.

Mikey and his therapist were able to formulate an understanding of how his mother's responses played a part in slowing down progress. They drew this up together and this led to the following Socratic Dialogue:

Therapist: Looking at this now, what do you see?

Mikey: I realize that Mum wants to protect me and she doesn't want to get upset either—but this actually stops me from properly testing my prediction in the way that we'd planned in our session.

Therapist: How do you think things might have to change so that you can properly test it?

Mikey: It might be better if someone else went with me.

Therapist: Ok—who could do that? Who would you trust?

Mikey: Teo has always been a good friend and I trust him to support me without getting too emotionally involved.

Therapist: What do you need to do to set things up so that Teo can do these behavioral experiments with you?

Mikey: First, I need to explain things to my mum, so that she is not hurt by this.

By asking a series of synthesizing questions, his therapist helped Mikey devise a detailed new behavioral strategy that stood a greater chance of helping him and which reinstated a sense of hope in both him and his therapist.

A final significant systemic factor to consider is ourselves. Therapist beliefs and behaviors can make or break the course of therapy. For example, some therapists fear moving too quickly with clients who are viewed as "fragile" and, as a result, unwittingly sabotage progress. Some therapists who are personally robust can feel overconfident in their client's ability to face challenges. It is vital to be aware of our own beliefs and the impact these can have on our therapy. Therapist beliefs are explored more fully in Chapter 9.

Keep in Mind

- Core beliefs and other tightly held beliefs can be expected to change slowly. Rapid change in beliefs only happens at the level of automatic thoughts or underlying assumptions.
- Psycho-education can help clients better formulate their difficulties and lead to hope.
- When inflexible beliefs are activated, experiential therapy methods are more memorable than discussion alone.
- Continually express realistic hope and do your best to instill this in your client.
- Consider the influence of systems in which your client is embedded.
- Identify any of your own beliefs that could have a negative impact on therapy.

Trap 5

Client inflexible beliefs trigger therapist (unhelpful) inflexible beliefs

---

Your client just isn't making progress; their inflexible beliefs aren't shifting. How often does this situation lead you to see client progress as hopeless and contribute to your own feelings of frustration, guilt, or shame? Along with your emotional reactions, unhelpful beliefs like these can get triggered:

"I'm inadequate—other therapists would have more success. I must try harder."

"I just *cannot* work with eating disorders/OCD/chronic depression …"

"This type of client just can't benefit from this type of therapy."

"This type of client always resists therapy/plays one therapist off against another/tries to manipulate the situation …"

These types of unhelpful beliefs often lead to unhelpful behaviors such as referring on to another therapist prematurely, getting caught up in a defensive or aggressive dialogue with your client, becoming passive in session, or holding onto a client when therapy really isn't working for them.

The key to managing this trap is supervision or consultation. Sometimes self-supervision will be sufficient. In any case, some form of systematic reflective practice is essential for managing this therapist dilemma. Chapter 9 offers an in-depth look at how to use guided discovery methods to tackle your own unhelpful beliefs. Please read that chapter now if this is a current concern for you.

Summary

Inflexible beliefs are commonly encountered in psychotherapy, especially when clients come to therapy to address more severe or chronic concerns. Fortunately, Socratic Dialogue and other forms of guided discovery are well-suited to help therapists manage the variety of traps that accompany rigidly held beliefs. Informational questions designed to unpack the origins of and evidence for inflexible beliefs sets a foundation for collaboratively conceptualizing these cognitions. A positive alliance has an opportunity to form when the therapist asks these questions with genuine curiosity and listens empathically to client experiences. Curiosity and empathy are centrally important in managing client mistrust of the therapist and beliefs that might otherwise interfere with a positive working alliance. In addition, therapists are encouraged to stay mindful that inflexible beliefs can be encoded in imagery, memories, and sometimes a physical "felt sense." These also need to be assessed on an ongoing basis.

Inflexible beliefs usually represent underlying assumptions or core beliefs. These levels of thought change more slowly than automatic thoughts, which are more situational. Thus, therapists need to be patient and also stay active, even in the face of slow progress. Therapist–client dialogues in this chapter illustrated the uses of imagery, active experiential learning, and humor as paths to keep therapy fresh over time. In addition, therapists are advised to use strategies such as a continuum and core belief log that accommodate the "all-or-nothing" nature of inflexible core beliefs.

The many guidelines offered in this chapter can foster progress over time and help reduce hopelessness in both clients and therapists as they work with beliefs that appear inflexible. The strategies illustrated can help therapists successfully engage clients' curiosity, identify and address fears about change, stay alert to systemic factors that maintain target beliefs, and patiently maintain a collaborative, investigative spirit for as much time as necessary to construct and strengthen more flexible and adaptive beliefs.

Reader Learning Activities

- Identify a current client who appears to have inflexible beliefs.
- Review the five traps in this chapter and consider whether any of these apply to your therapy with them.
- If so, review those sections and try out one of the interventions described that seems likely to be clinically appropriate at this point in your therapy.
- Use Socratic Dialogue to collaborate with your client and evaluate the usefulness of the approach you are trying.
- If you have been working with a client for a relatively long time on one or more inflexible beliefs, review the suggestions for Trap 3 on how to keep therapy "fresh."
- If it seems clinically appropriate, try out one or more of the strategies in that section and see whether that leads to greater therapy engagement for you and your client.
- If you can identify any clients with whom you are feeling hopeless about helping them, identify a supervisor or consultant who is skilled in working with inflexible beliefs. Book a session with that supervisor or consultant to see whether you can find a way forward.
- For interventions described in this chapter with which you have little to no experience, consider learning a bit more about it by doing follow-up reading from cited texts or articles. You can also look for further training in this area.

Appendix
Core Belief and Schema-Focused CBT Strategies[1]

Core belief logs (positive data logs) to collect information to support new beliefs
Continuum work or scaling techniques to address dichotomous thinking
Historical review of evidence
Socratic Dialogue
Responsibility pies
Core belief flashcards (with alternative beliefs written on reverse)
Role-play
Psychodrama/chair work
Transformation of meaning of early memories; complex imagery transformation
Body-image transformation

References

Arntz, A., & Weertman, A. (1999). Treatment of childhood memories: Theory and practice. *Behaviour Research and Therapy*, *37*(8), 715–740. https://doi.org/10.1016/S0005-7967(98)00173-9

Beck, A.T., Davis, D.D., & Freeman, A.(Eds.) (2015). *Cognitive therapy of personality disorders* (3rd ed.). New York: Guilford Press.

Greenberger, D., & Padesky, C. A. (2016). *Mind over mood: Change how you feel by changing the way you think (2nd ed.)*. New York: Guilford Press.

Hawley, L. L., Padesky, C. A., Hollon, S. D., Mancuso, E., Laposa, J. M., Brozina, K., & Segal, Z. V. (2017). Cognitive behavioral therapy for depression using mind over mood: CBT skill use and differential symptom alleviation. *Behavior Therapy*, *48*(1), 29–44. https://doi.org/10.1016/j.beth.2016.09.003

Kuyken, W., Padesky, C. A., & Dudley, R. (2009). *Collaborative case conceptualization: Working effectively with clients in cognitive-behavioral therapy*. New York: Guilford Press.

Mooney, K. A., & Padesky, C. A. (2000). Applying client creativity to recurrent problems: Constructing possibilities and tolerating doubt. *Journal of Cognitive Psychotherapy: An International Quarterly*, *14*(2), 149–161. https://doi.org/10.1891/0889-8391.14.2.149

Mooney, K. A., & Padesky, C. A. (2004, February). *Cognitive therapy of personality disorders*. 24-hour workshop presented at Palm Desert, California.

Padesky, C. A. (1991). Schema as self-prejudice. *International Cognitive Therapy Newsletter*, 6, 6–7. Retrieved from https://www.padesky.com/clinical-corner/publications/

Padesky, C. A. (1994). Schema change processes in cognitive therapy. *Clinical Psychology and Psychotherapy: An International Journal of Theory and Practice*, *1*(5), 267–278. https://doi.org/10.1002/cpp.5640010502

---

[1] Just as with classic CBT, some techniques are more purely verbal and "intellectual" and some are more experiential. Although there is evidence that experiential methods are more powerful, in that they can effect change more quickly (Arntz & Weertman, 1999), some clients cannot tolerate the emotional intensity of these interventions initially and the less emotionally evocative "intellectual" strategies should then be first choice.

Padesky, C. A. (2003). *Constructing new core beliefs* [Video]. Center for Cognitive Therapy. Retrieved from https://www.padesky.com/digital-padesky-store

Padesky, C.A. (2006). *Therapist beliefs: Protocols, personalities & guided exercises.* [Audio]. Center for Cognitive Therapy. Retrieved from https://www.padesky.com/digital-padesky-store

Padesky, C. A. (2020a). *The clinician's guide to CBT using mind over mood* (2nd ed.). *New York*: Guilford Press.

Padesky, C. A. (2020b). Collaborative case conceptualization: Client knows best. *Cognitive and Behavioral Practice, 27*(4), 392–404. https://doi.org/10.1016/j.cbpra.2020.06.003

Young, J. E., Klosko, J. S., & Weishaar, M. (2006). *Schema therapy: A practitioner's guide.* New York: Guilford Press.

7
Impulsive and Compulsive Behaviors

Helen Kennerley

> *Silvia's behaviors seemed so self-defeating that it was difficult to understand why she did them. Afterwards she was always so disappointed in herself: shameful and remorseful. People she loved suffered, and yet it was as if she were not able to stop herself.*

Some behaviors just seem irresistible: people feel compelled to do things or act on impulse even though the consequences can be dire. Sylvia was such a person. The terms "impulsive and compulsive" behaviors are used to describe these actions and they embrace a wide range of difficult-to-control reactions that are detrimental to the individual or to others: overeating, undereating, purging, overexercising, self-injuring, overspending, excessive drinking, drug misuse, online gaming, checking, touching, gambling, unsafe sexual practices, violent outbursts, stalking, watching pornography, hair pulling . . . the list really does seem endless. In this chapter you will learn:

1. How to understand and assess impulsive and compulsive behaviors,
2. Common traps and clinician errors in treating them, and
3. How to use Socratic Dialogue to minimize errors and manage the traps.

Understanding Impulsive and Compulsive Behaviors

Impulsive behaviors are "spur of the moment" actions, such as wolfing down a large amount of alcohol or food at a party, taking an unplanned overdose during an evening of intense loneliness. Compulsive behaviors are more considered and would include planned binge-eating or self-injury over a weekend of solitude, continued semi-starvation, and planned risky sexual contacts. The build-up to the behavior is sometimes savored and sometimes dreaded—or both at once, as was Frank's experience:

> Frank planned this night carefully so that he had no commitments: he would be free to drink—and drink. All day he anticipated the oblivion of that evening and he was distracted by thoughts of his drinking bout. He was excited knowing that he would be able to blot out the world in such an enjoyable way. He was concerned lest someone or something interrupted his ritual of buying a fine whiskey (only a very good one would do). He was scared that it would go wrong again and he would blackout and he was scared that—although he was planning the evening with relish—he was losing control.

Some behaviors are self-directed (such as hair pulling or excessive eating) while some focus on others (e.g., stalking, aggressive outbursts); some have a "positive" goal (e.g., relaxation and soothing achieved through substance misuse; gaining longed-for attention; stimulation from engaging in risky activities) while others have a "negative" function (e.g., self-punishment or the punishment of others). It is of note that impulsive and compulsive behaviors are very much cognitive–*behavioral* problems. In addition to tackling pertinent cognitions, clients are often helped by developing alternative ways of responding to distress, and then field-testing them. We will see this illustrated in some of the clinical examples in this chapter.

As shown in Box 7.1, therapists helping those with impulsive and compulsive behaviors need to be on the lookout for six common traps. Guided discovery methods will be illustrated throughout this chapter that can help therapists avoid or navigate these traps.

The first "trap" that we can fall into, when working with people struggling to manage impulsive or compulsive behaviors (ICB), is forging on with therapy despite not fully understanding the personal meaning of the behaviors. Linked to this is a second trap: not appreciating the level of risk that your client's behavior poses either to themselves or to others. Socratic enquiry helps us understand why behaviors make sense to a person, why they are so irresistible, and whether they are dangerous. Then we can build a meaningful conceptualization with our client and, of course, this then guides us toward relevant interventions.

Trap 1

Not understanding the personal meaning of problem behaviors

A key therapy task is making sense of unhelpful activities. Even the most bizarre, shocking, or damaging of behaviors *will* make sense to the client.

Box 7.1 Common Traps in Therapy for Impulsive and Compulsive Behaviors

---

Trap 1
Not understanding the personal meaning of the problem behaviors—an especially likely trap when key experiences don't readily map onto language.

Trap 2
Not appreciating the level of risk of serious harm to your client or to others.

Trap 3
Underestimating the risk of relapse.

Trap 4
Not appreciating your client's fluctuating motivation and so neglecting to work on it.

Trap 5
Overlooking the bigger picture: the wider and deeper world of your client.

Trap 6
The negative consequences of change.

Socratic Dialogue provides a process for discovering the understandable origins of a specific behavior for a particular person.

Insufficient exploration often happens when we assume that we understand the meaning behind an action and therefore we don't ask the necessary extra questions to check out our hunches. If we fully unpack the idiosyncratic *meaning* of problem behaviors it is possible to really understand why an ostensibly unhelpful action makes sense to our client. By doing this we can also more readily adopt an empathic and nonjudgmental stance.

In addition, truly appreciating the idiosyncratic significance of an act can also enhance our behavioral experiments. When we identify the particular reasons that make "sense" of an action, we can better construct a meaningful test for the problem activity. We can also use guided discovery methods to take things a step further by discovering meaningful alternative actions or benign substitutes for problem behaviors, actions that might take the edge off the urge or craving so that your client can resist (as is addressed later in this chapter).

It is worth noting that different forms of behavior can serve the same purpose or have the same function for a person. Thus, a woman might cut herself or binge-eat or drink to achieve a profound dissociated state. With several means of achieving her single goal, she might shift from behavior to behavior. Alternatively, a single action can simultaneously satisfy several goals and can therefore be particularly compelling. For example, the act of cutting could satisfy goals of self-punishment, catharsis, and achieving dissociation. Binge-eating might comfort, distract, and punish at the same time; unsafe sex might thrill, gain attention, and risk harm simultaneously.

Whether psychological or somatic, dissociation is commonly associated with impulsive and compulsive behaviors. Often, the purpose of self-injury, overeating/drinking/drug use, overspending, and so on is to achieve a dissociated state. Dissociation can be desirable when it promotes a profound distraction from psychological and/or physical distress or provides a gratifying state of elation or detachment. Interestingly, the very same acts are also used, by some, as a means of escaping from a dissociated state: interrupting depersonalization, derealization, or a flashback, for example. Clinicians need to be prepared to expect that some clients exhibiting ICB will "space out" in session or be triggered into a flashback. Recognizing these moments also provides an opportunity to teach your client skills for emotion management they can use themselves in these circumstances throughout their life. See Kennedy et al. (2013) for a guide for managing dissociation.

Keep in Mind

- ICBs are often multifunctional and your client could present with several different combinations of behavior. Therefore, Socratic enquiry needs to be gently thorough, teasing out all possible functions of the behaviors.

- Establish the personal meaning of the problem behavior(s) to help understand why it makes sense, guide the design of behavioral experiments, and generate possible substitute behaviors.

- Your clients may be prone to dissociation, so be aware of the forms that this can take and be prepared to help your clients manage detached states and flashbacks.

Useful questions that will help you elaborate personal meanings and discover the complexities of your client's actions include:

- And is there *anything else* that you find distracting/cathartic/soothing at this time?
- And if that were not possible *what else* might you do?
- Are there *any other ways* of feeling so relaxed/thrilled/alive/punished/etc.?
- Are there *other consequences* of doing this—other feelings or thoughts that you have as a result?
- And how do others react?
- And what happens in the longer term? How do you feel? What do you do?

Questions such as these can help you tease out the full spectrum of your client's practice and intent.

Central cognitions: What to look for

We often emphasize the behavioral aspects of ICBs but it is important to appreciate the cognitions that drive and facilitate engaging in an otherwise unacceptable act. As yet there is no cognitive model of impulsive and compulsive behaviors, although Marlatt and Gordon's Relapse Prevention model (1985) provides a ubiquitous understanding of lapse into unhelpful behaviors, and Kennerley (2004) suggested a framework for self-injurious behavior that might equally apply to impulsive and compulsive behaviors. This framework suggests that relevant cognitions fall into three categories, which interact to maintain the pattern of self-damaging activities (see Figure 7.1):

1. Fundamental cognitions and associated assumptions,
2. Facilitating beliefs, and
3. Reactions to the behavior.

1. **Fundamental cognitions and associated assumptions** are beliefs that are consistent with potentially harmful actions. These include thoughts such as "I'm bad and I deserve to hurt"; "I am nothing and it doesn't matter what happens to me"; "I matter and children don't"; "I am despicable—I should be punished"; "The world is cruel and spiteful—it's not for me"; "Others are superficial and selfish: no one is going to be there for me". These are the sorts of beliefs that support potentially harmful actions by undermining beliefs about oneself or others so that "unacceptable" acts begin to seem tolerable and acceptable. At times, these beliefs sanction the behavior directly. These cognitions can be the powerhouse driving impulses and compulsions.

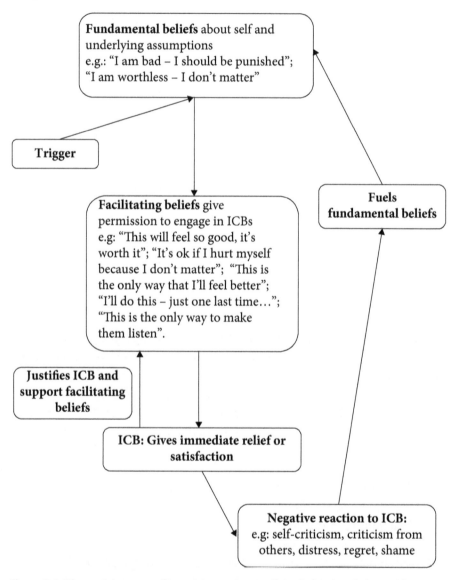

Figure 7.1 The maintenance of impulsive and compulsive behaviors (adapted from Kennerley, 2004).

2. **Facilitating beliefs** are "permission-giving" statements that enable a person to find engagement in a behavior acceptable. They include assumptions and predictions such as "I can't tolerate this feeling and there is no other way to deal with it"; "It's okay to do this because this is the last time that I'll hurt myself"; "Don't think about it—just drink. It will feel good"; "I have to do it, it's the only way to stop the urge"; "This will make her listen to me"; "This is the only way to show how I really feel"; "There is no other enjoyment in my life—I deserve this". Without such facilitating cognitions,

a person is unable to sanction an otherwise unacceptable act and it will not occur. The urge or craving might exist but it won't be transformed into action unless it can be endorsed. These cognitions often are ideally tested with behavioral experiments, a guided discovery method. Tackling facilitating beliefs can be a most expedient means of managing behaviors.

3. **Reactions to the behavior** are beliefs that fuel the person's problem either by feeding their negative fundamental belief system (e.g.: "This proves that I am bad/weird/weak/worthless") or by providing support for facilitating beliefs (e.g.: "It *does* feel good"; "This *is* the only way that I can cope"; "This *did* make them sit up and listen"). These thoughts often close a vicious circle, rendering a person vulnerable to further engagement in the problem behavior.

Keep in Mind

Identify all three relevant levels of cognition:

- Fundamental cognitions power the problem behaviors: without them the problem does not arise.
- Facilitating cognitions give clients permission to "release the brake": without this permission the behavior does not occur.
- Cognitive response to the behavior: this often "re-fuels the engine." Identifying and tackling these cognitions can reduce the drive to continue the behavior.

The following dialogue between Li and her therapist illustrates the interplay of these three levels of cognition. Li had struggled with an eating disorder since her early teens. She was now 21 and seesawed between overeating and undereating. Li used a wide variety of "compensatory" strategies when she felt that she had overeaten: strategies such as vomiting, excessive laxative use, overexercising, and fasting. She was painfully thin (her BMI was 15) and her health was now at risk. In this vignette, her new therapist is trying to understand why her binge-eating and purging episodes "make sense" given that Li is aware of the health risks involved.

Therapist: Can we look at last night's binge in more detail? When did you first decide that you would overeat?

Li: I had not eaten all day and I thought that it would be safe to have some pasta for supper. I was really looking forward to a "normal"

	healthy supper. While I was waiting for the spaghetti to cook, I began to taste the sauce in the jar because I was very hungry. Then I couldn't stop.
Therapist:	What was going through your mind at that time? When you couldn't stop, what were you thinking?
Li:	At first I thought: "This is OK because I have not eaten all day" (*facilitating thought*), and I even thought: "I deserve a treat for being so good" (*facilitating thought*).
Therapist:	So, these thoughts spurred you on and you kept eating the sauce. What happened next?
Li:	Halfway down the jar I felt full. Stuffed. Disgusted. But then I couldn't stop.
Therapist:	What was going through your mind then? What drove you on?
Li:	I thought that there was no point in stopping. I was fat, disgusting and this was all I was fit for (*central fundamental beliefs*). I felt bloated and ugly (*fundamental felt sense*) and I just wanted out. I wanted to feel nothing. I thought I'd binge my way through the bad feelings (*facilitating*) and then I'd starve tomorrow to make up for it (*facilitating*).
Therapist:	Let me see if I've understood this. Because you were hungry you began tasting the sauce but soon you felt bloated and just terrible. You predicted that binge-eating would help you feel better?
Li:	Yes
Therapist:	In what way better?
Li:	Out of it, relaxed, comforted.
Therapist:	So no wonder you planned to binge: you wanted fast relief and you anticipated binging would provide it. What happened next?
Li:	I had one of my "classic" binges: all the carbohydrates that I could lay my hands on.
Therapist:	How did you feel at this time?
Li:	Elated when I started because it's always liberating to be free to eat what I like (*confirmation of efficacy*). I felt numb while I was doing it (*confirmation of efficacy*) and wretched immediately afterwards (*confirmation of negative core beliefs*). I felt worse than when I started.
Therapist:	So at first it feels great and it seems to work but the effects are short lived?
Li:	Yes. I felt so bad that I couldn't bear it and I had to make myself vomit—it was the only way to get relief (*facilitating belief*).
Therapist:	With your permission, I'd like us to draw this up on the whiteboard.
Li:	Erm—ok then. Yes, it's ok.

Therapist: I can see that this isn't comfortable for you so just say if you want me to stop drawing this out. OK? Now, it started when you were hungry and began to eat … (They compile a simple conceptualization using Li's exact words.)

In the Therapist's Mind

Her therapist realized that Li found her behavior shameful, so he was particularly careful to be nonjudgmental and empathic. Throughout he was striving to be able to understand so that he could genuinely say: "It's no wonder that …" or "It's understandable that …" in response to Li's account. He kept in mind that there are often three key cognitive–emotional phases when people act on irresistible behaviors (pre-act/peri-act/post-act) and he attempted to tease out the relevant emotional and cognitive elements of each.

Therapist: (Looking at the conceptualization) How does this picture strike you?
Li: It's about right, that's what goes on.
Therapist: Looking at this, why might it be understandable that you began to overeat?
Li: I was hungry.
Therapist: And given what you believe about binging—why might you have been so vulnerable to binge-eating last night?
Li: I suppose I really thought that it would make me feel better—and it did initially (*confirmation of belief*) but not for long.
Therapist: That's interesting because the diagram shows how you go back to binge-eating even though it doesn't seem to help in the long term. What drives that? What's going on there?
Li: It gives me hope—and that's a powerful feeling—and I don't think of anything else at that time. I just think: "This will feel good—now!"
Therapist: So, no wonder you keep resorting to binging if it gives you hope of rapid relief. If you reflect on the diagram and what we've been talking about, do you have any additional thoughts about it?
Li: Well, I can see that I get hungry and then I'm vulnerable to overeating and when I've done that I feel terrible and believe that binge-eating will make me feel better. It does but only for a very short while, then I feel worse than ever. I feel like a sick, disgusting pig (*fuels fundamental beliefs*).

Li and her therapist studied the vicious cycles of her eating behavior and Li was encouraged to think of ways she might break the cycles. This formed the basis of behavioral experiments that altered her patterns of responding to food and distress.

Her therapist was also keen to help Li build up her ability to resist urges and cravings by developing a repertoire of alternative, benign substitute behaviors. This step in therapy is discussed in a later section of this chapter.

Hard to express meanings: Felt sense

Li was able to put into words her thoughts and feelings, but what about the person who struggles to do this, a person who has a "felt sense" or bodily sensation rather than tangible cognitions? It is not uncommon for the meaning that drives an act to be essentially visceral rather than verbal or visual and both client and therapist can struggle to put these types of meanings into words. This is well illustrated by a client with anorexia nervosa who maintains, "I just *feel* fat," or by the client with obsessive-compulsive disorder (OCD) who protests that "I still *feel* dirty. I simply *feel* that I could contaminate someone" or—as in the example below—the client who tries to explain that his self-injury is driven by an unbearable sensation that seems only to transform if he hurts himself.

In such cases, you can use Socratic Dialogue to first enquire about thoughts and visual images. If nothing is forthcoming (despite giving your client plenty of time to reflect), ask what emotions are present. Sometimes this is a useful "anchor" for clients to start their exploration. For example, someone who cannot readily identify cognitions might be able to describe emotions: "I feel scared, nervous ..." and so on. Once emotions have been identified, people frequently begin to add something like "I feel that ..." and then identify a cognition such as "I feel that something bad will happen." Some clients cannot even anchor their reactions in emotion and then questions can help to anchor it in sensation:

- Where is it in your body?
- What is happening in your body?
- Does it have a shape/color? and so on.

Again, some people will find that they can move from sensation to cognition (e.g., "When I get that feeling, I know I'm not safe"). When clients do not make this bridge from sensation to cognition, you can productively stay with their sensation and engage in a "visceral" transformation. For example, you can help your client substitute a soothing, satisfying physical experience for their distressing one.

Twenty-four-year-old Lucas had a history of both childhood and adult sexual molestation. With his therapist's help he had managed to reduce many unhelpful behaviors including binge-eating, overexercising, and overspending and he had stopped cutting himself in several situations. There was, however, one situation in which he felt absolutely compelled to self-injure but he could not put it into words. Attempts to encourage him to describe thoughts, images, and even emotions had failed; he would say: "It just is!" or "I just have to cut. I just need to."

Therapist:	Let's revisit the last time you felt this compelling urge to cut. Can you describe what was happening?
Lucas:	I was alone at home—nothing in particular had happened that day—and the need to cut just got stronger.
Therapist:	Can you stay with that feeling and tell me a little more about it? Where is it in your body? What is its color, texture, temperature, for example?
Lucas:	It's throughout my body—it's red and burning, spiky and cutting through my skin. I know the only way to switch it off is to cut.
Therapist:	Let's fast forward and imagine that you have switched off this awful sensation. What do you feel in your body now?
Lucas:	Green.
Therapist:	Can you tell me more about this "green" feeling?
Lucas:	It's a soft mossy green spreading through my body. It has flecks of golden.
Therapist:	Can you stay with that feeling and describe it to me in more detail?
Lucas:	It's soothing, it's comforting, safe.
Therapist:	Can you tell me more about the feelings in your body?
Lucas:	It's as if my muscles become spongy but strong. Every single muscle, even down to my fingertips and toes. Even in my face.
Therapist:	Tell me more about your face: what's in your expression?
Lucas:	I feel relaxed, serene. I can almost feel a smile.
Therapist:	That sounds good. Anything else?
Lucas:	I breathe easily, and it makes me feel relaxed and also strong.
Therapist:	And when you feel relaxed and strong—how do you feel or imagine your body position?
Lucas:	Well, I feel my shoulders lift up and back, but they are not tense. My posture feels more upright and confident.
Therapist:	Excellent. Let me check—are you feeling those strong, comforting sensations now?
Lucas:	Yes.

Therapist: That's interesting isn't it? You have managed to tap into that good feeling by simply using your thoughts. What do you make of that?

Lucas: Maybe I can get the green feelings without cutting?

Therapist: It's something to consider. Let's imagine that you were going to be able to do this in the future, what do you think might help you be good at it?

Lucas: Lots of practice I suppose.

Notice how Lucas's therapist got as much detail as possible from Lucas. Her goal was both to shed light on his soothing experience and to help build a vivid imaginal picture. As was discussed in Chapter 5, she enquired about multiple sensory parts of his experience, not just visual ones. The therapist asked about bodily sensation, body position, and facial expression in order to maximize the advantage of Lucas's positive awareness of multiple aspects of his desired state.

Thus, this part of their therapy focused on unpacking meaning at a visceral level and "replacing" a negative visceral experience with a constructive one. Lucas and his therapist then devised an assignment whereby he practiced accessing the "good" feelings without cutting. Once he was able to reliably do this in a fairly short amount of time, they planned a behavioral experiment to check out the validity of Lucas's belief that cutting was the only way to switch off the negative sensations. By engaging in the behavioral experiment, he discovered that he could imagine the green feeling and accompanying sensations vividly enough to soothe himself in a particularly painful situation, a situation in which he normally would have cut himself to get the same result.

Lucas and his therapist could only speculate about the origin of his powerful negative sensations. He had been sexually violated at an early age and there were medical records to substantiate this. They hypothesized that he had perhaps laid down the "meaning" of those physically painful experiences not in words or even pictures but as a body sense. Lucas accepted that he might never be certain of the origin of his terrible sensations, and he focused now on honing his skill in combatting them in his day-to-day life.

Physiological drives can also contribute to the maintenance of unhelpful behaviors. People experience a "high" when endorphins or adrenaline are released, calm after a drop in blood pressure at the sight of blood, and strong physical cravings for food, alcohol, or drugs. The drive behind impulses and compulsions cannot be fully appreciated unless you have also explored these physiological aspects. Ask questions such as:

"And how did that feel physically as well as emotionally?"
"And then what happens in your body or your mind?"

In addition, engagement in impulsive or compulsive behaviors is more likely following drug or alcohol use that disinhibits a person. Direct enquiry regarding the use of alcohol and prescriptive and non-prescriptive drugs is recommended in order to gauge direct and indirect risk to both the client and those around the client.

Trap 2

Not appreciating the level of risk of serious harm to your client or to others

---

ICBs often include risk of danger to self or others. It is important to remember that people who present in the emergency department with self-harm have a relative risk of suicide forty-nine times greater than the general population (Hawton et al., 2015). Socratic Dialogue can help you identify your client's level of risk, times of risk, and also ways of managing risk. Risk assessment is crucially important and a legal requirement in most parts of the world. Throughout therapy, make sufficient enquiries to enable you to gather enough information so you can make a judgment concerning risk of harm to your client and/or to others (adults and/or children).

Enquiries about suicidality or aggression towards others must reveal unambiguous responses and therefore therapists are encouraged to achieve clarity by asking direct questions such as:

"Do you have plans to kill yourself?" or
"Do you ever think that you could harm her?" or
"Do you ever see this happening in your imagination?"

Such risk assessment questions are only likely to initiate honest responses when they are asked within a framework of a good therapeutic relationship. We advocate using a combination of Socratic enquiries and empathic statements to help establish and maintain a positive therapy alliance.

> **Keep in Mind**
>
> - Risk assessment should be ongoing, not limited to your initial assessment.
> - Establish a trusting and safe relationship in order to maximize the likelihood of your client being honest about risk issues.

A mixture of direct Socratic informational questions will help you—and your client—appreciate whether risk is an issue. You can gently and sensitively assess the possibility by asking exploratory questions designed to prompt your client to consider and share feelings and thoughts about self-harm or harm to others. Follow-up questions can then be more direct. For example, observe the sequence of questions this therapist asks her gender non-binary client Misha who has a history of self-injury and attempted suicide:

Therapist: I realize that you have had a much harder week this week and that it's been really tough for you.

Misha: Yeah.

Therapist: When you feel this low, how do you cope, how do you get through the week?

Misha: I go out walking, just walking for miles and miles.

Therapist: Does this help?

Misha: Not really—I feel bad when I get home, only I'm too tired to do anything. So I guess it helps in that way—it stops me doing anything.

Therapist: Do anything? What sort of thing?

Misha: Drinking too much so I can't work properly next day.

Therapist: I see. Anything else?

Misha: Cutting myself—like really badly.

Therapist: Can you say a bit more about that?

Misha: Well you know, going deeper than usual.

Therapist: I'm wondering—how does that help at the time?

Misha: Well, I think that it might fix things for good.

Therapist: For good—how so?

Misha: I suppose I might bleed to death.

Therapist: I see. Misha, from what you are telling me, I can appreciate that things are much more difficult for you now—do you have thoughts of killing yourself?

Misha's therapist begins by asking empathic and curious questions about how they are managing a very difficult week. Rather than jumping quickly to direct risk assessment questions, this therapist listens to their client's statements and asks follow-up questions using the client's own words about what has been revealed each step along the way. For example, "Do anything? What sort of thing?" By patiently gathering information at the pace Misha is willing to reveal it, the therapist arrives at this point in the interview when it seems natural to ask direct questions to establish risk. Asking such questions prematurely could have led Misha to be less forthcoming and honest about their experiences.

Relapse Management

A further risk that we need to consider—and keep under consideration—is the risk of relapse. Irresistible behaviors are, by definition, difficult to resist and your client might remain at risk of lapse or relapse well into therapy and long after the behavior has apparently stopped. Urges and cravings can be extremely powerful—irresistible at times. That is why it is more realistic to talk of relapse "management" than relapse "prevention." Although you will probably support your client in abstaining from problem behaviors (indeed there might be legal and/or medical reasons for doing so) they are likely to remain very vulnerable to lapses because of the presence of strong urges and cravings and they need to be aware of the risk of relapses and the most helpful ways of managing them.

> **Trap 3**
>
> Underestimating the risk of relapse

Some years ago, I became complacent. My client and I had a contract wherein she had agreed not to self-harm. As she had not injured herself in several months, I jumped to the conclusion that she was in easy control of her urges. One session in October she arrived having inflicted serious self-injuries for one hour, precisely. On the previous Sunday morning, when the UK clocks changed from British Summer Time, she realized that there was one hour unaccounted for in our contract and therefore she could give in to the urges without breaking the contract. Only then did I appreciate that although her behavior had changed, her craving to self-harm had hardly shifted at all. Think how different the situation would have been if I had checked out my hunch that she was overcoming her urges; how I might have helped her work toward relapse management earlier.

It is helpful to introduce the concept of relapse management as soon as possible so that your client has plenty of time to develop the *skill* of relapse management. Good relapse management includes:

- Regularly checking in on urge levels; don't assume that the absence of the behavior means that the craving has gone;
- Helping your client identify personal risk of lapse or enhanced craving/urges;
- Helping them practice how to learn from setbacks; and
- Helping them develop a repertoire of relevant coping strategies.

Our clients are particularly vulnerable to ICBs if they only have access to an impoverished range of coping options because then the route to engaging in an unhelpful behavior will be relatively unobstructed. Therefore, we aim to help them develop a range of coping options, and keep in mind that alternative coping strategies must have credibility for them (see the later section on "Safer, substitute behaviors"). Thus, it is extremely important to use Socratic Dialogue to gain an understanding of a person's idiosyncratic strengths and vulnerabilities in order to build on those strengths and help craft alternative ways of coping that appeal to that person.

Damage limitation

It can also be helpful to employ an approach that embraces "damage limitation." This simply means minimizing the extent of harm to self or others in the event of lapse. Examples include a person who misuses drugs planning to use clean needles and not share them; someone who binge-eats agreeing not to combine the binge with alcohol—which would worsen it; a person who at present cannot resist the urge to self-injure using clean blades when cutting, and so on.

Teaching relapse management and damage limitation can be done didactically. However, Socratic Dialogue may prove a more useful approach for understanding your client's risk as demonstrated in the previous dialogue with Misha. Socratic approaches also can help people devise an individualized plan for how to anticipate setbacks and use their lapses to better understand their needs and to personalize their use of coping strategies. You can see this in action in the following example with Liz, which also illustrates how Socratic

Dialogue can be used to develop a client-driven solution to managing relapse at the same time it addresses absolutistic thinking, an Achilles heel for relapse.

Keep in Mind

- Check urge and craving levels.
- Relapse management is a fundamental life skill for those who are vulnerable to relapse, so start it as soon as possible. The earlier the training and practice, the better.
- Devise a number of alternative coping strategies; the more meaningful coping strategies your client has, the less likely is their relapse.

After nearly 20 years of abstinence, 45-year-old Liz began using drugs again after an emotional trauma. She returned to injecting heroin following a relationship breakup. Although at present she was using clean equipment and not mixing drugs, she was using it alone, which was particularly dangerous.

Therapist: Let me see if I've got this right. Last night when you got these really strong cravings, you found that you started thinking things like: "right now I *need* this: nothing else will do," and, "this is the last time and then I *will* go cold turkey tomorrow." You then telephoned one of your old contacts who supplied you in the past. Once a meeting was set up, you got increasingly excited about the fix and there was no ambivalence about taking drugs.

Liz: That's about right and that's how it is every time. Once I've got it in my head, there is no going back.

Therapist: Sounds like we have a chain of events here. How do you feel about us looking for places where we might break the chain?

Liz: I'm not sure that I can break the chain, but okay, let's look at it.

Therapist: Let's start with the cravings; what typically triggers cravings?

Liz: That's easy—two things. It's going to happen when my body tells me I need a fix and also when I'm feeling rotten. When I think of the mess I've made of my life and how miserable a specimen I am. I'm such a total failure.

In the Therapist's Mind

This therapist now must make a decision: focus on the cognitive bias of absolutistic thinking ("total failure") or on her self-criticism. It's the sort of decision that therapists have to make frequently. Knowing Liz, this therapist decided that there was perhaps more therapeutic mileage in tackling self-criticism because this was a primary trigger for her drug use. There is always the option of reviewing the "all-or-nothing" thinking later.

Therapist:	Let's try something. When you think of the mess you've made and how miserable a specimen you are; when you have those types of thoughts, how might a more compassionate side of you respond?
Liz:	We've been here before and you know it's not that easy for me to be gentle on myself.
Therapist:	I do appreciate that but *if* you were gentle on yourself, what would you be saying?
Liz:	I'd say: Come on Liz, it's not a *complete* mess, get some perspective here. You had fifteen really good years when you were clean and the relationship with Phil was actually bad for you and you are better off without him.
Therapist:	That's pretty supportive. Let's write that down so we remember it. (Writing.) How much do you believe it?
Liz:	9/10 right now; 1/10 when I'm miserable and alone.
Therapist:	Well, 9/10 suggests to me that there's more than a grain of truth to your more gentle perspective. What do you think?
Liz:	I suppose so. Those things are true enough. But it's hard to think that way when I'm alone and feeling low.
Therapist:	We can work on making it more believable when you are alone and low. Is there anything else that you could say to comfort yourself?
Liz:	I do beat myself up over losing my job and not turning up for interviews but I suppose I could remind myself that I did try my best to hold it together and if I can get clean again now I might well get another chance. It's not all over for me.
Therapist:	Take a minute and write those ideas down too. (Pauses, while Liz writes.) What do you notice about your perspective when you are kinder to yourself?
Liz:	It's not so extreme. I can see that I'm not totally washed up and a complete and utter failure.

Therapist: How does that help you?

Liz: I feel more hope and less desperate—so I might not feel so desperate for a fix.

Therapist: So already you have real insight into your vulnerability to relapse and some challenges to the first step in the chain. Let's both write these things down. (Pauses, while they both write in their notes.) The next step seems to be when you square it with yourself by saying things like, "I need this" and "This is the last time." How might you weaken these "permission-giving" thoughts?

Liz: Well, I know from my years of staying clean that I don't need the fix; I just feel as though I do. And it never is the last time—who am I kidding?

Therapist: Want to write those down, too?

Liz: Yes.

Therapist: Then you get in touch with someone who can supply you. How might you sabotage that part of the pattern if it goes that far?

Liz: That's really hard but I can see that I have to do this. I should get rid of all the telephone numbers. I know that I will remember one or two so I wonder if I should get rid of my phone—I never actually go downtown to find a fix; I set it up from home so it would be very difficult to get the stuff without my mobile. But life would be difficult without a phone. I'm going to have to think about this one.

Therapist: That's okay—we don't want to rush any part of this planning. It would be a good idea to think of what we are doing now as the foundation of a plan and you could "fine-tune" the plan over the course of this week. What do you think?

Liz: Sounds sensible. I'll do that before our next meeting and that will give me a chance to see if I can talk it through with Jake—he is my "addictions buddy" from years back and we've kept in touch. He's probably got lots of good ideas and he'll support me on this.

Together they then mapped out the steps in the chain of events leading to drug taking, and noted what they had so far identified to break the chain at an early stage. Now Liz and her therapist have a plan to minimize the likelihood she will lapse into drug taking in the upcoming weeks.

But relapses do happen, and that is why it is important that Liz has relapse management skills. It is not unusual for clients to shy away from these plans and if they do, you need to discover why. Perhaps they feel like it will somehow jinx their recovery if they think about lapsing; perhaps they are avoidant and don't like the discomfort of thinking about relapse; perhaps they are dichotomous thinkers so an urge or craving is enough to make them give up and abandon relapse management; perhaps they are ambivalent about giving up the behavior. Therapists should encourage thorough exploration of the obstacles to relapse management and be prepared to play "devil's advocate" as Liz's therapist does later in this session:

Therapist: So we have a preliminary plan and over time we will "fine-tune" it so that it better meets your needs. But let's just think of when things might go awry: let's imagine that you make a phone call to a dealer. How will you respond?

Liz: I'll probably label myself a failure, feel worse, and get the fix.

Therapist: And how would a gentle, compassionate you respond?

Liz: (Long pause.) I'd say we all have lapses—a phone call doesn't mean a hit. I am an addict not a failure.

Therapist: What is the difference for you?

Liz: We talk about this in my addict meetings. If I label myself a failure I give up. If I acknowledge I'm an addict, then I'm saying that it's no wonder that I have cravings but I do have choices—I could ring Jake straight away and I could try to refuse the drugs.

Therapist: So that's a good strategy for recovering from a lapse; let's remember that and write it down. Now—what if you took them, what if you took the drugs?

Liz: Do I have to think about this—I'm just beginning to consider coping again. I want to stay with positive thoughts.

Therapist: Of course you want to stay with positive thoughts; that's natural and I don't want to stress you unnecessarily, but can you see any advantage in us considering some other scenarios? Situations where you might struggle?

Liz: I suppose I'm prepared for the worst. My dad always used to say, "prepare for the worst and hope for the best" and I guess that's what we are doing. OK—so, even if I injected, I could really and truly try to make it my last time by getting help as soon as possible afterwards. I do want to kick this.

Therapist: How can you make it as easy as possible to get that help?

Liz: Speed dial. That's where I'll keep Jake's number—and my NA lead, and my community nurse link. I'll also add a couple of friends who I know would be there for me.

Therapist: Again, another good strategy for pulling out of a lapse—and again, let's write this down. This is really encouraging—you have good ideas for preventing a lapse from turning into a drug binge. (Pause).

	Now—do you have a sense of when you are vulnerable, what you need to look out for?
Liz:	I've discussed this a lot at with Jake in the past and I know that my high-risk situations are feeling lonely and being alone—especially at a time when my body is craving a fix. So I know that I need to keep up contact with friends and to make sure that I have activities at home. You won't believe how many jigsaw puzzles I have to distract myself! Luckily for me my current friends are not part of an active drug scene. My "clean" years have helped me build up a great social circle.
Therapist:	Excellent. Well done. You know what your high risk situations are and you are taking steps to minimize risk. Read your written plan and make sure you've reminders there so that if you do lapse, you will use strategies for recovering from lapses instead of reprimanding yourself and then feeling worse. (Pauses while Liz does this.)There is one thing that I would like you to add to you plan, though.
Liz:	What's that?
Therapist:	When you have a craving or a lapse, ask yourself: "Why is this understandable?"; "What have I learnt from this?" and "What will I do differently next time?" Write those three questions down so we can look at them together. (Repeats the questions while Liz writes these on her plan.) Any thoughts on why I might be asking this of you?
Liz:	I suppose the first question helps me to be caring and kind towards myself. The second helps me understand myself better so that I am better prepared and the third prompts me to update my plans so they will be more watertight.
Therapist:	That's right. It sounds like a cliché but we want every setback to be a useful learning experience. Do you think that you could summarize what we've discussed about managing relapse so far?

Systematically, Liz and her therapist built up a strategy for managing relapses that reflected her particular strengths and needs and which incorporated setbacks as learning opportunities. Although her therapist is initially didactic in recommending the strategy for learning from setbacks, their therapeutic interaction becomes Socratic when the therapist asks: "Any thoughts on why I might be asking this of you?" This analytical question directs the Liz toward personalizing the suggestion and generating a rationale that makes it more likely that she uses the strategy.

Although as therapists we—quite rightly—want to encourage and to emphasize strengths, when we carry out relapse management we must direct clients toward considering, and even dwelling on, their vulnerabilities. Sensitive Socratic Dialogue can help us do this. If we avoid doing so, or address vulnerabilities too lightly, we risk having inadequate plans in place.

Averting relapse is increasingly likely as our clients become more skilled in self-help strategies. A conceptually simple strategy that can also be introduced very early on, and one that helps fight urges and cravings, is substituting a safer behavior.

Safer, substitute behaviors

As a trainee many years ago, I observed a weight loss therapy group. The leader suggested that chocolate cravings could be curbed by eating a banana. Now, anyone who loves chocolate will realize that this is a poor substitute—but it has got quite a lot going for it. Just like chocolate, it is quickly accessible, it is sweet, and it packs a carbohydrate "lift" so it has similarities that can dull a chocolate craving. Sometimes an urge to engage in problem behavior can be resisted if a substitute action fulfills a similar function: a chocolate craving might well be dulled by eating a banana.

Substitute behaviors are ideal when they can "take the edge off" the urge. For example, if your client's goal is respite from stress, then forms of relaxation-training and developing soothing imagery can be helpful. If the aim is punishment, then benign forms of unpleasant activities such as uncomfortable exercises or cleaning a filthy shed can replace them. If the purpose is excitement, then adrenaline-provoking sports might be a good substitute.

The impact of substitute activities is rarely as immediate and as effective as the problem behavior and we must be honest about that with our clients—a banana will never perfectly substitute for a bar of chocolate. Nevertheless, substitute activities can interrupt what might otherwise seem like an irresistible urge to do something damaging. The continuation of the session with Li, who struggled to resist binge-eating, illustrates this.

Keep in Mind

- Substitute behaviors can take the edge of a craving.
- Be honest with your clients about their limitations.

Therapist: You said that binge-eating makes you feel good, powerful even, and that it gives you hope. Can you tell me a bit more about the "upside" of binging?

Li: I suppose I'm an expert on this, so here goes. When I decide to binge, I feel such relief because I don't have to fight the urge anymore. And I feel excited at the prospect of all the different foods I can treat myself to, really nice stuff so that I feel special. I start to feel "normal" because I can eat what I want. And then when I unwrap the cakes and the chocolate and there's no limit to what I can have—I feel so, well, joyful. I know it's a strong word but that's how I feel at first—before it all goes wrong. Then I panic and I hate myself and I'm so terrified of getting fat that I do whatever I have to do to get rid of the disgusting food and flesh. I vomit, I take laxatives, I starve, and I run and run until I feel that my insides could drop out.

Therapist: Listening to this helps me appreciate just why binge-eating is sometimes so irresistible despite the consequences and why you then feel compelled to take drastic action to make up for it. Binging seems to offer so much: you get a sense of relief when you make the decision to give in to the urge to eat; you feel excitement and you can feel as though you are special; you feel "normal" and also joyful. Have I understood you?

Li: Yes—all those things.

Therapist: Are there other ways that you could achieve these good feelings? Perhaps ways that don't involve binge-eating.

Li: Nothing works like binge-eating.

Therapist: Quite. So we are looking for activities that might in some small way recreate the powerful positive feeling that you have when you plan or engage in a binge. For example, is there anything else that gives you a sense of relief?

Li: Cutting does—but I don't want to start that again.

Therapist: I think that's a good attitude, but tell me a bit more about the relief you get from cutting or deciding to binge.

Li: It's a lovely "whoosh" of calm. All my tension flows away and I feel a bit unreal—in a nice way.

Therapist: Have you ever had even *something* of that feeling without resorting to cutting or binging?

Li: When I get back from a run I feel like that for a while and—although I think that they are lame—those relaxation exercises give me a bit of the feeling, but only a bit.

Therapist:	So that's a start—let's write these down. Running and relaxation exercises can recreate something of that feeling. Anything else? Anything at all, however modest?
Li:	Well there is something else that has a bit of that effect—holding a warm mug of milk, especially if it has honey in it. I love the smell of it and the warmth. I have to hold it with both hands, and it has to be a proper mug, not a little cup. You know, I also love the smell of vanilla and that gives me a mild "whoosh." And there are a couple of perfumes that will do it, too.
Therapist:	Good—more things to add to the list. Now we might be able to come up with even more "relief-giving" things to do, but at this point do you have any ideas about using this list of alternative behaviors?
Li:	I know where you are going with this and you are suggesting that instead of getting relief from planning a binge I should go for a run or relax or something. But it isn't that easy.
Therapist:	I'm sure that it's not easy at all; otherwise you'd be doing it without help. It might not work every time, and you've said that the relief will not be a great as it is with cutting of planning a binge, but how about we try to improve your relaxation skills and we do some planning so that it might be easier to take a run, smell vanilla, have a hot drink? Is there anything to lose?
Li:	No. I'll give it a go because it might just help me get over the urges.

Li and her therapist then made plans to take this forward. Her therapist also used Socratic Dialogue to help Li identify what substitutes might be appropriate to achieve a degree of the thrill, the feelings of being normal, the feelings of being special, and the joy that Li had identified earlier.

Trap 4

Not appreciating your client's fluctuating motivation and so neglecting to work on it

---

Impulsive and compulsive behaviors are, by definition, difficult to relinquish and your client is likely to be very ambivalent about doing so. It is important therefore to use Socratic Dialogue to help your client make a *genuine* decision to change before fully engaging in more "traditional" therapy methods for managing ICBs. As a start, we can draw on the motivational methods of Miller and Rollnick (2012) that emphasize nonjudgmental listening with reflections of dilemmas and choices.

Keep in Mind

- Irresistible behaviors are genuinely compelling: clients can thus slip in and out of motivation to change. Anticipate that they are at risk of relapse.
- Be your client's curious ally: support motivational statements, reflect dilemmas, and convey the message that you are not here to judge but to aid.
- Maintaining a stance of a nonjudgmental ally can be particularly difficult when a client's behavior conflicts with our own values. When this is the case, seek supervision or consultation.

Lars was a married salesperson in his early forties. A year ago his job began to take him away from home and he spent several nights each month in expensive hotels. This change enabled him to indulge in his fantasy of having casual sex. His wife had recently discovered this and had left him, taking their two children with her. His goal in therapy was to persuade her to return.

In the Therapist's Mind

Lars' therapist disapproved of infidelities and so was very aware that she needed to consciously put aside her own prejudices and she sought supervision to help make sure she did this. Discovering why Lars' behavior made sense to him was her most sure way of being able to find empathy for him, so this was her first goal. She knew that Lars was ambivalent about changing so she anticipated encouraging him to not only draw his own conclusions about the advantages of change, but to repeat and review these advantages so that they really hit home. She also aimed to explore troubleshooting early on in therapy as she saw that relapse was very possible.

Therapist: You know, there are no guarantees that your wife will return even if you work hard in therapy, so we need to think about what is achievable—what changes are within *your* control.

Lars: That's logical, yet it hadn't occurred to me. I've been thinking more about getting her to change her mind than me changing.

Therapist: Can you foresee any problems with that?

Lars: Yeah. My wife is smart and there's no hope that she'll return unless she believes I've made genuine changes in the way I think and behave. She's got to see that I'm different.

Therapist: So, genuine change is going to be central to our work?

Lars: Yes. I want to change.

Therapist: On a scale of 1–10, where 10 is maximum commitment and 1 is no commitment, how do you rate yourself?

Lars: 10.

Therapist: That sounds good, and I don't want to question your genuineness but I do wonder what, if anything, might undermine that commitment. Can you help me understand what made casual sex so compelling over the past year?

Lars: That's easy. First, there's the thrill of the chase: anticipating a conquest and fantastic sex, walking into the bar, making a choice, and enjoying the challenge of courting her. I feel like a lion looking to mate. Once we're in the hotel room we are strangers so I can be anyone I like and I can make her anyone I want. I can't tell you how exciting and liberating that is—it makes for the best sex I've ever had. And that leaves me wanting more.

Therapist: I can see that this is compelling for you. With that in mind, I wonder what your commitment to change rating is right now.

Lars: (Pause.) 3 at the most.

Therapist: What could this be telling us?

Lars: I know what I should do, and I yet want something different. If I'm honest I have to say that I want Viv and the kids back because I love them but I don't want to give up the best sex I've ever felt in my life.

Therapist: That's quite a dilemma: you want to share your life with the people that you love the most and you want to do the thing that will drive them away.

Lars: I guess so.

Therapist: In addition to losing your family, are there any other penalties for continuing to have sex with others?

Lars: Well the "cold light of day" is rarely fun. I never want breakfast with these women and sometimes it's hard work giving them that message. I don't feel too great the next morning either, if I'm honest. I have to admit I feel cheap and I worry that Viv might find out.

Therapist: Can you remember how it felt when she did find out?

Lars: Yeah—that has to be the worst feeling ever. My life flashed before my eyes—I'd blown everything that really matters. I'd lost my family.

Therapist:	Can you recall the feelings that went with that?
Lars:	Fear, panic, regret, devastation, anger with myself, sickness in my stomach. Oh God it was bad.
Therapist:	Can you stay with those feelings? Can you really recall just how bad they are?
Lars:	Yeah: I feel sick deep in my stomach. I'm so afraid. I hate myself. It's the worst—just the worst.
Therapist:	So, in trying to achieve the best feeling you ever had you experienced the worst?
Lars:	Yeah.
Therapist:	What is strongest right now: wanting to get the best feeling or wanting to avoid the worst?
Lars:	Wanting to avoid the worst—and I mean 10 out of 10!
Therapist:	That's good that you want to avoid that feeling; it means that you are making a commitment to change. You know people sometimes waver in their commitment during the course of therapy: how might you hold on to yours?
Lars:	Remembering that night and this conversation. And just what it feels like to think I've done something so devastating.
Therapist:	And how could you keep your memories vivid?
Lars:	(Quietly thinking for a minute.) I could make a voice recording on my mobile phone.

His therapist continued to help Lars become aware of, and then address, the real dilemmas that he faced. This is a key aspect of motivational work and it is crucial that the therapist is respectful and nonjudgmental to both sides of the dilemma—something that is not always easy when clients present with behaviors that seem reprehensible or shocking from the therapist's perspective.

The first task of therapy is to help clients appreciate their dilemma and hold the negative consequences of a behavior in mind to the degree they feel motivated to address it. Then there is a real possibility the therapist can use Socratic Dialogue to facilitate management strategies. In Lars's case Socratic enquiry revealed that he felt better about himself during episodes of illicit sex so his therapist hypothesized that he would benefit from working on his self-esteem—this led to some very fruitful work on self-esteem which actually diminished his urges.

Some clients initially engage in reducing target behaviors but they become ambivalent because the risk of giving up the compelling behaviors seems too much. When this occurs, motivation needs to be addressed anew as demonstrated in the next case example.

Thirty-five-year-old Hector had a ten-year history of health anxiety. He participated in therapy on a number of occasions and made progress only to become demotivated time and time again. He and his new therapist mapped out a formulation that explained why he felt compelled to self-check, almost constantly scanning his body for signs of ill health and scanning the media for health-related articles. He had made initial progress but had now returned to checking his body for signs of illness. Because she felt at a loss what to do next, his therapist sought supervision from a health anxiety specialist.

Her supervisor recommended that Hector's therapist needed to understand his engagement and disengagement in therapy (through more Socratic enquiry) and to provide Hector with an actual experience in order to consolidate his motivation to change (through behavioral experiments). In addition, her supervisor recommended that the therapist needed to "troubleshoot" in anticipation of Hector struggling to resist checking. Since Hector is so afraid to give up checking, as before, his therapist must remain empathic and non-confrontative, while identifying dilemmas for him to reflect upon. The following dialogue reflects how Hector's therapist used Socratic Dialogue to carry out these recommendations:

Therapist: Can we look more closely at this pattern of you feeling motivated to take the risk of changing, but then finding yourself less able to do this?

Hector: OK.

Therapist: Let's look at the checking problem, the one that we are trying to tackle at present. Is that OK with you, if we start there?

Hector: Yes, that is something that I have been struggling with for years now. There have been times when I feel I'm coping and then I just lose the will to keep struggling - because it is a struggle.

Therapist: And if it is such a struggle, no wonder you are tempted to give in to the urges to physically check your body for signs of illness every hour or so.

Hector: And after all that torment and worry—if I check and ask my partner to check, I get such relief and I relax. You've no idea. No more worry about my health and no more fighting the urges.

Therapist: I can see the upside of the checking, I really can, and I can see why you lose the will to keep up with therapy. How long does that sense of relief last?

Hector: When I check I do think that this time it will do the trick, but the relief is short-lived and I am soon worrying again.

Therapist: What do you make of this?

Hector: Well I can see that checking feels good in the short term but it doesn't last—but there's no way you're going to get me to stop. It's too hard and I can't keep it up. I can't stand the feeling that I could have a terrible illness and I'd miss it because I've not checked. Even though I stopped checking for a while, I didn't feel better for long. It soon began to feel too risky.

Therapist: Can you say a little more about it being too risky?

Hector: Well, I might waste some time checking for things that aren't there but if there is a chance of something really bad I can't afford to ignore it.

Therapist: Why is that?

Hector: Because it could kill me.

Therapist: It sounds as if there is another assumption—another "…if…then…"—there that helps explain your drive to check: how would you put that into words?

Hector: *If* I don't check, *then* I could die.

Therapist: That is a pretty sobering assumption, so again I can see why it became so difficult to resist checking. (Pause.) This might sound like an odd question but, for you, what's the worst thing about dying?

Hector: I've seen someone die from (pause) cancer and it's the most painful and undignified death. I'll do everything I can to avoid that.

Therapist: I see. That seemed very difficult to say, but thank you for saying the words as it really helps me to know more about your fear. Can I just check that I understand—it is dying of cancer in pain and without dignity you fear, not dying in other ways?

Hector: That's right I don't want to risk dying … that way.

This was a new revelation that helped the therapist appreciate why it was so hard for Hector to keep to the therapy plans and his reluctance to even say the word cancer had prevented her from learning this earlier. Not addressing his key fear had probably contributed to his difficulty in staying motivated, and Socratic enquiry had at last help reveal what he most feared. Now his therapist could target this fear of cancer.

Therapist: I see. That is certainly something anyone would want to avoid and I can see your reasons for wanting to continue checking. I don't want to sound unsympathetic but I am left wondering how certain can you be that if you don't check you'll die of cancer?

Hector: Not 100%

Therapist: So, maybe there's room for doubt?

Hector: Maybe.

Therapist: How much?

Hector: 1%

Therapist: Okay, I'm not going to say that your assumption is wrong—maybe you're right, maybe not. If you are right, perhaps we need to find a more efficient way of checking for cancer so that it doesn't take up so much of your time and if you are not right, then we could work on plans to help you give it up. How does this sound to you?

Hector: Logical I suppose but how on earth could you decide?

Therapist: We know that you have been living as though it is true that if you do not check you could miss a symptom and die, so let's set that aside just for now, and go with the hunch that if you don't check every hour or so you still won't be at risk of dying of cancer. Have you ever lived as if this hunch were true?

Hector: Up until a few years ago—yes. I didn't even look out for health-related articles. Then my friend died.

Therapist: I can see how that might make things look different. But let's go back, say, twelve years. How often did you check your body for signs of illness?

Hector: Once in a blue moon. (Smiles.) I can tell by the look on your face that you want me to be more specific—once a week at the most. We live in a hot climate, so I'd take a good look at moles and freckles every now and then. I'd never go checking for lumps and I wouldn't do the whole-body scan thing.

Therapist: And when you did check, what happened next?

Hector: If it seemed okay I'd forget about it.

Therapist: So you just checked the once and then let it go?

Hector: That's right.

Therapist: And during that time, did you ever miss anything significant?

Hector: No.

Therapist: How often did you find something that concerned you?

Hector: Once a year, maybe.

Therapist: ... and what happened then?

Hector: I saw my doctor and she reassured me or ran tests.

Therapist: So it sounds as though a weekly check seemed sufficient back then?

Hector: Yes.

Therapist: Has anything happened to change your own health status over the last twelve years?

Hector: Apart from getting older, no.

Therapist: Has anything actually assured you about your health?

Hector: My doctor is always at pains to tell me how fit I am—and she's a good doctor.

Therapist: So, your doctor tells you that you are as healthy as you ever were and, in the past, you found it sufficient to carry out a "home check" once a week. Where do you think I might be going with this?

Hector: I know where you're going, and I'm thinking about it. I can see that checking just once a week sounds sensible. But will I be able to do it? I don't know.

Together, they then listed the pros and cons of living as if his life weren't in danger and Hector looked at the lists he had made and decided that it was worth a try. Thus, the pros and cons lists served as an additional Socratic exercise in helping him reach his own conclusions and remotivate himself.

Therapist: Let's think about this in some detail. You are going to engage in a weekly health check—when would be a good time for you to do that?

Hector: Well, the idea is that I check and then move on so I'd probably do it when I know that I can't hang around dwelling on my worries. On the other hand, I don't want to feel rushed or I'll get frustrated.

Therapist: . . . and what happens if you get frustrated?

Hector: Then I can't stop thinking about things and my health worries will go round and round in my head until I'm compelled to check properly.

Therapist: "Properly"?

Hector: Yes . . .

By listening carefully and noticing his use of the word "properly," Hector's therapist wisely enquired for details about what he meant. These questions uncovered that Hector had a ritual associated with checking which dictated that he check body parts in a certain order so as not to miss anything. Hector and his therapist then negotiated the briefest routine that would be manageable at this time, which Hector estimated would take two minutes if carried out once. They determined that Sunday morning would be a good time for his weekly check as he had about half an hour between breakfast and his yoga class. By doing his check then, he would not feel rushed.

Therapist: Let's imagine that you finish checking in two minutes—what then?

Hector: I know that I'll be tempted to repeat the checking.

Therapist: What could you do to prevent that?

Hector: Distract myself by looking at the Sunday news.

Therapist: Anything else you might do to make sure you are focused on something neutral?

Hector: I know—I won't have my coffee until then. Reading the news and fresh coffee can be my reward for not checking again.

Therapist: That sounds really good, but we need to think what might undermine your new routine. For example, what thoughts might you have in the following week or after your checking that might increase your urge to check again?

Hector: I'm not sure—there are so many! One typical one is that I can't afford to miss something important, something that is an important symptom.

Therapist: How might you respond to that?

Hector: This is not easy—I feel nervous thinking of it—but I could try to remind myself that I will get a chance to check on Sunday and a day or two's wait won't make a difference.

Therapist: How does that sound to you?

Hector: It actually seems true enough.

Therapist: That sounds good, then. Take a moment and write that down so you don't forget it. (Pauses while he does so.) We can try it out and see what happens. Any other sabotaging thoughts?

Hector: There's the "One quick check won't matter" that gets me into trouble.

Therapist: And how might you respond to that?

Hector: I'll tell myself: "A quick check is the thin end of the wedge." I'll also look at my pros and cons list to remind me that it's worth sticking to the new regime.

Therapist: Excellent strategy: you are coming up with so many good ideas. Let's write those down as well so you don't forget. (Pauses while he writes.) Are there any other problem thoughts?

Hector: I'm sure there are but I just can't think of any right now.

Therapist: As we've said before, it's often easier to catch relevant thoughts and images as they happen, so perhaps you could keep a log of interfering

	thoughts and images over the course of the week. If you can counter them, that's great and if not, we can do it here in the session.
Hector:	OK (adding this idea to his written notes).
Therapist:	Now, it's seems that you've got a pretty good plan going; can you run me through it?
Hector:	OK, here goes. I will check my body once—and only once—a week on Sunday mornings before my yoga class. I will distract and reward myself with fresh coffee and reading the news afterwards. If I have thoughts that increase my urge to check I will note them and use the strategies I've written down to counter them.

The outcome of this behavioral experiment was a useful guided discovery process for Hector. To maximize his learning from it, his therapist used Socratic Dialogue in the next session to debrief and make a written summary of his learning. His therapist then asked Hector analytical and synthesizing questions such as:

- That's really interesting—although it was difficult at first you did find that the urges diminished as the week went on. What do you make of that?
- Your anxiety levels gradually fell. What might that tell you about the link between checking and how you feel?
- So overall, what have you learnt from doing this experiment?
- How could you take things forward?

Hector's responses helped him to refine his own understanding of his urges to check and to personalize his strategy for tackling his problem.

In this example, you can see how Socratic Dialogue was first used to unpack the assumptions that made sense of compelling urges and the facilitating beliefs that then allowed Hector to check. Next it was used to elicit a new possibility—that it would be safe to behave differently. Once Hector acknowledged this, his therapist enlisted his collaboration in developing a behavioral experiment to test out the validity of this new possibility. Before sending Hector out to do this experiment, Socratic enquiries were used to identify obstacles and troubleshoot these to maximize the likelihood Hector would be able to carry out the behavioral experiment. An alternative approach would have been for the therapist to take more of a lead in assigning an appropriate behavioral experiment but this can undermine the sense of choice and autonomy that is so crucial in remotivating a person.

Later in therapy, Hector and his therapist tackled his reassurance seeking as it transpired that his partner was unwittingly undermining his progress by subtle reassurance giving. This contributed to Hector making less progress than he'd hoped for, which reduced his motivation again. This is a good example of Trap 5, overlooking the "bigger picture."

Trap 5

Overlooking the bigger picture: The wider world of your client

---

In therapy we learn about our client's inner world: the feelings and cognitions that support a target behavior. However, the client's abilities to cope with their current life circumstances can be just as relevant in understanding why a behavior is so irresistible. Without the drug dealer, constant criticism from family members, and the endorsement of unhelpful beliefs by friends, your client might not give in to urges. So often our clients' living conditions are dysfunctional and this can play a significant part in maintaining their problems. On the other hand, there may be supportive elements in their lives and we need to appreciate the potential that these positive resources offer. You can see that we really need to get the "bigger picture."

Hector's partner undermined his progress by being "helpful" and colluding with his checking. Ultimately, his partner was caring and could easily become an ally in Hector's recovery. Remember Liz? Although her ready access to a drug dealer made her more vulnerable to relapse, her equally ready access to addiction buddy Jake could help her to resist her drug cravings. External factors entirely motivated Lars to change—he wanted his wife and family back. It is so important to explore our clients' wider world. Then we can better understand their vulnerabilities *and* their assets. It is a matter of good practice to enquire about social support as this is something that can protect your client's mental health. It is equally relevant also to identify dysfunctional and pernicious aspects of their circumstances.

Either Socratic Dialogue or direct questioning can be employed to discover information about interpersonal, social, and cultural aspects of someone's life. Pose simple information-gathering questions, such as:

- Who else is involved?
- Who else could be affected by this?
- How do you think that they might feel when that happens?

Questions like these can also help clients develop an appreciation of the wider, domestic, social, and occupational implications of their behaviors—a good life skill.

If Hector's therapist had asked earlier in therapy, "How do others respond when you do x?", his partner's reassurance-giving could have been identified and addressed earlier. For example, his therapist could have asked Hector Socratic questions to help him review the pros and cons of his partner's support and ultimately motivate him to give up reassurance seeking and enlist his partner's help in not giving it.

Other aspects of the bigger picture that we sometimes neglect are our clients' personal resources and strengths. The extraordinary or exaggerated nature of some behaviors can draw our full attention to their negative aspects, not least because we are concerned about safety. For example, we might exclusively pursue details about why a person engages in a potentially damaging act and what aspects of their internal and external world facilitate this. Keep in mind that it is just as crucial to discover what prevents a person from doing something, what helps them resist. We can ask questions such as:

- When you resist checking, what goes through your mind?
- What sort of things interrupt your spending sprees?
- What is happening on those occasions you don't give in to the urge?

Responses to questions like these give us deeper insights into the problem and can be written down to help our clients begin to construct a coping repertoire.

Keep in Mind

- Clients have internal and external resources.
- Make sure that you identify them and help your client use them to enhance recovery.

The following therapy excerpt illustrates how one therapist used Socratic Dialogue to identify both internal and external resources that helped a client resist problem behaviors. Jahon was underweight and struggled to eat. He feared weight gain because, although he disliked his body now, he predicted that it would be even less attractive if he gained weight. His therapist understood Jahon's very negative view of his body and his negative thoughts around eating. She hypothesized that it was also important to learn more about his ability to eat and about his positive attitudes as these could be developed to help him take charge of his eating and feel more comfortable with himself.

Therapist: You have described to me the satisfying things about not eating: the sense of control, the pleasant "spaced out" feelings, for example, and you've told me about the fears you have about eating. Today I would be interested in learning more about the good things (however small) that you might remember about eating. Do you have any positive recollections?

Jahon: Of course! I can remember enjoying my food before I went on the diet but now I see it as my beautiful enemy.

Therapist: Beautiful enemy. That's interesting, can you say more?

Jahon: Well I liked food. I really did. And although some fatty and starchy foods disgust me now, there are plenty of things that I would love to eat.

Therapist: And have you enjoyed any foods lately?

Jahon: I suppose.

Therapist: Can you remember a recent time? Can you describe it to me?

Jahon: I went to my friend's tea party. He's wonderfully proper and has really civilized gatherings with canapés and nibbles—I'm not so nervous around food if it's "small."

Therapist: So "small" is good. Anything else that made it possible to enjoy the food at the party?

Jahon: It was delicious—I mean *really* good. Then I'm not so tempted to wolf it down—I want to taste it. And there was no alcohol which helps me stay in control. I get more "bingy" and careless if I drink.

Therapist: Anything else that helped?

Jahon: The company—I was enjoying myself. I felt good about myself.

Therapist: What was it that made you feel good about yourself?

Jahon: The people there were interesting and seemed to find me interesting. I felt as though I could contribute something and that I mattered. It was such a fabulous afternoon that I've kept photographs on my mobile phone.

Therapist: That's really nice. Now, let me see if I've got this right. It is easier for you to relax and enjoy food if it is high quality and small quantities, if you don't drink alcohol, and if you feel good about yourself.

Jahon: That's true—and it helps if I can decide whether to eat or not. A buffet is easier than a "sit-down" meal.

Therapist: We have been working on your eating plans recently—how might this be relevant?

Jahon: I could try to only buy really nice food that I can enjoy—instead of buying larger quantities of cheaper products, and our discussion

has underscored what we have already said about it being important to avoid alcohol.

Therapist: It is really interesting that you said that you had more control if you
felt good about yourself—any thoughts on how you might remind
yourself how you felt at the party?

Jahon: I could look at my photographs—in fact, I could print the best—and
try to remember just what it was like and perhaps I could try to link
up with some of these people.

Jahon and his therapist used the information they gathered to revise his
plans for eating in a more healthy way. His therapist then returned to the formulation and reminded Jahon that another issue that he had wanted to discuss was the role of his dislike of his physical appearance.

Therapist: ... and is there anything about your body that you do like?

Jahon: Are you kidding?

Therapist: Well, perhaps there is a part of your body that you dislike less?

Jahon: Shoulders—at least they are never fat and they are quite square,
which I do like. And my back is okay, it's quite muscular but everything else—ugh!

Therapist: Let's just stick with what you like. I noticed when you described
liking your shoulders and back, you sat straighter, seemed a bit different in your body. How did you feel at that time?

Jahon: I'd never thought of it before, but I guess I feel a *bit* more okay
about myself.

Therapist: A bit? How would you rate that using one of our 1 to 10 scales?

Jahon: I'd say 4/10 instead of 1/10.

Therapist: To me that seems really interesting—what do you make of it?

Jahon: I suppose I can feel a bit better about myself if I focus on the
positive—but I still don't feel good.

Therapist: But you do feel a bit better and that's a start. Can you think of ways
in which you might use this new insight?

Jahon: I'm not sure what you mean. What do you want me to say?

Therapist: I wasn't thinking of a specific answer I was really just curious to
explore how this ability to feel a bit better about your appearance
might help you deal with some of the problems that we've identified in our formulation.

Jahon: Well, I've always said that the worse I feel about my appearance
the more likely I am to binge and the more I binge the more I am
disgusted by my appearance. So I'm guessing that you think that
I could break that cycle by trying to feel better about my body.

Therapist: Well it's a theory. In your view is it one worth testing?
Jahon: [Laughing.] If it will make you happy, I'll give a go.

In this example, Jahon's therapist entertained a hypothesis that visual and body imagery could help him access and generate good feelings that could then be used to develop new insights to inform his behavioral experiments. For Jahon, it was unlikely that focusing on his familiar negative critiques of his body would have so readily resulted in these new insights.

Trap 6

The negative consequences of change

A further trap that we can fall into if we fail to fully use Socratic exploration is the trap of not realizing the negative consequences of change. In considering the "bigger picture" we often ask about the benefits of relinquishing ostensibly unhelpful behaviors but we sometimes fail to check out the dangers or disadvantages of doing so. Helping a person shift a problem behavior or reaction can sometimes have unhelpful consequences. For example, someone might stop excessive eating only to replace it with a more dangerous drinking habit. Someone else might learn to be assertive only to suffer a beating from a partner who could not tolerate this change.

In each of these cases the unhelpful outcome might be identified and managed in advance if the therapist asks questions to investigate the likely implications of behavior change. It is helpful to ask if there could be a downside to change. This question paves the way to think about how to manage predicted negative effects *before* focusing on diminishing target behaviors.

Keep in Mind

- All change is stressful. Stress can deplete a client's coping resources. Make sure your client has the resilience to cope with change.
- Check that your client's surrounding social systems can cope with change.
- Change can promote danger. Get a comprehensive enough overview to ensure that you and your client are aware of potential dangers and prepared for them.

Sarah, a teenager, was undernourished and badly scarred from two years of self-injury. She began neglecting herself and cutting and burning her legs and arms after a boyfriend had ended a relationship. He had been hypercritical of her body shape and now she hated the way she looked and this drove her self-harm. Understandably, her therapist wanted to help Sarah recover as quickly as possible and he assumed that the best way to do this would be to help her accept her body. In this example, you will see how he pushed for cognitive and emotional change prematurely and almost lost his therapeutic alliance with Sarah.

Therapist: ... and, for you, what is the hardest thing about resisting the urge to hurt yourself?

Sarah: If I don't cut or burn, then I can't obliterate this disgusting body.

Therapist: Disgusting? In what ways do you find your body disgusting?

Sarah: It just *feels* disgusting. It just *is* disgusting. Fat, ugly, and disgusting.

Therapist: It's curious that you say "fat" and ugly because you told me that you are now below average weight, and you have had compliments from many of your friends. How does this make sense?

Sarah: Like I said—it *feels* fat and ugly. I can just feel it. It doesn't matter what the scales or the mirror say. I *feel* fat, ugly, disgusting.

Therapist: Tell me, if we could change the way that you feel in your body—change it to an okay feeling—how would that be for you?

Sarah: Sounds impossible but I suppose that would help.

At this point her therapist used body-image restructuring to help Sarah develop a pleasant nonthreatening physical sensation. Initially this seemed to be helpful. Sarah felt less repelled by the "visceral" sense of her body and she agreed not to self-harm between their meetings. The therapist was pleased with this rapid progress. However, when Sarah returned to the following session, she was very distressed by the work that they had done. She explained that she had become more accepting that her body was "okay" and that this had terrified her because she feared that she would attract attention and be ridiculed again and that she would relax her dietary restrictions and become obese. In addition, by giving up cutting, Sarah had lost a very powerful means of feeling good through dissociation and she had already begun to smoke cannabis to compensate for the loss. She also had grown wary of her therapist.

With hindsight, Sarah's therapist realized that he should have been more exploratory and asked sufficient questions to establish the functions of self-injury before leaping in with an alternative coping strategy. He also appreciated that, before teaching her a self-acceptance strategy, he should have asked questions that might have revealed the disadvantages to finding her body acceptable, questions such as:

- We've been talking very positively about your learning to feel okay in your body. How do you feel about this?
- Imagine that you are feeling okay about your body, you like it, and you are out with friends or at work ... what thoughts and feelings do you have?

Or more directly:

- If you began to like your body and feel at ease with it, what could go wrong?
- What would be the worst thing about feeling good in your own skin?

Once Sarah's fears were identified, her therapist could then help her review them before refocusing on body-image restructuring. This enabled reparation of their therapeutic relationship and established a much firmer basis for continued body-image work.

When Other Methods Are More Appropriate

As mentioned in Chapter 1, didactic approaches are often more efficient for imparting new information, information that the patient is unlikely to have. For example, an explanation of the neurobiological basis of urges and cravings or information concerning the physical dangers of self-injury or substance misuse is often most efficiently communicated didactically. Recommending reading materials and vetted websites can also be an efficient way of educating a client about important information. Socratic Dialogue then can help clarify what clients learn from this new information, their positive and negative reactions to it, why and how they choose to use or ignore this information, and how to manage any relevant roadblocks.

Direct questions are, of course, appropriate when gathering background information. This is particularly crucial when carrying out a risk assessment because the therapist needs to quickly, and clearly, obtain critical information. For example, direct questions are important when assessing suicide risk (cf. Jobes, 2012). When we know irresistible behaviors are potentially dangerous, we should ask direct questions to assess the dangers our clients, or others around them, might face. This can include direct questions about the amount a person eats, the number of vomiting episodes, specific information about where they cut, what drugs they use, how much alcohol they ingest, whether the children are at home during the behavior, and any other relevant risk details.

Summary

Impulsive and compulsive behaviors can seem irresistible to our clients, but we can help them develop strategies for resisting them. This largely rests on you and your client developing a shared understanding of the motivations behind their ICBs and your client gaining confidence in the strategies that evolve from therapy. These two therapy goals can often best be realized through use of guided discovery methods. However, therapists must do this in the context of seeing beyond cognitions to relevant felt-sense experiences; beyond the individual to the systems that they live within; and beyond the now to a future where relapse management skills will be essential.

Reader Learning Activities

- Identify a current client who is trying to reduce either impulsive or compulsive behaviors.
- Review the six traps in this chapter and consider if any of these apply to your therapy with them.
- If so, review those sections and formulate the details of that trap. Then try out one of the interventions described there that seems likely to be clinically appropriate at this point in your therapy.
- If target behaviors are dangerous, see if you can use Socratic Dialogue to help your client identify safer, substitute behaviors.
- If your own therapist beliefs and assumptions risk hampering therapy, then formulate this obstacle and, if necessary, take it to a supervision or consultation session.
- Interview your client to learn about their perceived risks and/or negative consequences of change.
- Be careful not to overlook and miss formulating the role of the bigger picture. Find out who else in their life will be affected if they successfully make and maintain changes. How do they think the other person(s) will react?

References

Hawton, K., Bergen, H., Cooper, J., Turnbull, P., Waters, K., Ness, J., & Kapur, N. (2015). Suicide following self-harm: Findings from the multicentre study of self-harm in England, 2000–2012. *Journal of Affective Disorders, 175*, 147–151. https://doi.org/10.1016/j.jad.2014.12.062

Jobes, D. A. (2012). The Collaborative Assessment and Management of Suicidality (CAMS): An evolving evidence-based clinical approach to suicidal risk. *Suicide and Life-Threatening Behavior, 42*, 640–653. https://doi.org/10.1111/j.1943-278X.2012.00119.x

Kennedy, F. C., Kennerley, H., & Pearson, D. G. (Eds.). (2013). *Cognitive behavioural approaches to the understanding and treatment of dissociation*. London: Routledge.

Kennerley, H. (2004). Self-injurious behaviour. In J. Bennett-Levy, G. Butler, M. Fennell, A. Hackman, M. Mueller, & D. Westbrook (Eds.), *Oxford guide to behavioral experiments in cognitive therapy* (pp. 373–392.). Oxford: Oxford University Press.

Marlatt, G. A., & Gordon, J. R. (1985). *Relapse prevention*. New York: Guilford Press.

Miller, W. R., & Rollnick, S. (2012). *Motivational interviewing: Helping people change, 3rd Ed.* New York: Guilford Press.

8

Guided Discovery with Adversity

Stirling Moorey

> *Adversity has the effect of eliciting talents which, in prosperous circumstances, would have lain dormant.*
>
> **—Horace, *Satires* Book II, 8, 73–74**

Given the choice most of us would prefer a comfortable life, but when challenged it is remarkable how we can find strengths we never thought we possessed. On her 50th birthday the Swedish journalist Ulla-Carin Lindquist was diagnosed with amyotrophic lateral sclerosis—an incurable degenerative neurological condition. As she says in *Rowing without Oars* (Lindquist, 2006), her remarkable account of her final year of life:

There is only one end: death. No cure. No recovery.

What happens to a person in this situation?

A year ago I was a full-time TV reporter. Today I cannot eat without help, walk or wash myself.

I feel profound sorrow about everything I am not going to experience. I am devastated that soon I will leave my four children.

At the same time I feel great joy and happiness about everything I am experiencing at the moment. Several times a day my house is filled with laughter.

Does that sound strange?

(Lindquist, 2006, 1)

Her book is a moving story of how she lived with her condition, solving practical problems, maintaining some quality of life in the face of an inexorably shrinking world, and preparing herself and her family for her death. It is also an account of her emotional journey of anticipatory mourning—of letting go—of "rowing without oars." It exemplifies in a particularly vivid way the dilemma facing anyone coping with adversity: how do I keep a sense of control of my life, while still recognizing there are things I no longer have control over? This is summed up succinctly in the famous Serenity Prayer:

> Grant me the serenity to accept the things I cannot change,
> The courage to change the things I can,
> And the wisdom to know the difference.

Helping people cope with adversity is very much about supporting them in the process of decision making about what to accept and what to change in their lives, about finding ways to exert control over seemingly uncontrollable situations, and about living with uncertainty and uncontrollability. Ulla-Carin Lindquist found depths of resilience within herself. Many others when faced with significant challenges such as degenerative illness, disability, loss, or social or financial deprivation also negotiate these challenges naturally.

However, for some people, the challenges of adversity are so great they feel overwhelmed and experience clinical anxiety or depression. For these people cognitive behavior therapy (CBT), with its use of guided discovery, may be a particularly appropriate model for several reasons. First, CBT is based on the assumption that we are all doing our best within our unique cognitive world: it is the therapist's job to help us explore whether our thoughts and coping responses are as realistic and useful as possible. It is a normalizing rather than pathologizing model. The collaborative empiricism of CBT offers a supportive and respectful approach for clients who face significant life challenges, because it allows them to discover for themselves what works and what doesn't work.

Second, CBT is based on the assumption that the therapist allies with the client's strengths and resources, helping them rediscover talents, which have "lain dormant" in Horace's words, which have not been needed because "the buzz of life has been too loud" (Lindquist, 2006, 128). This work may actually be easier than CBT in general psychiatric settings, because many people facing adversity have coped effectively all their lives and then only decompensated under extreme stress. This means that the therapist often does not need to teach new skills, but to empower the client to rediscover old coping approaches, or use them more skillfully. CBT draws on the client's existing knowledge about how they managed situations in the past and helps them think through how they can apply this to their current problems.

This chapter describes how Socratic Dialogue can be applied in a range of adverse life situations. It begin with a presentation of some of the questions therapists can ask clients to help them cope better, illustrated from Lindquist's story. It then uses examples from clinical practice to demonstrate how Socratic approaches can help address some of the common difficulties encountered when working with this client group.

I have found it clinically helpful to divide coping into three areas of focus. In *problem-focused coping* we do things to remove or reduce the effects of the problem we are facing. In *life-focused coping* we engage in meaningful activities that may not be directly related to the problem but which might support us in dealing with it, or just in getting on with our life and maintaining its quality. In *internal-focused coping*, we attend to the emotional effects of the problems we are facing, through either managing difficult emotions or allowing space for natural feelings of sadness, grief, etc. to be experienced.

Ulla-Carin Lindquist's account illustrates all three of these types of coping:

> A year ago I carried a tripod along Svearagen in Stockholm.
> Today I am fed strained food.
> A year ago I asked questions about travel insurance.
> Today I'm checking over my life insurance.
> But.
> I can laugh.
> Hug my four children, or at least lift my left arm so that I can touch them.
> Hug my husband and kiss him with my semi-paralysed mouth.
> Read.
> Listen to music.
> Breathe fresh air.
> Wander in the labyrinth of my memory.
> Listen to friends.
> Peace … ?
> Feel peace within me!
> (Sometimes.)
>
> **(Lindquist, 2006, 130–131)**

When she checks her life insurance and discovers how to give cuddles with a weakened body she is engaging directly with her illness and mitigating its impact on her life (problem-focused coping). By finding activities that can still give her pleasure, such as reading and being with friends, she is focusing on areas of her life she can still control rather than on the areas she cannot (life-focused coping). At the same time, she is also allowing herself to experience the sorrow arising from the loss of control over her life and the future of her family (internal-focused coping).

Questions to Help Unlock Clients' Strengths

This section offers tips on how guided discovery can be used to:

- Help clients appraise their problems realistically and helpfully (Box 8.1),
- Build strengths in each of the three areas of coping (Boxes 8.2–8.4), and
- Find a balance in their coping (Box 8.5).

The core of any cognitive model is the assumption that our appraisals shape our feelings and behavior. Before we can select coping strategies we need to be able to appraise the situation in a realistic and hopeful way. Ulla-Carin Lindquist assessed her situation with searing realism, and did not hide from the fact that she was going to die. She did not respond with denial or wishful thinking, and yet she also did not fall into hopelessness and helplessness. She did not assume that her life was over, or that there was nothing to give life meaning while she still lived. This does not mean she did not sometimes experience anger, despair, and even self-pity. Coping is not about sailing through adversity without any storms, but rather, Lindquist made use of her resources and support to anchor her appraisals in reality. She made a decision about what, for her, was the most helpful way to approach her life:

> There are two roads I can take. One is to lie down, be bitter and wait. The other is to make something worthwhile of the misfortune. See it in a positive light, however banal that sounds. My road is the second. I have to live in the immediate present. There is no bright future for me. But there is a bright present. Nothing coming afterwards. Therefore I laugh like a child.
>
> (Lindquist, 2006, 72)

Not everyone can show this level of resilience. The realistic appraisal of a negative situation can easily lead to a spiral of distorted automatic thoughts that magnify and catastrophize, making something that is bad even worse. Sensitive and compassionate enquiry can help clients separate realistic negative appraisal from distorted and unhelpful thinking. Questions therapists can ask clients, or that clients can ask themselves are listed in Box 8.1.

Research has consistently shown *problem-focused* (Lazarus & Folkman, 1984) coping is associated with better adjustment across a range of stressful situations. Questions that facilitate problem-focused coping revolve around the theme—"Can I do anything to resolve or reduce the effect of the stress?" Lindquist's illness was terminal, but she was able to mitigate its effects to some

---

Box 8.1 Questions to help evaluate the situation

- Can I separate realistic negative thoughts from unhelpful critical or catastrophic thoughts?
- Am I catastrophizing or overestimating any aspects of the problem?
- Am I underestimating my ability to cope?
- Am I jumping to conclusions? What will things look like in 6 months or a year's time? Am I foreclosing on the future?
- Can I see this as a challenge?
- Is there anything good that might come out of it?
- If the situation is as bad as it seems, what are the implications? Am I making assumptions about what this means for my value and worth in my own and others' eyes?

---

degree. She, like many people with terminal illness, was able to plan for the future, do things to prepare her children for her death, and use practical aids to maximize her control over her life. One of the most striking examples is how she wrote the latter part of her book using a reflector on the tip of her nose to press down the computer keys. Questions clients can ask themselves to help promote problem-focused coping are found in Box 8.2.

Box 8.2 Questions to help with problem solving

- What strengths and resources do I have to deal with the situation?
- Have I faced similar difficulties in the past? How did I deal with them?
- What practical help or advice is available to me?
- Are there things I could deal with that I am avoiding?
- What can I do to remove the stress/problem/difficulty?
- If I can't eliminate it, what can be done to minimize or manage it?
- Can I break the problem-solving tasks down into manageable steps?
- What do I need to get started?
- What obstacles will I face?
- How can I overcome these obstacles?

Box 8.3 Questions to help with life-focused activities

- What is important to me in life?
- Am I spending time on activities that move me toward my valued goals?
- Can I find activities that give me a sense of mastery or pleasure?
- Can I find activities that I find supportive and nourishing?
- What can I do within the restrictions of my situation that is still rewarding?

Life-focused coping is, like problem-focused coping, an active, change-based coping method. It is not possible or desirable to spend all our time managing adverse life situations. Life goes on and there are duties and responsibilities, and also joys and dreams. It is therefore important not to lose sight of what makes life meaningful, so continuing to move towards valued goals can happen alongside problem-focused coping. Lindquist engaged in activities she could still manage like reading, listening to music, listening to friends. Most of all, in her paralyzed state, she was still able to "wander in the labyrinth" of her memory, going through actions in her head like knitting, cooking, and rowing: memories that were a bitter sweet mix of pleasure and sadness. Life-focused coping for her was very much about living in the present moment and finding things she could still manage to do even when she had little mobility. Some questions to help clients focus on quality of life can be found in Box 8.3.

So far we have discussed evaluating the situation, solving problems relating to it, and ensuring that other rewarding areas of life are not sacrificed. It is also important to sometimes turn towards and accept painful feelings as part of the process of adjustment (*internal-focused coping*). If we are grieving the loss of a loved one we cannot spend all our time on the practicalities of the funeral, or throwing ourselves into work. We need to allow ourselves space for grieving. This third focus of coping should not be ignored. Throughout Lindquist's book she describes how her laughter is interspersed with tears at the loss of what she had lost and was about to lose. Some suggestions for questions to help clients pay attention to their internal experience and to accept and manage emotions are listed in Box 8.4.

Finally, coping can be understood as a balancing act: problem-focused, life-focused, and emotion-focused coping can all be helpful in the right

---

Box 8.4 Questions to help attend to and manage emotions

- Have I accepted the reality of the situation?
- Am I accepting that strong feelings are a natural part of coping with adversity?
- Can I allow strong feelings to come and go, knowing they are signs of adjustment?
- Am I making sure that I don't criticize myself or catastrophize about feeling upset?
- Have I allowed myself to express my feelings?
- Is there anyone who can give me emotional support through these difficulties?
- Am I giving myself permission to take time out to look after myself?
- What can I do to look after myself? For example, getting enough sleep, finding "down time," relaxation, meditation, yoga, doing things I can still enjoy.

---

circumstances and doses. Questions to help clients find a balance in their coping efforts are listed in Box 8.5.

Guided discovery can be used to help people answer all these questions. Even so, sometimes guided discovery will need to be complemented by more

---

Box 8.5 Questions to help find a balance

- How much time am I spending on trying to solve the problem and how much on living the rest of my life? Am I getting the balance right?
- Am I putting my efforts into what I can control, or trying to control what I can't?
- Is there a balance between problem solving, chores, and pleasure in my life?
- Is the thought of facing the problem leading me into avoidance and distraction? What can I do about it?
- Is there anyone who can help me face my fears?
- Am I allowing myself to experience realistic sadness about the situation, or am I trying to escape from thinking about it?

---

direct interventions. If the client cannot figure out the answers or put them into practice, other approaches may be more appropriate. For example, there may be times when therapists need to be more psycho-educational, such as when a client lacks skills in problem solving, assertiveness, or stress management.

Common Traps in Working with Clients Facing Adversity

In my experience, the main challenge of working with people facing adversity comes less from the need for any technical changes to therapy, but more from the doubts that arise in the therapist and client about the applicability of CBT to their real difficulties. Handling the therapeutic relationship well and using guided discovery are essential if therapy is to be successful. We will consider two common client-based traps that are often encountered:

Trap 1
Clients find it hard to accept that the cognitive model is relevant to their situation, especially the assumption that our thinking affects the degree of distress we experience. To them, the cognitive model appears to invalidate the seriousness of the problems they face.

Trap 2
The client believes that either things have to be as they were or it's not worth it.

We will also look at two therapist-based traps:

Trap 3
The therapist experiences a strong emotional reaction and is overwhelmed by their empathic reaction to the client.

Trap 4
The therapist overemphasizes the "rational" aspects of cognitive therapy.

Finally, we will examine how the adverse environment itself may interfere with effective treatment:

Trap 5
The constraints of the situation limit the opportunities for problem solving, such as when physical illness, disability, or social impoverishment restricts options for problem solving or behavioral activation.

Trap 6

A long history of adversity wears the client down and makes it hard for them to draw on constructive beliefs and experiences or to identify alternative possibilities.

Client traps

Popular literature about CBT and even some of the self-help materials available can give the impression that CBT is about thinking positively or challenging irrational beliefs. This misrepresents CBT and can seem overly simplistic to clients facing adversity who know only too well that their circumstances are negative. A problem-solving approach can also seem irrelevant when there is widespread social or cultural agreement that the adversity faced is overwhelming.

Trap 1

Client finds it hard to accept that the cognitive model is relevant to their situation, especially the assumption that our thinking affects the degree of distress we experience. To them, the cognitive model appears to invalidate the seriousness of the problems they face.

Therapists who are novice or have less experience in working with adversity may inadvertently exacerbate this. Common mistakes include:

- giving the client self-help pamphlets that are not tailored to their situation;
- presenting the cognitive model in a very didactic fashion, rather than guiding client understanding via guided discovery;
- presenting a simplistic explanation of "distorted thinking";
- introducing problem-solving or automatic thought records too quickly.

Preventing Trap 1: The role of Socratic Dialogue

Tailoring our approach to the client's needs is particularly important for people experiencing losses or major life challenges because overly simple formulae do not do justice to the realistic basis of their problems. Collaborative, sensitive, and empathic questioning helps the therapist understand the client's world and helps the client to feel understood. This provides the groundwork for shaping how we introduce therapy interventions. For instance, a client exhibiting borderline personality disorder traits may feel overwhelmed, angry, and hopeless after losing a job:

Client: It's all over! It's awful!

Therapist: This was a real blow for you. You just said it feels like the end of the world. We'd all feel upset if something like that happened to us. I'd like to really understand what it is about losing that job that is especially terrible for you.

This client will benefit from some help with problem solving but the therapist first needs to validate her distress and find the idiosyncratic meanings that makes it feel so overwhelming and hopeless. Jumping to problem solving too quickly can lead someone to conclude their therapist doesn't appreciate how difficult it is for them to deal with their current adversity.

When people face a significant change in their fortunes, they often go through an initial phase of rapidly fluctuating emotions as they process the experience. It may be necessary to employ more validating and supportive interventions at this time rather than launch immediately into problem solving (Moorey & Greer, 2012). Giving the client time to tell their story, normalizing emotional reactions to their situation, and simply listening are all ways to facilitate emotional expression and acceptance. Socratic Dialogue can be helpful by demonstrating curiosity about the client's experience in order to elicit emotions and cognitions that may be confusing or avoided. Written summaries prove extremely important for people who have poor memories because their adversity includes neurological challenges or they are on strong medications. As with all clients, the language used in summaries and the other stages of Socratic Dialogue should be as simple as possible and reflect the client's own language style and vocabulary.

Carol recently separated from her partner because of domestic abuse. She feels depressed and is still emotionally numb and minimizes the seriousness of the control and violence to which she was subjected. Her therapist in the dialogue below helps her access some of the feelings she might be avoiding by paying attention to emotionally relevant cues when they arise. Notice how her therapist identifies material that feels upsetting to them but is expressed without emotion by Carol. Asking questions about a client's feelings in relationship to experiences that would normally evoke emotional reactions can help overcome experiential avoidance:

Therapist: That sounds really awful. As you describe what you went through, I find myself feeling quite upset. How do you feel right now? What is it like for you to describe the things that happened to you?

If Carol describes that she is unable to feel anything, it can be a sign she is numbing out as some people do when a depressive disorder is severe or during and after trauma. This can be an indication her therapist should assess for the presence of post-traumatic stress disorder or detachment disorder, and adjust the treatment plan accordingly. Alternatively, Carol may disclose negative beliefs about emotional expression, such as, "People will think I'm weak and vulnerable if I show them my emotions." The therapy session can be used as a safe place for identifying and testing out these sorts of beliefs about feelings:

Therapist: Do you think I will think less of you if you get upset here?
Carol: I suppose not.
Therapist: What's the worst you can imagine might happen?
Carol: If I start I won't be able to stop crying.
Therapist: It will be difficult for you to move forward without us looking at some of the feelings of anger and sadness you're feeling. How might we make it safer for you to feel those things?
Carol: Maybe if we could stop talking about upsetting things if I cry for more than 10 minutes.
Therapist: Shall we try that as an experiment?
Carol: OK.
Therapist: To make it a proper experiment, let's make a prediction. You said you are afraid that once you start crying, you won't be able to stop. That is one prediction. What would be another possibility?
Carol: I suppose I would be able to stop?
Therapist: Would that be helpful for you to find out? That is, whether or not you would be able to stop crying if you do cry for 10 minutes about things that happened?
Carol: Yes.

Another useful and nonjudgmental way to conceptualize emotional reactions during the early phases of therapy is the five-part model (Greenberger & Padesky, 2016; Padesky & Mooney, 1990) which demonstrates reciprocal interactions among life events, thoughts, moods, behavior, and physical reactions. It is particularly applicable to adverse life situations and can be generated in a personalized way using Socratic enquiry (Padesky, 2020).

One way to engage the client in constructing this model is to collaboratively generate a description of the interactions between their life events, thoughts, feelings, behaviors, and physical symptoms. The five-part model gives equal weight to all five elements so there is no assumption that the client's emotional distress is caused by "faulty thinking" or that any one part of the system is driving the client's distress. This is a major advantage over the simpler ABC model which describes how thoughts (B) about a situation (A) shape emotions and behavior (C). The ABC model places primacy on the interpretation of events but immediately invites the response, "Yes, but I really do have something to be worried about!"

The five-part model also allows the therapist to acknowledge the importance of external stresses, through its inclusion of environmental and situational components. Financial, interpersonal, and social stresses can be placed on the model, as can losses such as divorce or bereavement, ongoing disability or illness, and even future threats of deterioration or death. Writing these down in the client's own words contributes to the sense of being understood and to the feeling that the immensity of the problem is not being underestimated. The inclusion of physical state in the five-part model can be very helpful for people with a medical condition, because it allows the complex interactions between body sensations, emotional state, thoughts, and behavioral reactions to be disentangled.

The following dialogue with Mary who had metastatic bone disease from breast cancer illustrates use of the five-part model as a simple form of CBT case conceptualization. Analgesics worked to relieve her pain when Mary was in the hospital but when she went home, the pain seemed to break through the medication and she felt she needed to take extra. The therapist empathized with Mary's pain and distress and began by asking questions about the most compelling part of the model for Mary, her pain.

Therapist: I'm sorry to hear that you've been having so much trouble with pain since you've been home.

Mary: Yes, it's unbearable. I just can't stand it.

Therapist: You say the medication isn't working as well as it was when you were in the hospital?

Mary: I need to have a higher dose, I think. I don't know that you can be of much help; I need to speak to my doctor.

Therapist: You may be right, but what I may be able to help with is how you are coping with the pain. Would you be willing for us to look at how you're managing when the pain gets worse?

Mary:	I'll try anything.
Therapist:	We often find it helpful to draw a diagram of how different aspects of the situation fit together—how the pain interacts with your thoughts and feelings, and what you do when you're in so much pain. Would it be OK if we did that together now?
Mary:	If you think it would help.
Therapist:	Where in your body do you get the pain?
Mary:	I always have a pain in my back, and when it's worse it goes all down my side.
Therapist:	How do you feel emotionally when that happens?
Mary:	I get anxious the cancer's spreading even more.
Therapist:	So you feel anxious, and it sounds like you have some anxious thoughts about the cancer getting worse.
Mary:	Yes, and then I can't stop worrying about what's going to happen next.
Therapist:	That must be very upsetting. How does that affect your mood?
Mary:	I get more worried and can't stop myself.
Therapist:	What do you usually do when the pain gets worse like that?
Mary:	I take more tablets, but they just make me drowsy. They don't seem to help. Then when I feel tired I have to go to bed.
Therapist:	Does that help the pain?
Mary:	I don't know. If anything it seems to get worse.
Therapist:	How is that?
Mary:	The pain in my side comes on when I'm in bed.
Therapist:	Do you find it's easier to take your mind off the pain when you're in bed?
Mary:	Only if I sleep. If I'm awake I can't stop thinking about it.
Therapist	(Showing patient the five-part model in Figure 8.1.) I've been writing some of this down as you've been describing your pain. From the physical perspective, you are in a lot of pain and notice new pains arising. I've also put down that you feel drowsy a lot of the time from the medication. Is that right?
Mary:	Yes.
Therapist:	(Pointing to the relevant sections in Figure 8.1.) When you get the pains you start to think, "My cancer is getting worse" and "Why am I getting new pains?" You also mentioned that you have the pain all the time. Is that something that you think about a lot?
Mary:	Yes. I worry why it never goes away. (Therapist adds this to the diagram.)

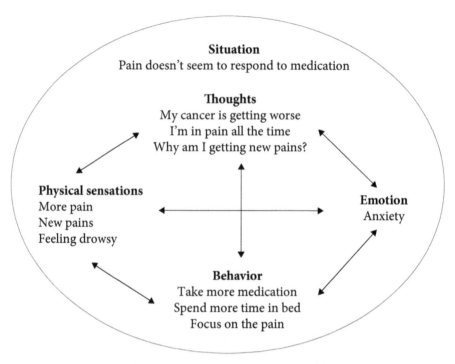

Figure 8.1 Descriptive conceptualization of Mary's pain using the 5-part model. (Model adapted with permission of Christine A. Padesky, copyright 1986).

Therapist: If we look at what you do when you are in pain, we see that you take more medication, and you go to bed. I can understand why you would do that. When you look at this picture (indicating Figure 8.1), how do you think going to bed might affect these other parts?

Mary: (Looking at diagram.) It makes me feel more tired . . . and I seem to get more pains.

Therapist: And what about those negative thoughts?

Mary: I think I just have too much time in bed to dwell on things.

Further enquiry helped Mary re-evaluate her decision to go to bed when she was in pain. Mary could see that while in bed she had nothing to take her mind off the pain and so she focused on it even more, making it seem to get worse and worse. Being in bed for long periods was uncomfortable and she noticed new pains and started to worry about them as more evidence that the disease was progressing faster.

Socratic Dialogue and the use of the five-part model as a written summary of the information gathered helped Mary break her pain reactions into their constituent parts. A visualization like this often helps enhance the Socratic process. Empathic questioning acknowledged the reality of her physical symptoms and helped create a nonjudgmental space in which Mary could explore the effects of her thinking and behavior on how she felt, without feeling her pain was being discounted.

When clients think their therapist doesn't understand

There are many reasons clients can conclude their therapist doesn't understand them or their situation. Sometimes clients get the sense that their therapist is not appreciating the enormity of their problems. Some people frequently find themselves in adverse situations because of poor problem-solving skills or poor choices of friends and partners. If they also believe they are intrinsically unable to cope, they can hope the therapist will rescue them. They can become angry if they feel the therapist doesn't understand how hard it is for them to cope with life problems that arise during therapy.

People with chronic or recurring illness sometimes have been facing challenges for years and they can become worn down to the point they just want to be looked after. Another setback or relapse during therapy can seem like the last straw. They can feel angry if their therapist fails to acknowledge how hard they've been trying and how tired they have become.

Client: Do you think it's easy to keep dealing with this? I'd like to see you manage half of what I have had to deal with for half the time!

Therapist: No, I understand it is not easy at all. You've been through a lot and I can understand why you want to give up. Shall we think together about how we can make some changes in our therapy so we are helping your challenges rather than adding to them?

An empathic comment like this coupled with a Socratic enquiry can lead to collaboration in finding a balance between supportive and problem-focused components of therapy.

When a client thinks you just don't understand how hard it is for them and demands understanding rather than change, there are four basic steps to take:

1. Validate their emotions.
2. Ask questions to understand your client's perspective.
3. Reflectively and empathically summarize to check out your understanding of their perspective.
4. Then, explore how you can work more effectively together.

These steps are illustrated in the following example.

John was a successful barrister who had come from a very impoverished single-parent Black British family. He felt he had always had to work twice as hard as his white colleagues in order to prove himself, many of whom had progressed in their careers more quickly. His driven and sometimes adversarial style served him well in overcoming discrimination and in fighting for justice for his clients, but it also contributed to feelings of dissatisfaction, self-doubt, and irritability. He felt that his white female therapist could not really understand what it was like to face prejudice on a daily basis; he was also concerned that she would try to persuade him that he should be able to rationalize all this away and not make a fuss.

She began by acknowledging that her experience of life had been very different from his, and that she could never fully understand what he had been through. She told him it wasn't surprising that he had doubts about her ability to empathize and about the therapy (Step 1). She emphasized that therapy was a collaborative process in which he needed to test whether it had anything helpful to offer. She then focused on understanding what aspects of the model seemed unsympathetic, and worked with John to develop a conceptualization that took account of the severity of the discrimination he had experienced in his childhood and beyond (Step 2).

In the Therapist's Mind

John's therapist asked herself: "If I were in the John's situation, how would I think and feel? What are the meanings of this therapy situation for John?" At times she felt frustrated and irritated by John's rejection of interventions she thought were promising. By asking herself, "Can I see John's behavior as his best attempt to cope, given the way he is seeing things?", she was able to recognize that his "resistance" was based on a skepticism that had been a useful coping strategy throughout his life.

John's therapist summarized some of the rules that had been helpful for John to live by:

Don't trust anyone until they prove themselves.
If you don't stand up for yourself, no one else will.
If I take control of a situation I'm less likely to get abused.

She reflected that she now understood even more clearly why it was hard for him to accept therapy (Step 3), and asked what he needed to see happen before he would be willing to commit to it (Step 4). Therapy was formulated as a behavioral experiment in which John agreed to try some of the methods such as thought monitoring to see whether they gave him any useful information about himself. His feedback also helped the therapist to move the initial focus of therapy away from identifying distortions in John's thinking and on to ways in which he could manage his anger and act assertively rather than passively or aggressively in difficult work situations. This problem-focused approach gave him confidence that CBT had something to offer.

When clients are skeptical it sometimes helps to stop asking questions. Hold off from Socratic Dialogue when questioning is seen as one of the components of therapy that is irritating! In this instance it is safer to stay with empathic comments until a collaborative alliance is achieved.

Managing Trap 2: Test and evaluate all or nothing thinking

Trap 2

The client believes that either things have to be as they were or it's not worth it.

It is an almost universal experience that, no matter how confident we are in our abilities, when faced with a major life change we doubt ourselves and our resilience. Under pressure we revert to more primitive emotional processing such as all-or-nothing thinking. We can flip from seeing ourselves as competent to seeing ourselves as completely unable to cope. At some point in life, most people will shift from their usual belief that they are competent, able to exert control and that the future has some hope, to the opposite position where they feel helpless and hopeless.

Fortunately, most people come out of this quite quickly and find ways to access their past strengths. A minority become fixed at the negative pole. A common example of this is the person who asserts that because the gap between where they are and where they used to be is so large, it's not worth doing anything. If the client has a physical illness the focus may be on all the things they are no longer able to do on a day-to-day basis. If they have lost a loved one, they may dwell on all they have lost.

A business man had always believed that you can only be worthwhile if you are making a contribution, and had applied this rule both to himself and other people. When he retired he became depressed because he was no longer able to make a contribution as he did in the past. Other activities such as hobbies or looking after his grandchildren were perceived as second best.

Socratic Dialogue can be helpful in eliciting the pros and cons of such an "all-or-nothing" style of thinking. Using visual aids such as drawing a continuum and locating points along the way to record information gathered is also quite helpful. A continuum helps break down the dichotomy, and seeing the possible stages between the extremes might well motivate the client to take some small steps towards their ultimate goal.

Karen was a 27-year-old unemployed woman who was moderately depressed. She had a diagnosis of bipolar disorder. Her father had left when she was only 3 and her mother had brought her up alone. They had a close relationship in which they did many things together and Karen believed that she could not cope alone with the pressures of everyday life. When she had been in a hypomanic phase she had run up debts of £15,000 and her mother was in debt too. When Karen looked at her present life situation it seemed so far away from where she wanted to be that she just gave up. This was compounded by the fact that she thought that the only way she could be happy was if she had a lot of money so that she could live on a farm with her mother. She had an elaborate fantasy of what her life would be like, but this further emphasized the discrepancy between her ideal and current situation. Notice how Karen's therapist uses Socratic Dialogue to unpack the pros and cons of this fantasy:

Therapist: How do you feel when you think about where you would like to be in your life?

Karen: I get a warm feeling when I think about being with my mum and having lots of money.

Therapist: Do you spend a lot of time daydreaming about it?

Karen: Usually before I go to sleep at night.

Therapist: How do you feel when you think about it during the day?

Karen: Not always so good, because I can't get away from what life is really like, and then I feel hopeless and it's not worth going on.

Therapist: Does there seem a gulf between where you are and where you want to be—does it seem huge?

Karen: Exactly. It's so big I can't think about it without becoming suicidal.

Therapist: At the moment it seems like you either have all the things you want and are happy, or you don't have them and you're miserable. You mentioned your friend Teri; does she have more in her life than you?

Karen: I suppose not; she's unemployed and a single mum. I don't know how she does it.

Therapist: Is she unhappy?

Karen: No. She finds it hard sometimes.

Therapist: Would she like to be rich and comfortable and supported?

Karen: Of course.

Therapist: I wonder why she isn't unhappy?

Karen: She doesn't think about it like me.

Therapist: Do you know what she does think about when she looks into the future?

Karen: I don't know … maybe she just thinks about the next day?

Therapist: Does she look forward to things?

Karen: Yes. But they're just small things. She seems not to mind that she doesn't have the big things.

Therapist: We often find that if people set their sights very high compared to where they are they can get very discouraged. It's like wanting to climb a mountain and always keeping our eyes on the summit. Sometimes focusing on the base camp can get us further and motivate us more.

Karen: I don't know. I see what you're saying …

Therapist: What could be a first step?

Karen: Perhaps I could talk to Teri about how she copes.

Therapist: That sounds a good idea. She might have some better ideas than me because she has to face a lot of difficulties like you do. Let's see if we can plan how you're going to do this—what you want to know from Teri, how you're going to ask her, when you're going to do it …

In the Therapist's Mind

Her therapist uses Socratic questions to understand the impact of Karen's wishful thinking on her life. Formulating this as a problem of dichotomous thinking, the therapist steps outside the Socratic framework and asks a leading question: "Does there seem to be a gulf between where you are and where you want to be?" This is meant to express empathy and convey a non-judgmental attitude. The therapist then returns to Socratic questions to learn more about how her friend copes with a similar situation. Often people are more able to think flexibly about other people than they are about themselves. While the therapist thought the metaphor of climbing a mountain would make a good example of the demotivating effect of all-or-nothing thinking, he notes that Karen returns to the comparison with her friend when she thinks about taking a first step. Therefore, he follows her lead and begins to plan with Karen what questions she would like to ask her friend.

This dialogue would only be the beginning of a process of engagement and motivation, testing whether giving up the daydreams and focusing on day-to-day objectives might help Karen feel less depressed. Box 8.6 summarizes the guided discovery methods proposed in this section to deal with common client traps that arise when working with clients experiencing adversity.

Box 8.6 Common Client-Based Traps and Recommended Guided Discovery Methods

Trap 1
- Clients find it hard to accept that the cognitive model is relevant to their situation, especially the assumption that our thinking affects the degree of distress we experience. To them, the cognitive model appears to invalidate the seriousness of the problems they face.

Guided Discovery Methods
- Use Socratic Dialogue to collaboratively develop a compassionate conceptualization, using warmth, understanding, and empathy, which validates the client's experience and identifies some ways of coping.
- The language used by the therapist can be very important in the engagement of skeptical clients, so it is necessary to tailor this to the client's situation. This also applies to the vocabulary and phrasing used, especially when a client's attention or memory are compromised.

Trap 2
- The client believes that either things have to be as they were or it's not worth it.

Guided Discovery Methods
- Use questioning, continuum, and behavioral experiments to test all or nothing thinking.

Therapist traps

We cannot help but be affected by the sadness of someone who is facing death, or the limited life of a single unemployed mother with a child with an autistic spectrum condition, or the frustration of an asylum seeker who has no benefits and no way of getting good legal representation. This emotional identification can lead us to feel hopeless about our skills in dealing with their problems. It can go further to the point that we also buy in to the client's helpless and hopeless view of the situation. This viewpoint that it is perfectly appropriate for the client to be depressed, angry, or paralyzed with anxiety can also be reinforced by the expectations of partners, carers, and other professionals.

Trap 3

The therapist experiences a strong emotional reaction and is overwhelmed by their empathic reaction to the client. For example, "I would feel depressed/terrified/angry if I was in this situation."

This trap arises when the therapist empathizes with the emotional and/or cognitive aspects of the client's experience, and then becomes paralyzed. Allow yourself to experience your client's emotional distress and show them you understand. But at the same time, remind yourself not to make assumptions. The fact that a situation generates almost universal feelings of fear or sadness does not mean that everyone feels sad or anxious for the same reasons.

A first step when feeling overwhelmed by emotion in reaction to client adversity is to use Socratic enquiry on yourself to tease out and clarify your thoughts and feelings. Second, ask Socratic questions to elicit the actual meaning of the situation for your client. You can then compare the two. You may discover that the client's cognitions are completely different from what yours would be in the same situation, and this may free you up to be more objective. Establishing the client's actual thoughts and feelings sometimes reveals biased thinking and helps identify potential ways out of the seemingly hopeless situation. Therapists are well advised to consider writing their own thought records, and seeking supervision when they feel hopeless or overwhelmed by a client's problems. Further tips on how to manage empathic overinvolvement can be found in Chapters 1 and 12 of Moorey and Lavender's (2019) *The Therapeutic Relationship in Cognitive Behaviour Therapy*.

Managing this trap: Don't make assumptions

One of our excellent cognitive therapists working in palliative care (Kathy Burn, personal communication) recalls a client she worked with as a novice. The client was experiencing panic attacks, which the therapist assumed were connected with her fear of dying. Fortunately, she checked out this assumption:

Therapist: When the panic is at its worst, what do you fear will happen?
Client: I think I won't get enough oxygen. I'll suffocate.
Therapist: You think you'll die?
Client: I don't know. Worse than that. I might end up a vegetable.
Therapist: How do you mean?
Client: Well if you don't get oxygen, your brain dies doesn't it? But you're still alive. It's like a living hell.

This woman's fear was that she would run out of oxygen and so become brain damaged. The ultimate catastrophe was to be in a living vegetative state. It emerged that she had spent many years caring for her husband who had been disabled by a cerebrovascular accident and this was the reason for this idiosyncratic interpretation of her panic symptoms. Having used Socratic enquiry to identify the woman's belief, the therapist was able to give her some basic information about respiratory function. That is, the brain and lungs function automatically and it is not possible for a panic attack to cause brain damage.

Keep in Mind

The revelation of this client's idiosyncratic belief was unexpected. Unless the therapist had asked, she would never have guessed that this was the fear underlying the panic attacks. It is important to check our assumptions about what underlies our clients' emotional reactions.

The therapist and client then moved beyond discussion, to gathering information. As a homework assignment the patient searched the Internet for independent information about panic attacks and brain function. They then took the guided discovery one step further by setting up a behavioral experiment to test out her belief by inducing symptoms of breathlessness to see whether it led to brain damage. This action-oriented guided discovery increased her confidence even more that her fears were unfounded.

Trap 4

The therapist overemphasizes the "rational" aspects of cognitive therapy.

In an earlier section we discussed what can happen if the client believes CBT is too simplistic. This problem can be iatrogenic. Therapists can deliver CBT too simplistically. Examples of this include when:

- Therapist pushes client into problem solving too soon (see Trap 1),
- Therapist fails to discriminate between realistic and biased negative thinking, and
- Therapist sticks too rigidly to techniques like looking for evidence for and against negative thoughts when thoughts are negative but realistic.

At least in part, each of these therapist errors results from neglecting an empathic consideration of the client's experiences. There are several reasons behind a therapist's failure to recognize the need for a more empathic approach:

- Novice therapists try to adhere to evidence-based practices and sometimes try to fit their clients into disorder-based models and follow protocols without fully understanding the "cognitive and emotional world" of the person in front of them.
- A second reason, which applies particularly to therapists who move from general psychotherapy settings into health settings, is the failure to adapt the model from one of testing distorted thinking to one of collaboratively examining the helpfulness of thinking patterns.
- Finally, the emotional challenges of working with people's disability, degenerative conditions, or ongoing social deprivation are considerable. Some therapists take refuge in a more emotionally distanced style that can alienate clients or lead to unproductive interventions.

The negative automatic thoughts of people facing adversity often contain the same cognitive biases seen in any people with anxiety or depression, e.g., "Because I have lost my partner I can never have any happiness again" or "Being unemployed means I have no worth in anyone's eyes." These thoughts can certainly be examined by looking at the evidence that supports and does not support them. However, there will also be many thoughts that are negative and realistic. Taking too "rational" an approach may confirm the client's view that they are not being taken seriously. Questions that aim to demonstrate that a thought is distorted can seem patronizing in this context. This is where a style of "curious questioning" to really understand the facts of the situation can be helpful. Clients can be asked questions to help them explore whether they are:

- overestimating the severity of the stressful event,
- underestimating their ability to cope,
- missing possible avenues of support, and
- drawing overgeneralized conclusions about the meaning of the stressor for self, others, or the future.

Sidney had worked in the same firm for 40 years and needed to retire because of the onset of mild dementia. He was depressed and could not see any future. He said, "My life is over now, I've got nothing to look forward to, I'm on the scrapheap." Through curious questioning, his therapist helped Sydney see that he had already mapped out his future with the assumption that there were no options for anything to be different from a life "on the scrapheap."

Exploring Sidney's past revealed that he had experienced a number of significant losses (his mother died when he was 12 and he lost his first wife to cancer) with which he had coped extremely well. His therapist asked him how he had managed to get through these troubles and discovered he had coped with deep grief in the past using social support and a keen interest in making the world a better place for others. Next, his therapist asked whether and how he could bring any of these resources to bear on his current situation.

She also asked him what his wife thought about his dementia and retirement and discovered that she had several ideas about what they could now do together.

With Sydney's agreement, his therapist brought his wife into their sessions. His wife introduced a source of support and became a "co-therapist"—helping set up experiments to test whether he got any pleasure and meaning out of doing things with her. This proved helpful, but it was more important to him to regain a sense of being useful, so he agreed to ask his children if they wanted any help with the grandchildren. Sidney and his wife began to pick them up from school twice a week and this improved his mood considerably. Through Socratic Dialogue, Sidney's therapist helped him redefine his sense of worth and what it meant to "useful" beyond the rigid confines of his work identity and in this new phase of his life when he needed to begin coping with the beginning stages of dementia.

When negative automatic thoughts are realistic, questions that explore the helpfulness of beliefs and behaviors are often the best strategy. Rather than asking "what's the evidence?", asking "what's the effect of thinking this way?" can be more productive. This can then lead to experiments to test the effects of these thoughts. Similarly, questions that generate an alternative perspective are valuable. People who cope well with objectively awful situations frequently focus on areas of their life that they can still control and on what hope remains for the future. The therapist in effect says to the patient:

> "You are in a realistically difficult situation. My job is to help you to explore how you are coping, and together we can find out if there are other ways of thinking or acting that might help you cope even better."

Despite being blind and deaf, Helen Keller considered herself an optimist and made a conscious decision to focus on what she had in her life and what she could achieve rather than what she had lost:

> If I regarded my life from the point of view of the pessimist, I should be undone. I should seek in vain for the light that does not visit my eyes and the music that does not ring in my ears. I should beg night and day and never be satisfied. I should sit apart in awful solitude, a prey to fear and despair. But since I consider it a duty to myself and to others to be happy, I escape a misery worse than any physical deprivation.
>
> Helen Keller (1903, 21)

An approach that we have found useful in our work with people in palliative care, and which can also be applied to any type of adversity, has been to use Socratic Dialogue followed by behavioral experiments to explore the benefits and costs of pursuing current beliefs and behaviors compared with an alternative coping model. We use "Plan A" and "Plan B" first described in the context of depression by Melanie Fennell (1989). Plan A is to continue with the present coping style. The therapist discusses this, asking detailed questions about the present consequences of the behavior and enquiring into the future effects. This may involve time projection: imagining what it would like in 1 or 5 years' time if the current coping strategies are maintained. Plan B is to investigate alternative ways of approaching the problem, which usually involve more active, instrumental problem solving, more constructive thinking, and a more hopeful view of the future. The following example illustrates this approach.

Jim was a 35-year-old man experiencing depression along with avoidant and paranoid personality traits. He had been physically abused throughout his childhood by his father who was a quixotic bully. His mother was uninterested in caring for him and gave him the message that he was a nuisance by his very presence. He developed the belief that the world was a hostile place where no one could be trusted. Small injustices done to him or others would trigger a rage that he could not express openly. He spent hours on end pacing the rooms in his small apartment ruminating about the state of the world. Within a short time this escalated to include thoughts about his father and he would then shout out angrily as he paced. He believed that once this process had started there was no way of stopping it until it ran its course over 2–4 hours.

Therapist: I'd like us to look at how you're coping with these memories of your father, and whether there are any other ways to manage these angry feelings. We've talked a lot about your pacing and rumi-nating. Would you like to sum up what we've discovered?

Jim: I suppose I know already that it winds me up more. Once I get started it has to go on for hours till it burns itself out. But after-wards I feel exhausted.

Therapist: Let's call this current coping your "Plan A." At the moment you feel this is about the best way of dealing with it.

Jim: It's the only way.

Therapist: If we were to imagine a "Plan B" what might it look like?

Jim: Well, we've talked about how I just make myself worse by ruminating.

Therapist: Are there any times that you can break into the cycle?

Jim: Very occasionally I can nip it in the bud.

Therapist: How do you manage that?

Jim: Sometimes I can stop it by going out for a walk, though that has to be in the dark or I get worried about being near other people.

Therapist: OK so part of Plan B might be to do something active, like take a walk, when you start to ruminate. What else might an alternative plan contain?

The components of Plan A and Plan B were further developed, written down, and examined side by side. Plan B was then set up as an experiment which Jim tried over the next few sessions. He came back after the first week rather despondent:

Jim: I was ruminating as much as ever.

Therapist: Were you able to try Plan B?

Jim: My anger just took over before I could do anything.

Therapist: Can you remind me what we put on the list for Plan B? Do you have the list with you?

Jim: (Looking at the list.) It says going for a walk, watching a DVD, making a cup of tea, and phoning a friend.

Therapist: Were you able to try any of these?

Jim: No. I didn't even think of them at the time.

Therapist: So we haven't really given Plan B a trial yet. It seems there might be two problems with our current plan B. First, you get angry pretty quickly and that makes it hard because ... ?

Jim: Partly, I start Plan A without thinking. I also didn't remember Plan B.

Therapist: Hmmm. So what could we add to Plan B to make it more likely you would think of it and give it a try?

Jim: (Pauses, thinking.) I could put some post it notes up.

Therapist: How would that help? Wouldn't you still just get angry and start pacing?

Jim: I tend to look in the mirror and shout at my face there first. Maybe I could put a post it there.

Therapist: Good idea. What about your mobile phone?

Jim: I suppose I could put in a reminder?

Therapist: Yes. What would that reminder say?

Jim: I could put in a reminder every morning and afternoon to read Plan B and remember to try it if I get angry.

Jim found the reminders helpful and also experimented with more activities—he found that tasks that took up his attention, like cooking or shopping, were more effective at breaking the cycle of rumination than more passive activities. He added these to his notes in his phone about Plan B.

See Box 8.7 for a summary of the guided discovery methods proposed in this section to deal with common therapist traps experienced when working with clients experiencing adversity.

Environmental traps

Problem-focused coping is consistently associated with better psychosocial adjustment, so one of the best ways to improve well-being in adversity is through problem solving. This will often, though not exclusively, involve taking some physical action: doing something to make the situation better. For example, when people are feeling depressed and see life circumstances as hopeless, behavioral activation enhances self-efficacy and improves mood. This is an example of life-focused coping that may not directly change the adverse situation and yet may improve the quality of life around it. However, adverse life circumstances can limit opportunities for problem solving and action.

Box 8.7 Common Therapist-Based Traps and Recommended Guided Discovery Methods

---

Trap 3

The therapist experiences a strong emotional reaction and is overwhelmed by their empathic reaction to the client. For example, "I would feel depressed/terrified/angry if I was in this situation."

Guided Discovery Methods

Clarify your own beliefs and emotional reactions. Don't make assumptions that these match your clients' experiences. Use curious questioning to understand the reasons and beliefs underpinning their emotional reactions. Test these out as appropriate.

Trap 4

The therapist overemphasizes the "rational" aspects of cognitive therapy.

Guided Discovery Methods

Listen empathically to your clients' circumstances. Then ask questions to help them explore whether they are:

- overestimating the severity of the stressful event,
- underestimating their ability to cope,
- missing possible avenues of support, and
- drawing overgeneralized conclusions about the meaning of the stressor for self, others, or the future.

Trap 5

The constraints of the adverse situation limit the opportunities for problem-focused and life-focused coping.

For example, physical illness or disability may prevent certain energizing activities like going to the gym or even going for a walk. Financial impoverishment can reduce options for socializing. Refugees may have extra burdens related to fighting for asylum, learning a new language, and poor access to culturally familiar paths of action. Discrimination against marginalized groups can make some actions more difficult or even dangerous. There are three ways to tackle this obstacle:

1. Use graded task assignments to break the task down into smaller steps. When it is not possible to achieve the full goal, the steps along the way may in themselves prove rewarding.
2. Identify achievable activities that still give a sense of pleasure and mastery.
3. Identify the values and meanings underpinning clients' previously rewarding activities and devise new activities that provide similar satisfaction.

Graded task assignment

Dora was experiencing heart failure. She used to be very active and, even at 89 years old, enjoyed going to the shops round the corner every day and meeting with people. Since a recent heart attack she was breathless when she walked any distance and now spent much of her time sitting at home and watching TV. Graded task assignments will be familiar to CBT therapists who have worked with clients who feel depressed. Tasks are broken down into small, manageable steps. For Dora, this meant creating a series of journeys of increasing length, starting with just getting out of her chair and standing for a minute and building up her stamina and strength until she could walk to her front gate. This plan was approved by her cardiologist as part of a healthy recovery.

Her therapist presented this as an experiment, "We don't know how far you'll be able to get, but we can try and find out." Dora was able to start with a few small journeys around her living room and surprised herself. As she grew in confidence she found she could go for slightly longer walks, resting as she needed, and eventually managed to get to her garden gate. Although disappointed not to be able to get further than this, she felt a sense of achievement and a small degree of independence. In this approach, care needs to be taken to ensure the steps are not disqualified because they are too insignificant (see Trap 2). Socratic enquiry can be used to identify tasks that are achievable yet relevant to the overall goal:

Therapist: What would you really like to be able to do?
Dora: To get round the shops.
Therapist: I don't know if we'll be able to get you that far, but we can have a go. Would you find meaning in anything less than getting to the shops?
Dora: I'd like to be able to get about the house a bit more than I do. And perhaps reach a chair in my garden so I could enjoy sitting outside on a pleasant day.
Therapist: What would be the very first thing you could manage?
Dora: Well, I could get up from the chair more. The physio said that if I don't use my legs I'll get weaker.

Therapist: How long could you stand for?
Dora: I don't know.
Therapist: Shall we find out?

Rather than waiting for Dora to test this out at home, her therapist invited her to do a behavioral experiment and stand right then, during the appointment. He asked her to predict the likelihood she would be able to stand and stay standing for even one minute. Dora expressed doubt that she would be able to do this without assistance. She discovered that she could stand for three minutes, resting her hands on the back of a chair until she regained her confidence. Her therapist showed curiosity about what Dora had learned from each small experiment, beginning with this first one in the office:

Therapist: That was three minutes. How did you feel doing that?
Dora: I'm a bit surprised I made it that long.
Therapist: How difficult would you say that was, physically?
Dora: It was hard to stand up. But once I got there, the standing wasn't too bad although my legs began to feel quite tired in the final minute.
Therapist: How tired do they feel now that you are sitting again?
Dora: Oh, they feel alright now.
Therapist: I wrote down your prediction before you tried. You only gave yourself a 15% chance that you would be able to stand without assistance. And you predicted you would only be able to stand for one minute if you got up.
Dora: Yes, I'm surprised how well I did.
Therapist: Let me write here the results of your efforts. You did stand without assistance and stayed standing for three minutes.
Dora: I did rest my hands on the chair while I stood. But I think that was smart because I could catch myself if I started to fall.
Therapist: I'll add that to our summary of your experiment here. (Writes it down.) What does it mean to you that you were able to stand for three minutes, with your hands on the chair?
Dora: I feel a bit of hope, actually. It's a start. A bigger one than I expected.
Therapist: If you were to rate this achievement from 0, not much at all, to 10, the best you could hope for, how would you rate this achievement today?
Dora: I'd give myself a 7. I really did well and hope I can do more in the weeks ahead.
Therapist: So what do you think would be the next step you want to take this week?

Dora was not very good at writing down a record of her experiments in the following weeks, but her therapist was attentive and thoroughly debriefed Dora's sense of fatigue, strength and mastery each week. Synthesizing questions such as "What does that mean to you?" and "Do you feel more or less independent this week?" helped Dora see that each step could be rewarding in its own right even though there was only a slim hope she would reach her ultimate goal of her previous level of independence.

Identify activities linked to mastery and pleasure

As was already discussed for Trap 2, sometimes people believe if they can't do what they could in the past, then current activities are worthless. For other people it may simply be that they are not thinking about the whole range of activities available to them, but just what they usually do. When questioning a client does not generate ideas, including their partner or carer in the discussion sometimes reveals a range of enjoyable activities they used to do. Sometimes giving a person a list of pleasurable activities will help jog their memory or free their mind to be able to brainstorm new ideas. Guided discovery is all about inducing a sense of curiosity in the client, so what can they still do that they may have forgotten, what new activities might they try? Therapist and client can then test whether these activities lead to a sense of mastery or pleasure.

Identifying new activities consistent with client values

The third approach is influenced by Acceptance and Commitment Therapy (ACT; Hayes et al., 2016). It establishes the values that underlie behaviors that are rewarding for people. Once values are identified, there can be a discussion about alternative ways in which these values could be pursued. Within ACT, a value is seen as giving a direction of travel. Achieving objectives along the way is not the goal, since once we achieve one goal we usually set another. It is more important to feel we are acting in ways that are consistent with our values. For some people that might include seeing oneself as kind, constructive, contributing, strong, or other valued characteristics.

Trevor had a spinal injury from a road traffic accident and was now in a wheelchair. His therapist helped Trevor identify his values in the following way:

Therapist: We've been talking about things you might look forward to doing in the future that would help you feel good about yourself. Before your accident you were a very good tennis player. What did you enjoy about tennis?

Trevor: It was just great being able to know you were fit.

Therapist: What was it about being fit?

Trevor: It felt good, and now look at me. What good am I in a wheelchair?

Therapist: Was there anything else about tennis that you're missing?

Trevor: I was champion of the club 3 years running. I guess I'm a pretty competitive person.

Therapist: So there's something rewarding about beating an opponent?

Trevor: Definitely. I don't like to lose. That's why I've done so well with my rehab.

Therapist: Yes, I hear you've surprised the physios with how quickly you're recovering.

Trevor: Yes, but I know I'll never walk again.

Therapist: Was it the physical fitness or the winning that mattered to you?

Trevor: Both ... well I think it was the winning mostly.

Therapist: So competing and overcoming an opponent is something that gives you a great sense of achievement. If that's the thing that's important to you, I wonder if there are other areas you might branch into?

Trevor: I'm not going to be one of those Paralympic athletes—you won't get me in a wheelchair race.

Therapist: Are there any non-physical sports you used to enjoy.

Trevor: Chess, but that's not a sport ... well, actually I was the school chess champion ... yes ... I haven't played for years.

Therapist: Did you get sense of achievement from beating an opponent at chess?

In the Therapist's Mind

As a first step, the therapist has learned Trevor is competitive so together they can look for competitive activities he can do and consider the pleasures these might bring him. The therapist is also aware that competition is not always a good thing, especially in relationships. So the therapist wants to also find out what values brought Trevor pleasure outside of competition. What values did he have outside of tennis? Were any values sacrificed along the way to becoming a top tennis player? Which of these did he most regret not having time for? Are any of these aspects of life ones that might be a meaningful focus now?

Factors limiting action are not only physical, they can also be psychosocial. Social stigma may limit the opportunities for refugees or people with a chronic mental health challenges. Families sometimes hold unrealistic expectations or express so much criticism that people struggle to thrive. Socratic Dialogue can be used to help people question where these cultural beliefs came from, and ask themselves whether they really need to ascribe to them. Jane was unemployed and her family had unreasonable expectations of what sort of career she should aspire to:

Therapist: So your family all believe that you're nothing unless you've got a professional job.
Jane: Absolutely.
Therapist: Do you believe that?
Jane: I don't know.
Therapist: Do other people believe that?
Jane: I never really wondered that before.
Therapist: I wonder how we might find out? For example, sometimes we do surveys to find these things out.

Jane and her therapist constructed a survey that asked what sort of job people thought was an acceptable achievement, what they would think of someone who did not have a job, what things they might value in someone other than achievement in their career, etc. She gave this survey to a number of friends and to people in a chat group she attended online. The results helped her see that her family's rules were not universal. The next challenge for Jane was to find her own rules and live them in the face of her family's negative judgment. Socratic enquiry helped her find her own set of values and to experiment with what living by them would be like.

In a similar way, people who experience social stigma may find it hard to maintain a sense of worth when many in society consider them to be inferior. Here again Socratic Dialogue can be employed to question whether these values are morally acceptable or helpful in any way. Finding social contacts who are compassionate, supportive, and accepting is often an important component of helping people cope with social or family stigmatization.

> ### Trap 6
> ___
> A long history of adversity wears the client down and makes it hard for them to draw on constructive beliefs and experiences or to identify alternative possibilities.

We've examined how external circumstances limit some people in the *behaviors* that are available to them. People who have experienced extensive adversity throughout their lives may live in a *cognitively* impoverished environment. They do not have a database of coping and good fortune to draw on, so using Socratic questions to gather evidence for alternative, more adaptive beliefs can be very difficult. These are sometimes people who have experienced physical, emotional, or sexual abuse as children or severe deprivations due to refugee or marginalized group status, and then gone on to live in socially deprived or abusive environments as adults.

Jim, whom we met earlier, had been severely physically and emotionally abused as a child. He not only believed that no one could be trusted but that if he got into any conversation it might be used against him. For example, he would not even consider starting a conversation with his local newsagent in case they found out things about him and used the information to burgle his house. He had very little evidence to counter these beliefs. His early life had been spent with people who were violent, his neighborhood was subject to frequent robberies, and in recent years he had only seen two friends. His long years of social avoidance prevented him from gathering information that contradicted his negative beliefs.

Empathic questioning and listening are needed to understand the extent of someone's deprivation, abuse, or hurt and to help them understand how their belief system has developed. Sometimes a compassionate conceptualization will help them achieve some distance from their core beliefs. Questions can be used to identify exceptions, strengths, and coping abilities. Jim had spent ten years as a traffic warden and had done this quite successfully. In this session, Jim's therapist used that information as a springboard to uncover information that could help him:

Therapist: I was surprised to hear that you had been a traffic warden. How did you manage that with your fear of people?

Jim: It's not as bad as people think. You don't get too much trouble. Most people are OK if you explain why you're giving them a ticket.

Therapist: How did you cope with them when it's so difficult for you to talk to people?

Jim: You have a script. You know what the rules are. And you've got the uniform, so you can just fit into the role.

Therapist: How well did you cope?

Jim: Not too bad for the first few years. I ended up as a trainer and then I had 16 people under me.

Therapist: How does that fit with your belief that you can't safely interact with people?

Jim: I suppose I can interact if I know the rules.

Therapist: Would you say someone who had spent 10 years doing a job where they had to cope with motorists in upsetting situations had some social skills?

Jim: I suppose so.

Therapist: Do you think they promoted you because they thought you had social skills?

Jim: I suppose so.

Therapist: You don't need to agree with me. Honestly, what do you think?

Jim: I have been able to do the social stuff in the past.

Therapist: Especially if you knew the rules.

Jim: Yeah.

Therapist: Do you think we could figure out some rules together that you could use to help you now?

Jim: Well ... I suppose so.

Therapist: If we could, do you think that would make a difference?

Jim: I have been able to do the social stuff in the past. So I guess if I had some rules to go by, I might be able to do it again.

His therapist's interested, empathic enquiry allowed Jim to begin to recognize that there had been times in his life when he had been able to trust work colleagues enough to interact with them. The therapist used this as a starting point for testing his belief that he could not get on with people, and that no one could be trusted.

See Box 8.8 for a summary of the guided discovery methods proposed in this section to deal with common environment-based traps experienced when working with clients experiencing adversity.

Box 8.8 Common Environment-Based Traps and Recommended Guided Discovery Methods

---

Trap 5

The constraints of the adverse situation limit the opportunities for problem-focused and life-focused coping.

Guided Discovery Methods

Use graded task assignments to break a task into smaller steps. Focus on the rewards of what can be done rather than what cannot be done at this time. Identify achievable activities that give a sense of pleasure and mastery. Identify the values and meanings underpinning previously rewarding activities and devise new goals and activities that provide similar satisfaction.

Trap 6

A long history of adversity wears the client down and makes it hard for them to draw on constructive beliefs and experiences or to identify alternative possibilities.

Guided Discovery Methods

Use empathic questioning and listening to understand the extent of someone's deprivation, abuse, or hurt and help them understand how their belief system developed. Ask questions designed to identify exceptions, strengths, and coping abilities.

Summary

This chapter has considered the application of cognitive and behavioral techniques with clients facing real life adversity. Although much of the work can follow standard CBT approaches, there are a number of traps for therapists. Client and therapist traps tend to mirror each other. Clients can feel that CBT is too rational and does not pay attention to the seriousness of the problems they face, and this is sometimes exacerbated by anxious or inexperienced therapists applying techniques too simplistically or rationally. The solution here is to emphasize warmth, understanding, and empathy and to use Socratic enquiry to understand the client's unique perspective on the world. Other clients may see their situation as hopeless and view it in all or nothing terms. In reaction to this therapists can become disheartened and buy into the client's helplessness and hopelessness. Guided discovery methods are particularly valuable in understanding and testing client beliefs and behaviors that fuel hopelessness and helplessness. External circumstances can themselves impinge on therapy through limiting the scope for behavioral and cognitive work. Socratic enquiry can be used to identify alternative behaviors which meet valued goals, and to identify strengths that might be overlooked.

Once therapists are aware of the traps addressed in this chapter, working with people facing major life difficulties is often not as challenging as one might expect. There are frequently more rapid gains than with other clients. Clients facing adversity often have coping skills that have simply been submerged, and Socratic Dialogue prompts their rediscovery. If therapists approach clients' problems with compassion and respect, they will find working with this group very rewarding. The experience of adversity is universal, but so is the capacity for hope and for living life in its fullness. As Ulla-Carin Lindquist ends her story:

> A fresh wind is blowing from the shore when I untie the half hitch and put out to sea.
> The sea is choppy, with little white horses.
> I settle myself comfortably on the deck and wait.
> The wind rows me out and I am at peace.
> When it slackens at dusk I will have reached my haven.
> Every second is a life.
>
> **(Lindquist, 2006, 197)**

Reader Learning Activities

Based on what you learned about using guided discovery methods with clients who experience adversity:

- Which of the six traps addressed in this chapter do you see in your work?
- Which of your clients fit with these traps?
- Which of the guided discovery methods illustrated might be helpful with them?
- What do you need to learn or practice before you can try this out with those clients?
- How will you make this happen?
- What do you need to do to increase your understanding of these issues or your skills base (e.g., reading, training, supervision, or consultation)?

Acknowledgments

I am grateful to my colleagues Kathy Burn and Lyn Snowden who provided clinical material from supervision, and for their helpful comments on an earlier draft of the chapter.

References

Fennell, M. (1989). Depression. In K. Hawton, P. M. Salkovskis, J. Kirk, & D. M. Clark (Eds.), *Cognitive behaviour therapy for psychiatric problems: A practical guide* (pp. 169-234). Oxford: Oxford University Press.

Greenberger, D., & Padesky, C.A. (2016). *Mind over mood: Change how you feel by changing the way you think*, 2nd ed. New York: Guilford Press.

Hayes, S. C., Strosahl, K. D., & Wilson, K. G. (2016). *Acceptance and commitment therapy: The process and practice of mindful change* (2nd ed.). London: Guilford Press.

Keller, H. A. (1903). *Optimism: An essay.* New York: T. Y. Crowell and Company, 21.

Lazarus, R. S., & Folkman, S. (1984). *Stress, appraisal, and coping.* New York: Springer.

Lindquist, U-C. (2006) *Rowing without oars.* London: John Murray.

Moorey, S., & Greer, S. (2012) *The Oxford guide to CBT for people with cancer.* Oxford: Oxford University Press.

Moorey, S., & Lavender, A. (2019). *The therapeutic relationship in cognitive behaviour therapy.* London: SAGE.

Padesky, C. A. (2020). Collaborative case conceptualization: Client knows best. *Cognitive and Behavioral Practice, 27*, 392–404. https://doi.org/10.1016/j.cbpra.2020.06.003

Padesky, C. A. & Mooney, K. A. (1990). Clinical tip: Presenting the cognitive model to clients. *International Cognitive Therapy Newsletter*, 6, 13–14. [available from: http://padesky.com/clinical-corner/publications].

9

Chasing Janus: Socratic Dialogue with Children and Adolescents

Robert D. Friedberg

Janus is a figure in Roman mythology who represented change, growth, and progress, as well as the capacity to see multiple perspectives. In fact, Janus is often depicted with two heads. While Janus is occasionally seen as being duplicitous, he can also be viewed as open-minded. More specifically, Janus is also remembered as the god of doors and gateways. Effective Socratic Dialogue opens up doorways, pathways, and gateways to new thought, feeling, and action patterns. As truncated perspectives broaden, problem-solving strategies emerge and new light is shed on young people's assumptions and beliefs. Good Socratic Dialogue can fashion the art of the possible and clear the path for young people to walk through fresh perceptual doors.

Common Traps in Therapy with Children and Adolescents

Distressed children and adolescents operate under precarious illusions about themselves, their world/experiences, and their future. These misinterpretations contribute to a variety of dysphoric emotions such as depression, anxiety, anger, frustration, shame, and guilt. Skillful fashioning of a Socratic Dialogue with these young clients can shepherd them away from their misleading assumptions. Through guided discovery, new options and perspectives emerge.

Three clinical traps that therapists encounter and can fall into are presented in this chapter. First, therapists have fallen into a trap when Socratic Dialogue resembles interrogation, coercion, or quizzes aimed at disproving children's thinking. Therapists can also fall into related traps such as trying to argue or debate rather than initiate guided discovery. At their worst, therapists can adopt an adversarial stance, resulting in vituperative exchanges, especially with argumentative children or adolescents. Children can react angrily to perceived power struggles; alternatively, they sometimes withdraw or obsequiously defer to therapists. Some children and adolescents emotionally distance themselves entirely from the therapeutic enterprise.

A second trap occurs when dialogue is an intellectual colloquy rather than a sensitive, emotional task. Some therapists even adopt a stuffy professional role, which can seem patronizing to children and adolescents. Finally, a third trap is encountered when working with children whose tolerance for ambiguity, abstraction, and frustration is so low that Socratic Dialogue is burdensome.

The chapter begins with thoughts on the differences between young people and adults when using Socratic Dialogue. This first section, "Differences between Children and Adults When Scaffolding a Socratic Dialogue," provides a general orientation for the rest of the chapter. Next, our three traps are described ("Navigating Three Common Traps using Socratic Dialogue") and uses of guided discovery methods to manage them are illustrated with clinical examples. "Keep in mind" boxes throughout this chapter steer therapists toward guiding principles helpful in these sticky situations. Finally, numerous therapy dialogues and examples of experiential exercises designed to unite the head and heart are presented.

Differences between Children and Adults When Scaffolding a Socratic Dialogue

Children enter cognitive therapy in fundamentally different ways from adults. At the most basic level, children rarely seek psychological treatment on their own. In most cases, someone else decided they need treatment and should come to psychotherapy. Therefore, few children are truly self-referred. When they come for initial sessions, they would prefer to be somewhere else (for many, anywhere else would be preferable!).

Since these children are brought to treatment by powerful others, they hold implicit beliefs about the process. Some see cognitive therapy as punishment. Others think coming to therapy makes them weird, freaky, damaged, defective, or weak. Young children can even think they are going to get a shot or be forced to swallow a pill.

Children's cognitive set influences how Socratic Dialogue will be interpreted. If treatment is viewed as punishment, young people are primed to interpret the dialogue as reprimand. Children who believe coming to the mental health clinic means they are weird and damaged are prone to hypervigilance to any line of questioning that smells like blame or pathologizing. Younger children are notorious yay-sayers and they may "go along to get along," passively agreeing with therapists in order to shorten treatment and/or avoid disapproval.

Woody Allen (2007, 127) wrote, "physics, like a grating relative has all the answers." Pedantry rarely catches fire in children and adolescents' minds. As is the case with any of our clients, psychotherapists should not presume to have all the answers for young people. When escorting children through the guided discovery process, remember they are not tiny adults (Kingery et al., 2006; Piacentini & Bergman, 2001). Keep developmental variations in mind. Sensitivity to language, perspective taking, reasoning skills, and verbal regulation/mediation abilities is mandatory, or therapy will not go well.

Attention to typical developmental struggles is another important requirement for effective therapy with youth. While the stereotypical teenage mantra that life is about "sex, drugs, and rock and roll" is an overgeneralization, it is not completely untrue for adolescents. Jim Morrison, leader of the iconic rock group The Doors, said, "Each generation wants new symbols, new people, new names. They want to divorce themselves from their predecessors." From a neuroscience perspective, Dahl (2004, 7) remarked that "adolescents like intensity, excitement, and arousal. They are drawn to music videos that shock and bombard the senses. Teenagers flock to horror slasher movies. They dominate queues waiting to ride the high adrenaline rides at amusement parks. Adolescence is a time when sex, drugs, very loud music, and other high stimulation experiences take on great appeal. It is a developmental period when an appetite for adventure, a predilection for risks, and a desire for novelty and thrills seem to reach naturally high levels." Adolescents experience emotion passionately and frequently these passions overwhelm their reasoning skills (Dahl, 2004; Daniel & Goldston, 2009).

Teenagers possess an urgent calling for independence and autonomy coupled with immature coping capacities. Respectfully balancing their exigency for self-determination and liberation from parental/adult authority with an appreciation of their half-grown capacities is a difficult dialectic. Nonetheless, achieving this balance in therapy with teenagers is vital.

In *Sense and Sensibility*, Jane Austen (1908) wrote, "There is something so amiable in the prejudices of a young mind, that one is sorry to see them give way to the reception of more general opinions." Children's relatively naïve views are at times endearing and often reflect an unblemished perspective on life and can inoculate them from pernicious self-criticism. For instance, younger children show a self-enhancing bias when they distance themselves from failure and take credit for successes (Zuckerman, 1979). Indeed, this normal bias protects them from self-critical depression (Leahy, 1985). However, this inoculation ostensibly wears off by middle childhood. Consequently, there is a cost to greater cognitive development.

Navigating Three Common Traps using Socratic Dialogue

> Terry Malloy: *So what happens? He gets the title shot outdoors—And what do I get? a one-way ticket to Palookaville . . . I coulda had class, I coulda been a contender, I coulda been somebody instead of a bum, which is what I am.*
>
> —*On the Waterfront* **(Schulberg, 1954)**

Trap 1

Child/adolescent sees Socratic Dialogue as interrogation and/or attempts at control/coercion

---

The legendary scene from the American classic film *On the Waterfront* demonstrates deep personal regret, absolutistic, and almost fatalistic thinking. A similar thinking process plagues many depressed adolescents. Casting doubt on these types of cognitive patterns through a Socratic dialogue requires considerable flexibility, patience, and creativity. Changing personal views is especially arduous for teenagers struggling with independence and identity issues.

Logically slugging it out with young people is generally unproductive. The dialogue morphs into a punch–counterpunch interaction. Children and adolescents bob and weave to avoid being pummeled. They side-step verbal fisticuffs, so they are not cornered against the ropes. Teenagers are wary about potentially being jabbed and knocked down. Resist the urge to argue and battle so you won't buy a one-way ticket to Palookaville and find yourself down for the count.

Keep in Mind

- Take a stance of championing advocacy for young clients rather than an adversarial role.
- Maintain cultural alertness to issues of ethnicity, gender, socioeconomic status, sexual orientation, gender identity, able-bodiedness, religion/spirituality, etc.
- Embed Socratic Dialogue within collaborative case conceptualizations.
- Adopt a collaborative hypothesis testing approach.

- Remember stuck points in therapy are data points and opportunities to be curious and ask new questions.
- Invite children or adolescents to write summaries of what you and they learn or write summaries for them.

Socrates is recognized for his passion for self-examination and questioning assumptions (Lageman, 1989). James et al. (2010) explained, "Within cognitive therapy, questions are used to explore issues from different angles, create dissonance, and facilitate re-evaluation of beliefs whilst at the same time building more adaptive thinking styles (83)." Nonetheless, as illustrated throughout this book, Socratic Dialogue is composed of more than questions.

Pounding away at inaccurate beliefs until a youngster submits is rarely effective. Mixing empathic statements with questions provides a respite for the young client and also communicates understanding. Active listening vitalizes Socratic questioning (Padesky, 1988, 1993). Varying the type of question asked or mixing questions with statements is another helpful component of pacing. For example, you can nudge Socratic Dialogue along with declarative comments such as "Tell me how losing a swim meet makes you think you are unacceptable."

The following dialogue with 12-year-old Jeff, a Euro-American male, who struggles with anxiety, illustrates good pacing and the therapist adopting a role of advocate.

Jeff: I don't want to talk about my anxiety.
Therapist: I understand you prefer to keep these feelings and ideas to yourself. What do you expect will happen if you share them?
Jeff: I don't know . . . it will make them worse.
Therapist: Tell me, what makes you think it will make them worse?
Jeff: When I think about it, I feel worse.
Therapist: That certainly makes sense, then. No wonder you want to keep it to yourself.
Jeff: Yeah.
Therapist: You really want to hold onto it.
Jeff: Yeah.
Therapist: And if you let go of it and told me . . .
Jeff: I wouldn't control it anymore.

Through pacing, his therapist was able to discover Jeff's private thoughts. The therapeutic mix included empathic statements (e.g., "You want to keep these feelings and thoughts. That makes sense. You really want to hold onto it."). Additionally, the therapist varied the type of question used with Jeff (e.g., "What do you expect will happen if you share them? Tell me, what makes you think it will make them worse?"). Finally, the therapist invited Jeff to fill in the blank in an incomplete sentence (e.g., "And if you let go of it and told me … ").

Adolescents can be tough customers in therapy. They are often adept at getting under a therapist's skin. When Socratic dialogues turn adversarial, favorable outcomes become less certain. Consider the example of Bailey, a 16-year-old depressed female with a history of cutting behavior who owned first-class skills in turning interactions into arguments.

Bailey:	This is a f***ing waste of time (chewing gum loudly and blowing a bubble).
Therapist:	Take the gum out of your mouth, please.
Bailey:	No … Why?
Therapist:	It takes away from the session.
Bailey:	No it doesn't!
Therapist:	Put the gum in the waste basket.
Bailey:	Screw you! It's my session …
Therapist:	(Hands waste basket to Bailey.) Spit it in here.
Bailey:	Make me!

This contentious dialogue raises several points. First, the therapist made an issue of what is essentially a non-issue. The gum chewing is not likely a therapeutic interference and more than likely increases her comfort in the session. If the therapist really believed gum chewing was an interfering behavior, an experiment could be set up (e.g., chew gum for half the session, rate the effectiveness of that portion of the session, spit it out, work without the gum for second half, rate the effectiveness, and then compare the two halves). Finally, the therapist slid into a pseudo-parental role with Bailey and entered a control battle.

This scenario reminds us of the importance of keeping tuned into the cognitions of the therapist—what was driving this therapist's anti-therapeutic behavior? Where was his curiosity? Therapists' assumptions are explored further in Chapter 11.

Ask for permission to test thoughts

Changing strongly held beliefs can be scary. Even beliefs that are connected to painful emotions can make the world understandable and predictable. Familiar private truths sometimes hold a degree of comfort for youngsters despite their distressing nature. Therefore, obtaining permission to test a thought is a respectful habit to develop. The following dialogue with 15-year-old Paula, an African-American female, who presents with depressed mood shows one way to obtain permission to test thoughts.

Paula: I feel like my mother is constantly judging and evaluating me. She can't let me go and I resent the hell out of her!

Therapist: You sound furious with your mom.

Paula: I am! She gives the gift that keeps on giving!

Therapist: I am not sure what you mean.

Paula: I see the look of disapproval in her eyes. I just know what she is thinking . . . I'll never measure up in her eyes. So f*** it! I'll prove to her what a f***-up I am.

Therapist: You are determined. Those are some powerful feelings and thoughts.

Paula: I'm used to them.

Therapist: Would it be OK if we test out some of these thoughts?

Paula: Test them out? What does that mean?

Therapist: Maybe shed a little light on the thoughts to see if they are totally accurate.

Paula: It's in my head. I know what is true or not. So I don't get what you mean by the testing thing.

Therapist: I totally agree that these are your thoughts, and it is crucial that you decide on their accuracy. By testing, I mean talking about the thoughts so we can take a fresh look at them from all sides. How willing on a scale from 1 to 10 are you to give it a try?

Paula: Maybe a 5.

Therapist: What part of you is unwilling?

Paula: I don't want you to take my mother's side and I am sick of being blamed.

Therapist: That is really reasonable. No one wants to be blamed. Testing isn't about assigning blame. It's about looking at the whole picture and then you can figure out what conclusions are best fits for you. How does this sound?

Paula: Well, when you put it that way I guess it would be OK.

Children and adolescents feel in control of little in their lives. Anytime you find a chance to empower adolescents, take it! Obtaining permission is a simple means to increase their perceptions of control. The therapist assiduously authorized Paula to maintain control in the dialogue. The therapist asked an open-ended question about Paula's willingness to test thoughts (e.g.,

"How willing are you on a scale from 1 to 10 to give it a try?") instead of a closed yes/no question. This created some therapeutic wiggle room in which the therapist could maneuver. Consequently, the therapist was able to process the unwillingness from a dimensional rather than an all-or-none perspective (e.g., "What part of you is unwilling?"). Indeed, this question led to an extremely meaningful response ("I'm sick of being blamed.").

Keep in Mind

- Use flexibility, patience, and creativity in your communications.
- Remain an advocate: Don't slug it out with the person.
- Create a good therapeutic mix in the dialogue by sprinkling in empathy and varied question formats.
- Collaborate and ask permission to test thoughts.
- Resist the urge to enter control battles.

When and why adolescents want to hold onto thoughts

Wednesday Addams, the gothic, sullen, and iconic daughter of Morticia and Gomez Addams created by cartoonist Charles Adams and further immortalized in the musical *The Addams Family* (Brickman, 2010), warned, "Don't analyze me, it's a deep dark hole and you don't want to go there!" Many children and adolescents share this view, holding tight and hard to their inaccurate thinking patterns. Making their private thoughts public and subjecting them to empirical testing is at times an excruciating crucible for these young people. Not surprisingly then, Socratic Dialogue with these clients can be a challenge.

In the following dialogue, Stacy, a depressed 16-year-old Euro-American girl who just lost her relationship with her boyfriend, gives her therapist a "don't go there" message.

Stacy: I just feel so crappy. No one understands how crappy I feel. People just don't listen.

Therapist: What is it that makes you feel so crappy?

Stacy: I just lost my boyfriend! What is so hard to get?

Therapist: Can you tell me some more about what happened?

Stacy: Why? You don't really want to know. I don't want to say it because it makes me feel bad and I don't want to feel worse. So we're even.

Clearly, this dialogue is a struggle at this moment. Stacy holds beliefs about revealing what is going through her head, how it will help her to express them, and what the therapist's reaction to the disclosure will be. Her therapist needs to switch the focus to the beliefs that mediate the "don't go there" stance.

Therapist: You are telling me a lot of things. Let's see if we can break them down together. What makes you say I don't want to hear what you have to say?

Stacy: Nobody does … It makes them feel uncomfortable and sorry for me. I don't need their pity. I have plenty of that on my own.

Therapist: I see. You think I will see you as pitiful and almost be scared off by what you say.

Stacy: Yeah … Kind of.

Therapist: What part am I missing?

Stacy: I don't even want to hear myself saying it … It makes me feel bad about myself.

Therapist: Sure. If you guess that I'll be scared off and you'll feel bad about yourself—then of course you wouldn't want to tell me what's going through your head.

Stacy: That's what I have been saying!

Therapist: Would you be willing to test a part of that out?

Stacy: What do you mean?

Therapist: Well, let's see … tell me the safest part about what you see as pitiful about you. Then we'll check in after a time to see if you are feeling bad or worse. How does that sound?

At this point, the therapist is engaging in a difficult calculus and making real-time adjustments in session. Collaboration is being assiduously sought (e.g., the use of the word "together"; "What part am I missing?"). Empathic responding is integrated into the dialogue (e.g., "If you guess that I'll be scared off and you'll feel bad about yourself yourself—then of course you wouldn't want to tell me what's going through your head."). Finally, the therapist floated the idea of a non-threatening graduated task which offered Stacy increased control.

Young people's beliefs often represent a form of boundary marking. They may see their emotions and cognitions as possessions (e.g., "These thoughts are mine."). Moreover, in their mind, these attitudes may preserve their identity (e.g., "I am a scenester. This is how we think and feel. I wouldn't expect you to understand it."). Their identity makes them different, unique, and separate from others, especially family. These youngsters may equate change with coercion. Accordingly, they may think that changing their beliefs means they are selling out and conforming to adult/parental authority.

In these instances, the dialogue can explore their absolute reasoning (e.g., "My thoughts define who I am. Giving them up means I lose who I am."). It is best to couple gentle questioning with explicit acceptance and nonjudgmental understanding of their longing for independence and identity.

The following dialogue is between her therapist and Kat, a 16-year-old Latina, whose beliefs are locked into place by boundary formation.

Therapist: You are sounding pretty depressed, Kat.

Kat: I know you and my parents are worried about me. But this is just how I am. It is really who I am.

Therapist: What do you mean that this is who you are?

Kat: Let's face it, I'm an emo.

Therapist: An emo?

Kat: Don't you know what emos are? We all sit together at lunch. The other kids stare at us. We all have *issues.* We kinda freak the other kids out especially the jocks and populars.

Therapist: So, it's your group.

Kat: Yep. We have the same interests and lots of the same emotional issues. We understand each other ... we help each other.

Therapist: It sounds like this group is helpful to you. How does it figure into your depression?

Kat: We're all depressed ... I don't cut but a lot of my friends do.

Therapist: I'm learning a lot about your friends but not so much about your depression.

Kat: Look ... we feel depressed about the same things. School is pointless ... parents are clueless ... and focus on the wrong things... we don't fit in ... we're lost, misfits. Rejects ... the things people chew up and spit out... we're roadkill.

Therapist: How much do you believe these things about yourself?

Kat: A lot. It pisses me off when people are really perky and think everything has to be fine. Like my mother, she always tells me to look on the sunny side of life ... she is so ... out of it. She like invented the pink side of life.

Therapist: And your color is black.

Kat: She doesn't get it ... but I feel for her ... she wanted this perky pretty cheerleader for a daughter like she was ... now she is stuck with me ... that must suck for her.

Therapist:	You are tuned into other people's thoughts and feelings like your mother and your group. What about you? Tell me what you predict will happen if your depressed feelings and thoughts began to change?
Kat:	It's who I am! I don't want to change who I am.
Therapist:	I can understand how you feel and how torn you feel and how annoying therapy is for you sometimes. You believe that if you are less depressed you risk losing who you are . . . Your true self.
Kat:	Yes.
Therapist:	What is clear is that you define yourself by your depression. What other things make up who you are?
Kat:	I love heavy metal music. I am really into anime. I like graphic novels.
Therapist:	How about your personality?
Kat:	I've got a kind of sick sense of humor . . . I am a deep thinker sometimes. I've got a . . . funky sense of fashion.
Therapist:	Anything else?
Kat:	No, I don't think so.
Therapist:	I'm going to draw this pie and I want you to slice it up giving each of these factors a percentage based on how much you think they determine your personality.
Kat:	. . . OK . . . metal music (fills in about 15%) . . . anime, that's a lot maybe a quarter of the pie (25%) . . . Graphic novels (fills in about 10%), humor (10%), deep thinker (5%), fashion (5%) . . .
Therapist:	So that last piece is depression (about 30% of the pie remains).
Kat:	. . . Yeah.
Therapist:	What does that mean about depression totally defining who you are?
Kat:	Hmm . . . Maybe it is less than I thought.

In this dialogue, the therapist did a good job adopting nonjudgmental stance while gently questioning Kat's sense that depression defined her. Using empathy (e.g., "And your color is black. I can understand how torn you feel and how annoying therapy is for you. You believe that if you are less depressed, you will risk losing yourself."), Socratic questions (e.g., "What do you predict will happen if some of your depressed thoughts change?") and a collaborative stance helped to engage Kat. Summary statements moved the dialogue forward. Finally, the synthesizing question was purposefully open-ended to propel guided discovery ("What does that mean about depression totally defining who you are?").

Keep in Mind

- Respect boundary marking thoughts, feelings, and behaviors.
- Balance explicit acceptance, a nonjudgmental attitude, and gentle, systematic questioning.
- Adopt a graduated task approach.
- Make real-time adjustments in session.

Trap 2

Socratic Dialogue resembles an intellectual colloquy rather than an emotionally meaningful task

---

Socratic dialogues are interpersonal enterprises that can pack an emotional punch. Dialogues that resemble intellectual debates or lectures fall flat with adolescents and children. While there may be earnest Socratic questioning occurring in session, when it becomes intellectualized or abstract or is accompanied by an aloof stance on the part of the therapist, it will be met with the deafening sounds of emotional silence.

Remaining clear about the difference between rational analysis and rationalization is a way to keep you on track. Rationalization is a defense mechanism which protects individuals from experiencing anxiety. Shapiro et al. (2005, 108) summarized, "when the need to avoid anxiety and distress outweighs the need for reality-based adaptation, people use defense mechanisms to avoid being conscious of some painful aspect of their internal or external world." Rationalization causes distortions in reality testing and consequently gets in the way of seeing clearly. Defense mechanisms fog awareness and stall psychological growth.

Rational analysis, on the other hand, is a skill set that helps people see themselves, others, and their experiences more accurately. Rational analysis is a logical reasoning process that can be applied to firmly held, albeit inaccurate, beliefs in order to foster more adaptive emotional functioning and productive action. Seminal cognitive therapists (Bandura, 1986; Beck, 1976) concluded that a person's illogical thinking patterns are a function of misleading appearances, insufficient evidence, overgeneralization, selection biases, flawed inductive reasoning, and faulty deductive analyses. Rational analysis, propelled by Socratic dialogues, serves to clarify and modify these thinking errors (Friedberg et al., 2014).

Two different dialogues with a 14-year-old African-American female named Ciara serve to illustrate the distinction between rationalization and rational analysis. In the first dialogue, the therapist reinforces rationalization.

Ciara:	I am so worried that the kids in my class will laugh at my project. I know it is going to be horrible.
Therapist:	How do you know this, Ciara?
Ciara:	I just do. It seems right.
Therapist:	Does it help you to worry about this?
Ciara:	No ... I guess not.
Therapist:	So it's not helpful. Have they ever laughed at you before?
Ciara:	No ... I don't think so.
Therapist:	So, although it seems like they will laugh, they haven't in the past and thinking about it is not helpful. So maybe it is a good idea not to worry about things that will not happen.

To the misinformed eye, this may look like some rudimentary cognitive restructuring or "reframing." However, the message to Ciara is Pollyannaish and "Don't worry about it," which is a rationalization. The therapist is unwittingly colluding with Ciara's style of avoiding anxiety and dreading fears of negative evaluation.

In the following second dialogue, read how the therapist spurs rational analysis with Ciara instead of rationalization.

Ciara:	I am so worried that the kids in my class will laugh at my project. I know it is going to be horrible.
Therapist:	These thoughts pump up your anxiety and so of course you want to put off the project. What makes you guess that the kids will laugh?
Ciara:	I just do. It seems right.
Therapist:	Because it feels right to you it convinces you the laughter will happen.
Ciara:	Yes!
Therapist:	That's the way it works with anxiety and the thoughts that surround it. May I ask you something else?
Ciara:	OK.
Therapist:	When in your past have the kids laughed at your project?
Ciara:	... Never ... but I have seen it happen to others.
Therapist:	It scared you and you worried the same thing might happen to you.
Ciara:	Exactly.

Therapist:	I see. Now, so I can get a clear picture of how this is for you, what would be so horrible if they laughed at you?
Ciara:	It would be embarrassing, I couldn't stand it.
Therapist:	You would feel really uncomfortable. What runs through your mind?
Ciara:	They'll think I'm stupid. It would be awkward and stuff. I would feel jittery and I'm a chill person.
Therapist:	If this horrible thing happened, what does it mean about you?
Ciara:	If they don't like me or think I'm stupid, then I'm a fake. They'll see right through me.
Therapist:	Wow, so the oral presentation is a threat because they could see the real you who is stupid and uncool.
Ciara:	(Teary.) Yes.
Therapist:	Can we look at this belief more closely?
Ciara:	I guess.
Therapist:	The real you is stupid and uncool. What convinces you of that?
Ciara:	I don't know.
Therapist:	Let me ask it in a different way. What makes you believe you are stupid and uncool?
Ciara:	I look at all the other kids and they seem to have it together. They don't stress out about little things. I freak out over everything.
Therapist:	So one thing is that you feel stressed a lot. And you don't notice the other kids being, as you say, freaked out.
Ciara:	Yeah.
Therapist:	I'll write that here under facts that say you are uncool and stupid. What else goes here?
Ciara:	… Um … I just don't know about all the popular movies and cool TV shows.
Therapist:	I'll list that. What else?
Ciara:	I don't joke around with kids much at school.
Therapist:	I see. That's a third piece of information. What else is there?
Ciara:	… I think that is pretty much it.
Therapist:	OK … Now what makes you doubt that you are stupid and uncool?
Ciara:	I can't think of anything.
Therapist:	I wonder, can you think of something about you that shows you are not stupid?
Ciara:	I'm in honors classes, I guess.
Therapist:	Okay. Now, what is true about you that could not be so true if you were uncool?
Ciara:	Like what?

Therapist:	Let's take a step back. What does cool mean to you?
Ciara:	You know … popular … having lots of friends … being chill.
Therapist:	So, tell me about your friends.
Ciara:	Well, I have a few really good friends.
Therapist:	How much do you hang around them?
Ciara:	Pretty much, I guess.
Therapist:	What do they think of you?
Ciara:	I guess they think I am chill.
Therapist:	Do they know you pretty well? I mean, the real you.
Ciara:	Yeah.
Therapist:	So, if they think you are chill, would you say that makes you doubt a little that you are uncool?
Ciara:	Sort of.

The second dialogue does not pre-empt Ciara's inaccurate beliefs. The thoughts are unpacked and examined. Additionally, Ciara completes the difficult work of questioning her own mental myths. The therapist guided Ciara's self-reflection by asking specific questions (e.g., "What is something about you that shows you are not stupid?" "What does cool mean?" "What is true about you that could not be so true if you were uncool?").

Therapist-created barriers

In the movie *The Wizard of Oz* (Fleming, 1939), Professor Marvel proclaims about himself, "Professor Marvel never guesses, he knows." Sometimes therapists confuse Socratic Dialogue with persuasion and lecturing. When therapists try to lecture, they engage in long-winded monologues. A reliable indicator of this trap is the young person's face glazing over with confusion and/or boredom.

Being a know-it-all like Professor Marvel is typically off-putting to young people. Indeed, a pedantic and dogmatic clinical stance may reflect therapeutic narcissism. Freeman et al. (2008, 369) wrote, "Therapeutic narcissism may take the form of telling rather than asking clients how they feel. It may show up in other ways; deciding what the client needs without consulting the client, believing that change should take less time than it does, setting goals for change that are distal and grandiose, or labeling clients as resistant for continuing to believe the dysfunctional ideas taught by parents and significant others."

Therapists sometimes slip into the trap of showing off their talents. When working with young people, they demonstrate their well-developed reasoning

skills and hypothesis testing abilities and forget they are working with individuals who are hypervigilant to evaluation. Children and adolescents often
are prone to seeing dialogues with adult authorities as battles in which adults
say, "I win, you lose. I'm right, you're wrong. I'm smart; you're dumb." When
therapists show off, children will likely plead no contest and submit rather
than join in the guided discovery process. Further, they may also passively act
like an audience and listlessly watch the therapist perform. Therefore, keep in
mind it is OK for therapists to be dumb.

The first dialogue with Davis, a 12-year-old Euro-American male, illustrates the version of this trap in which the child surrenders and resigns himself to the therapist's logic.

Therapist:	So, you see your brother as thinking he is the king of the family and wanting to make you a slave.
Davis:	Yes, I'm not going to be his slave.
Therapist:	I think seeing him as a king and trying to make you his slave causes you problems and you get into trouble with your anger. What is king-like about your brother?
Davis:	I don't know.
Therapist:	Maybe it's because he has his own ideas.
Davis:	I guess.
Therapist:	Can he have his own ideas and not be your king?
Davis:	I guess.
Therapist:	Maybe he just wants a chance to do what he wants.
Davis:	Maybe.
Therapist:	So, it would be more helpful to you if you stopped seeing him as a king and just a guy who has his own ideas. Is that right?
Davis:	Right.

In this flawed dialogue, the therapist unilaterally works diligently to decrease
Davis's all-or-none thinking that lead to his labeling his brother as "king."
There is conspicuous absence of collaboration and forced feeding of new
interpretations. Davis's reaction to this one-sided discussion was to shut down
and outwardly yield to the therapists' thinking.

This next dialogue with Blake, an 11-year-old Euro-American male, illustrates another aspect of this trap.

Therapist:	You certainly have a lot of worries about bad things happening to you if you stop worrying. I have an idea of something that might help.
Blake:	OK.

Therapist:	I've listed some of the bad things that could happen. Look at this list. Here's a tornado, car accident, house fire, being bullied at school, mom and dad getting sick, flunking a test, mom and dad getting robbed, and your dog running away.
Blake:	Those are bad.
Therapist:	They are bad but they are not very likely. Some even will never happen to you, right?
Blake:	Some of them.
Therapist:	But you still worried about them, right?
Blake:	Yeah.
Therapist:	OK. If worrying about them stops them from happening, none of them would happen if you worried about them. But still they did happen. So that means that worrying does not have any effect on whether bad things happen, right?
Blake:	I never thought about it like that before.

In this example, Blake observed the therapist debunk his belief that "If I worry, bad things won't happen." While the therapist's logic may be impeccable, Blake had no opportunity to test his own thought. The data came almost exclusively from the therapist.

A Socratic Dialogue is fundamentally a creative enterprise (Greenberg, 2000; Mooney & Padesky, 2000). In a very simple sense, children and adolescents come to therapy "stuck." They persist with maladaptive and unproductive patterns. These youngsters sometimes become frozen in place due to their psychological inertia and sense of hopelessness. Creativity can unlock their frozen assets.

Keep in Mind

- It is OK and sometime preferable for therapists to be dumb.
- Genuine two-way dialogue can enhance creativity and that can unlock the young person's frozen assets.

Socratic use of games

Games are great ways to facilitate Socratic Dialogue with younger children. Therapists can use board games, video/computer games, electronic hand-held games, and so on. Box 9.1 offers a partial list of potential games.

Box 9.1 Games Useful as Prompts for Socratic Dialogue

Checkers
Chess
Jenga
Card Games
Connect Four
Battleship
Operation
Mouse Trap
Hungry Hippos
Memory Game
Password
Nerf Basketball
Naughts & Crosses or Tic-tac-toe
WII games

One therapist used games to help Kashmir, a 9-year-old African-American male who became angry and aggressive when he believed his self-esteem was assaulted. Losing in a game, getting a poor grade, or being scolded were typical triggers. Since written and purely verbal Socratic Dialogue was somewhat unproductive, Kashmir and his therapist decided to use video game play as a way to test his thoughts. The following dialogue demonstrated the way games can be used as prompts for Socratic Dialogue.

Kashmir: You sit in here and practice all day! That's why you are winning!

Therapist: I am getting more points than you right now.

Kashmir: This isn't my favorite game anyhow. I hate this! (Throws the game controller.)

Therapist: OK, Kash, let's stop here. Look up here at this white board. How are you feeling?

Kashmir: Pissed.

Therapist: Good that you can let me know that you're pissed off, but throwing something is not an OK way to show your anger. We have to find out what's going through your mind when you throw things. So, what went through your mind just then?

Kashmir: I hate losing!

Therapist: I see. What does it mean about you if you are losing?

Kashmir:	I'm not good! I don't want to be a loser. Losers suck! You are making me be a loser!
Therapist:	No wonder why you are so mad. Sounds like you feel a little ashamed too.
Kashmir:	I should win against you all the time!
Therapist:	Kash, now I can understand how angry you get. You think when others beat you they are shaming you and causing you to believe you suck.
Kashmir:	I guess so.
Therapist:	Can I ask you something?
Kashmir:	OK.
Therapist:	What might be some other reasons people win or beat you in a game?
Kashmir:	I don't know ... They cheat?
Therapist:	OK ... possible. How about they are lucky?
Kashmir:	OK.
Therapist:	What else? I'll write them down for you.
Kashmir:	... They're older ... They play more ... I guess they might be better.
Therapist:	So you came up with three other explanations. If you thought you lost because they are older, play more, or even are better than you, how much do you believe they are purposely trying to make you feel bad?
Kashmir:	I don't know.
Therapist:	Is just being better at a game the same as trying to make you feel bad about yourself?
Kashmir:	I guess not.
Therapist:	So how about this idea? Would you be willing to write about the question, "What are some reasons people win other than trying to make me feel bad?" on a card and keep it with you and read it over before you explode.
Kashmir:	... I will if you write the card.

The therapist used the emotion elicited through the game play to launch Socratic Dialogue. The therapist processed Kashmir's thoughts and feelings as well as setting limits in the session (e.g., "Throwing something is not an OK way to show your anger."). Since Kashmir was a younger child, the therapist simplified the task by writing down the summary ideas for him. It is unlikely Kashmir will use the card on his own outside of therapy unless he and his therapist practice using the card in session when he loses future games. Use of the card in session also gives both of them a chance to see whether it helps or not.

Foster fun in therapy

Humor in therapy requires spontaneity and is consistent with the notion of experiential learning (Franzini, 2001). Martin and Ford (2018) concluded that humor in therapy fosters a positive alliance, promotes cognitive flexibility, alternative thinking, and broader perspective taking. Moreover, humor sparks coping and minimizes criticism (McGraw & Warren, 2010).

Therefore, avoid becoming stuffy and stiff in your clinical manner. At the very minimal level, be mindful about using adult vocabulary and jargon. The following example with 10-year-old Isiah illustrates a dialogue marked by overly sophisticated language.

Isiah:	I know I can't let myself have friends. It will turn out bad. They'll tease and bully me.
Therapist:	You seem afraid of being vulnerable and worry your friends will abandon you.
Isiah:	. . . Um . . . I guess but I don't know what these words mean.
Therapist:	Vulnerable means being hurt and abandoned means you feel like your friends will leave you. Do you understand now?
Isiah:	. . . I think so
Therapist:	So, let's do a test of evidence.
Isiah:	. . . I don't know what evidence means.

In this brief exchange, the therapist erred by using both overly sophisticated language and jargon. Words such as vulnerable and abandonment are not commonly used in lay conversation. A preferable approach would be explaining the constructs in everyday language children understand. (e.g., instead of saying "abandoned," say "feel like you are all alone"). Additionally, evidence is a technical term. A better option might be to explain the process (e.g., "Are you willing to check out whether your guesses about your friends will come true?").

Fun is an underappreciated concept in Socratic dialogues with children. When children see therapy as playful, they are apt to forget they are in therapy. In this way, they may be more likely to approach emotionally powerful material. Stories, games, cartoons, humor, metaphor, and exercise are the "stuff of childhood." Therefore, including them during guided discovery is developmentally sensitive and contributes to the fun.

Workbook exercises can foster Socratic Dialogues and offer clinicians several advantages (Friedberg, 1996). Workbooks walk therapists through guided discovery processes. They provide structure and direction to dialogues. Exercises are inherently interactive so children's participation is encouraged. Finally, workbooks typically include written assignments, which allow for making summaries and review. There are a number of workbooks available for children and adolescents that are fun for children to use (Kendall et al., 2013; Stallard, 2019). For adolescents, there are a number of workbooks that include cartoons and graphic novel characteristics. These address a number of issues such as shyness and social anxiety (Shannon, 2022); anxiety, worry, and panic (Shannon, 2015); procrastination and perfectionism (Shannon, 2017); and mindfulness approaches for managing depression, anxiety and trauma (Scarlet, 2017).

Despite these advantages, remain mindful of several cautions. First, for children with reading, writing, or attention difficulties, workbooks may be off-putting. Second, over-reliance on workbooks can distance therapists from children. These tools can be used when they move the treatment alliance forward rather than get in the way. In sum, therapists are encouraged to work diligently to make the exercises come alive and not stagnate on the page. Make sure you find a way to engage children in any written work.

Using puppet play as part of Socratic Dialogues is beneficial with many children (Friedberg & McClure, 2018). One puppet character can voice the thoughts linked to the child's distress and the other can use Socratic Dialogue to guide the first puppet's discovery. The practice could start with the therapist playing the Socratic role and then progress to the child assuming the role of a wise friend expressing alternative ideas to the struggling puppet.

Metaphors also can help free youngsters from unyielding thoughts that emotionally handcuff them. They provide psychological distance from problems and facilitate alternative thinking. A metaphorical Socratic Dialogue is a style of questioning used with children (Beal et al., 1996). Grave and Blissett (2004) emphasized that metaphors with children simplify sophisticated reasoning processes involved in tests of evidence, reattribution, and decatastrophizing.

For example, a line from the Disney movie *Mulan* (Bancroft and Croft, 1998) provides basis for a favorite metaphor. In this charming film, the Emperor of China explains, "The flower that blooms in adversity is the most rare and beautiful of all." This metaphor could be used to help children realize the importance of tolerating and persisting despite negative emotional arousal. For older children plagued by debilitating regrets and remorse over minor flaws and setbacks, Don Draper's, the protagonist from the US Television Series *Mad Men* (Veith, 2008) mantra, "I live life in one direction ... forward!" is apropos. Therapists can initiate Socratic Dialogue focusing on how that metaphor could apply to them.

Embracing immediacy in session is a pivotal way to mobilize Socratic Dialogues with children. In general, immediacy refers to attending and responding to moment-to-moment reactions in sessions. Mood, physiological, behavioral, and cognitive shifts are clues for immediacy. Coupling Socratic questions with experiential learning is another option for avoiding being too intellectual in session. Kraemer (2006) recognized that psychotherapy is an intense encounter and often resembles live theatre. In line with this idea, improvisational theatre games are excellent vehicles for experiential guided discovery with children and adolescents. Improvisational theatre games are unscripted, occur in real time, and involve decreased verbal demands and keep clients present focused (Fink, 1990; Weiner, 1994). Improvisation games can feature situations similar to those that trouble the child or ones that evoke similar moods or thoughts.

Monsterpiece Theatre (Weiner, 1994) is a fun, experiential method of guided discovery that can help children objectively view their problems and gain added perspective. In this game, a list of monstrous attributes is generated. Weiner recommends these attributes include emotions, mannerisms, hygiene habits, and interpersonal strategies. The child then plays the "monster" in the scene and the therapist helps process both their internal experiences (e.g., thoughts/feelings) as well as their effect on others.

Monsterpiece theatre fits nicely with the talk back to OCD approach espoused by March and Mulle (1998). Essentially, Monsterpiece theatre concretizes an objectification process. For example, the monster could assume the characteristics of OCD (e.g., demanding, bossy, controlling, harsh, punitive, etc.). The therapist and child take turns playing the monster. Initially, the child plays the OCD monster and the therapist models talk-back strategies during the dialogue. During "intermission," the therapist and child process the first act (e.g., "What was it like to play the OCD monster?" "What ran through your head when I argued back?" "How did the monster feel then?" "When did you as the monster feel more powerful?" "What did you see as the best ways to talk back?"). The best counter thoughts should then be written on index cards.

During the next phase in act two, children play themselves in a scene with the OCD monster. The child may elect to keep some cue cards handy to help construct the talk-back strategies. Similarly, after the second act is completed, the therapist and patient process the exercise. The therapist will help the young client record productive coping thoughts and provide helpful feedback in order to develop additional strategies.

Experiential guided discovery

As described in Chapter 1, Socratic Dialogue can readily be coupled with experiential procedures. Rigidly held beliefs require powerful disconfirming experiences in order to change (Bandura, 1977). Adding an experiential component can make discussions more emotionally rich and genuine. Linking concrete experiential exercises with Socratic Dialogue fosters consensus between head and heart (Padesky, 2004).

Consider the following example with Brandi, a 9-year-old Euro-American girl who frequently thought she was not good enough. This thought was associated with sad and anxious moods. Just talking about this belief did not lead to any cognitive dissonance. Therefore, her therapist introduced an experiential task, Label Fable (Friedberg et al., 2011). Label Fable teaches three crucial principles. Children learn that false labels do not determine content. Moreover, content is sometimes independent of labels. Finally, testing the accuracy and validity of labels is important.

In the first phase of the task, the therapist brought out two cans of soda. In this example, one can was cola and the other was root beer. The therapist then labeled one styrofoam cup "Cola" and one cup "Root Beer." Then, he asked Brandi to close her eyes. The therapist then put root beer in both cups. The following dialogue picks up the session at this point:

Brandi: Hey, they are both root beer!

Therapist: (Smiles.) But they weren't labeled that way, were they?

Brandi: You tricked me!

Therapist: Yes I did. That's kind of the same way your mind tricks you. Sometimes the labels you put on yourself don't match what is inside you. Do you think that could be true for some of the labels you put on yourself?

Brandi: Maybe.

Brandi: How did you know the label on this cup wasn't right?

Brandi: I could taste what was inside.

Therapist: So you knew what root beer was made of. You could taste the ingredients. Would it help if you were sure about what goes into your label of being good enough?

Brandi: I kinda think so.

Therapist: So let's test the stuff that goes into your being good enough so you are sure about the label. What things are good enough about you?

Brandi: I'm a good student ... I am on student council ... I place usually at my swim meets ... I am a good friend ... I don't get into trouble with my parents.

Therapist: Great. I just wrote down the things that go into your label of being good enough.

The work with Brandi show how experiential tasks make abstract material more concrete. Brandi learned from a real-life experiment that labels can be arbitrary and even inaccurate. The therapist worked diligently to help Brandi apply these ideas to her own label making. Finally, the therapist simplified the task by writing summary ideas down for Brandi.

Santana was a 10-year-old highly anxious Latina girl who feared disapproval and subsequently erected harsh standards for herself. She believed that she should never criticize anyone or break any rule, however minor. While Socratic Dialogue alone was modestly successful, her beliefs remained relatively entrenched. Therefore, an experiment was collaboratively designed. Santana filled out a negative comment card and put it in the suggestion box. She also put an empty soda can in the trash rather than the recycling bin while in full view of clinic staff. Prior to conducting these experiments, Santana made predictions (e.g., "People will think I am irresponsible and I'll be punished."), completed the task, and then processed the experience with her therapist ("Which predictions came true?" "What do you make of them not coming true?" 'How do you account for that?").

Keep in Mind

- Be clear on the distinction between rational analysis and rationalization.
- Embrace immediacy in session.
- Repeatedly check in with the child and adolescent.
- Don't show off and express "therapist narcissism."
- Integrate experiential exercises, workbooks, play materials, humor, and fun with Socratic Dialogues.

Trap 3

Children's tolerance for ambiguity, abstraction, and frustration is low and therapists struggle to handle this

---

Children's who have low tolerance for ambiguity, abstraction, and frustration provide a third trap for therapists. Children with a high need for certainty can find abstract, open-ended questions aversive. Fear of loss of control can lurk behind children's high needs for certainty. Additionally, ambiguous questions often sail over the head of youngsters who are earth bound by concrete thinking processes. Finally, children and adolescents with low frustration tolerance seek immediate gratification. In short, they want answers, not more questions. Consequently, they may boycott the guided discovery process.

Match the informational processing level of the child

Matching guided discovery methods to the information processing level of the child minimizes frustration. For children and adolescents whose abstract reasoning is less well-developed, guided discovery methods that include cartoons, graphics, and other simplifying materials are indicated (Kingery et al., 2006; Piacentini & Bergman, 2001). Further, guided discovery methods emphasizing behavioral experiments and other experientially based procedures are good ideas. Written tests of evidence are only beneficial for children whose logical and sequential reasoning skills are well-developed.

There are a number of strategies that can make Socratic Dialogues more accessible to these youngsters. First, breaking down questions into their simplest form is imperative. Using short, crisp questions can jump start stalled rational analysis. Being pithy is good. Youngsters get lost in rambling, vague, and diffuse questions. Try to match task demands to children's response capacities.

Jake is a 12-year-old boy diagnosed with autism spectrum disorder (ASD). Similar to other youngsters with ASD, Jake is chained to rigid rules for himself, others, and the way the world should work. His therapy provided an excellent illustration of navigating this third trap, working with children who have low tolerance for ambiguity, abstraction, and frustration. You can see how Jake balked in the early part of the following Socratic Dialogue. See if you can discern errors his therapist made as she fell into the trap of his frustration.

Jake: I can't believe how stupid and boring my language arts teacher is. I tell her my opinion of the book and she sends me to the office. All the kids call me a brainiac and laugh at me; I hate that!

Therapist: So, what did you say to get you sent to the principal?

Jake: I told the teacher we shouldn't be spending our valuable time reading books like this. That's all.

Therapist: I see. How were you feeling at that time?

Jake: Really mad.

Therapist: Mad? What went through your mind?

Jake: I hate language arts. This class is sucking the life out of me.

Therapist: Those are strong words. What do you mean sucking the life out of you?

Jake: I shouldn't have to take that class.

Therapist: You really have some clear rules for yourself.

Jake: I don't know what you mean.

Therapist: There are ways you think people should be and the way the world should work.

Jake: Doesn't everyone?

Therapist: Of course they do.

Jake: So what's the big deal?

Therapist: Do your rules work for you?

Jake: Sure they do. Why wouldn't they?

Therapist: Let's take a look at the evidence that the rules work for you.

Jake: Why?

Therapist: Do you think it will be helpful?

Jake: I don't think so

Therapist: Why not?

Jake: The rules are mine. I don't want to change my rules.

Therapist: I wonder why you don't want to change your rules.

Jake: I like them. Why should I change them?

Therapist: If we look at possible advantages and disadvantages perhaps we could see whether language arts would be easier if you change the rules?

Jake: Why is it me that has to change? Why shouldn't Mrs. Promer change and assign us a different book?

Jake started his boycott early in the dialogue. (e.g., "Doesn't everyone?" "So what's the big deal?" "Why wouldn't they?"). The therapist became frustrated and drifted toward unproductive "why" questions (e.g., "Why not?" "I wonder why you don't want to change your rules."). The why questions seemed to drive Jake further into justifying his rules and sunk the dialogue. Perhaps, a more productive dialogue would emerge if the therapist adjusted her stance to address Jake's unwillingness to change his rules (e.g., "You are determined to keep your rules. What's the reason you are so determined?" "You seem to be fighting for your rules. What's that about?" "What do you think would happen if you loosened your rules?"). The following dialogue shows how these "What" questions are more productive than "Why" questions, especially when they are paired with empathy for Jake's viewpoint:

Therapist: You are determined to keep your rules. What's the reason you are so determined?

Jake: I feel calmer when the rules make sense.

Therapist: I can understand that. That fits with why you begin to fight your teachers when they insist on a different rule—one that doesn't make sense to you.

Jake:	Their rules are stupid. I shouldn't have to take language arts.
Therapist:	I hear you. And I worry about you, too.
Jake:	What do you mean?
Therapist:	I somehow think because there's a law that every student has to take language arts, this is a rule you won't be able to change. But I see how upset it makes you and I worry about how you will be able to deal with feeling so upset all the time.
Jake:	Yeah. That sucks!
Therapist:	I wonder if we could figure out a way for you to not be so upset, even when a rule doesn't make sense to you.
Jake:	I don't know what you mean.
Therapist:	I'm not sure either. I think we would need to figure it out together. Would you be willing to see if we could come up with some ideas to help you feel better with rules that don't make sense?

Dose Socratic Dialogue with empathy and optimal doubt

Dosing Socratic Dialogue is a productive strategy. Simply, dose the dialogue so the process is on the cutting edge of learning rather than overly frustrating. In the previous dialogue, Jake's therapist mixed questions with expressions of empathic understanding of Jake's replies. Expressions of concern balanced the introduction of a new and somewhat challenging idea, "I wonder if we could figure out a way for you to not be so upset, even when a rule doesn't make sense to you." The Yerkes–Dodson law leads the way here. As a refresher, Yerkes–Dodson (1908) stated that in a situation, there is an optimal point of arousal. If the arousal is either too low or too high, performance will suffer. Therapists want to ensure that their Socratic Dialogues are sufficiently arousing to stimulate doubt but not so overstimulating as to create frustration or discouragement.

Creating doubt is a dimensional task rather than a categorical one. Therefore, therapists should embrace the question of how much doubt is necessary to create with Socratic dialogues.

The issue of whether sufficient doubt is aroused is ambiguous. Learning to tolerate ambiguity is essential for therapists (Mooney & Padesky, 2000; Padesky, 2007). An absolute criterion for sufficient doubt is construction of a completely new thought that accurately reflects multiple aspects of one's experience. A relative criterion is decreasing the person's degree of belief in a negative automatic thought. Accepting relative criteria can leave therapists with an unsettling sense of incompleteness. However, adopting a therapeutic perspective that incorporates a range of doubt is prudent. Over time and with repeated sessions, therapists can revisit distorted thoughts and work to further decrease their believability.

The following dialogue with a 16-year-old Asian-American female named Sydney is an example of adopting a dimensional view of doubt and dosing the dialogue. In addition to experiencing depressed and angry moods, Sydney was caught between her parents' desire for her to adhere to their traditional Korean cultural values (e.g., strict deference to elders/authority, de-emphasizing autonomy, maintaining a degree of emotional stoicism, etc.) and her own desire to assimilate into dominant United States teen culture. Accordingly, the therapist needed to introduce a cultural context into their Socratic Dialogue:

Sydney: My parents treat me like I'm a baby or some kid who just stepped out of a short yellow bus. (Laughs.)

Therapist: You're laughing but you've told me that makes you really furious.

Sydney: Yeah. So what that I skip out on school. It's so boring at school anyway. What do I need that s*** for? Yeah, I am angry and depressed but I'm not a f***ing child.

Therapist: How much do you think your parents trust you?

Sydney: Not at all.

Therapist: I am sure that hurts. How is it that you think your parents see you?

Sydney: You'd have to ask them.

Therapist: Fair enough. But what is your guess about how they see you?

Sydney: A disappointment . . . A f***-up . . . an infant who has to be watched so she won't put a fork in the toaster.

Therapist: So you see your parents' protection as due to them seeing you as a baby and a f***-up.

Sydney: Yep.

Therapist: How do you want them to see you?

Sydney: Not like that. Like someone who knows what they doing. Someone who is in charge of their life.

Therapist: You want them to see you as capable . . .

Sydney: And they see me as a total screw up!

Therapist: OK . . . I see . . . How sure are you that that see you that way?

Sydney: 100%.

Therapist: Wow, you're convinced. It is certainly possible that your parents' overprotectiveness is due to seeing you as a baby. I wonder what could be some other reasons?

Sydney: Like what?

Therapist: I'm not sure yet. Let's see if together we can think of some things. For instance, how much of a worrier is your dad?

Sydney: A big one … He freaks out over everything!

Therapist: Could that make him overprotective for any reason?

Sydney: I guess. He always worries bad things will happen to me.

Therapist: Let's write that down. What else?

Sydney: … Well my mother is a control freak.

Therapist: And you think that could be a reason she is overprotective?

Sydney: For sure.

Therapist: Anything else?

Sydney: … They think the world will f*** you over … I guess that comes from watching the news too much.

Therapist: I'll write that one too. (Writes.) How much do you think they want the best for you?

Sydney: … Pretty much

Therapist: I'll write what we have so far. So we have your dad is a worrier, your mom is a control freak, they think the world will f*** you over and they might want the best for you. How much do you believe each one?

Sydney: … On a scale of 1–10. Let's see … Dad a worrier 10, Mom a control freak definitely a 10, the world will f*** you over 8, wanting the best for me 4 or 5.

Therapist: Let's just pause and look at what we've written so far, because I think that it's really interesting. At first it seemed that your parents' overprotectiveness was 100% due to them thinking you were a screw-up. Then you came up with some really interesting observations—your dad's a worrier (10/10), your mother's a control freak (10/10), they think the world will f*** you over (8/10), and they want the best for you (4–5/10). When you take all that into account, I'm wondering what you make of this?

This long dialogue illustrates the merits of patience. The therapist used belief ratings repeatedly to chip away at Sydney's absolute reasoning. These ratings allowed the therapist to lay the foundation for doubt with the synthesizing question (e.g., "I'm wondering what you make of this?"). Indeed, in order to shift her cognitive set, Sydney did not have to believe her parents saw her as 100% competent; she only needed to decrease her certainty that the overprotectiveness was absolutely determined by her parents' poor view of her.

Keep in Mind

- Use short crisp questions.
- Match task demands to children's capacities.
- Dose the dialogue so learning is facilitated.
- Emphasize the child's capacity to help themselves
- Champion a dimensional view of doubt by liberal use of belief ratings.

Summary

Children and adolescents who experience emotional difficulties can hold darkly subversive thoughts about themselves, their future, present experiences, and other people. Developmental trajectories and productive behaviors can be blocked by those private stories. Proficient use of Socratic Dialogue guides children toward identifying, testing, and eventually doubting their undermining assumptions. This chapter presented common traps encountered when applying guided discovery methods. Keep in mind principles guided the way.

Remember that expertise in Socratic Dialogue is more of an ongoing process than an attained skill. Socratic Dialogue competence is dimensional and movement along the continuum is fueled by supervision, experiential learning, and self-reflection that appreciates both successes and failures. While patience when working with children and adolescents is a must, patience with oneself is a cardinal virtue. A perfect dialogue is an impossible standard. Inevitable stuck points can be fortuitous in that they may lead to robust arenas for investigation. Like Janus, as cognitive therapists, we seek to open up multiple doors and explicitly value wide exploration. Therapeutic values such as flexibility, creativity, patience, self-reflective practice, collaboration, and learning to embrace negative emotional arousal as well as to tolerate ambiguity fosters good Socratic Dialogue with children and adolescents.

Reader Learning Activities

- What traps do you see yourself falling into in your therapy with children and adolescents?
- For each trap, review those sections and this chapter and formulate your unhelpful pattern. Then try one or more of the interventions

described that seems to be clinically appropriate for your clients taking into account their ages and reasoning levels.

- Consider what experiential activities you could add to your therapy with children and adolescents. Try one of these out that is promising as a means to guide your client's discovery and pair it with Socratic Dialogue.

- If you hold any therapist beliefs or assumptions that risk creating barriers in your therapy, identify these. Consider how to address these in self-supervision or with a supervisor or consultant.

References

Allen, W. (2007). *Mere anarchy*. New York: Random House.

Austen, J. (1908). *Sense and sensibility*. London: Cassell.

Bancroft, T., & Croft, B. (Directors). (1998). *Mulan* [Film]. United States: Walt Disney Feature Animation.

Bandura, A. B. (1977). *Social learning theory*. Englewood Cliffs, NJ: Prentice-Hall.

Bandura, A. B. (1986) *Social foundations of thought and action*. Englewood Cliffs, NJ: Prentice-Hall.

Beal, D., Kopec, A. M., & DiGuiseppe, R. (1996). Disputing patients' irrational beliefs. *Journal of Rational-Emotive and Cognitive Behavioral Therapy, 14*, 215–229. https://doi.org/10.1007/BF02238137

Beck, A. T. (1976). *Cognitive therapy of the emotional disorders*. New York: International Universities Press.

Brickman, M. (Writer). (2010). *The Addams Family Musical* [Musical theatre]. United States: Stuart Oken, Roy Furman, Michael Leavitt, 5 cent Productions and Elephant Eye Theatrical Productions.

Dahl, R. E. (2004). Adolescent brain development: a period of vulnerabilities and opportunities. *Annals of the New York Academy of Sciences, 1021*, 1–22. https://doi.org/10.1196/annals.1308.001

Daniel, S. S., & Goldston, D. B. (2009). Interventions for suicidal youth: A review of the literature and developmental considerations. *Suicide and Life-Threatening Behaviors, 39*, 252–268. https://onlinelibrary.wiley.com/doi/abs/10.1521/suli.2009.39.3.252

Fink, S. O. (1990). Approaches to emotion in psychotherapy and theatre: Implications for drama therapy. *The Arts in Psychotherapy, 17*, 5–18. https://doi.org/10.1016/0197-4556(90)90036-P

Fleming, V. (Director). (1939). *The Wizard of Oz* [Film]. United States: Metro-Goldwyn-Mayer.

Franzini, L. (2001). Humor in therapy: the case for training therapists in its uses and risks. *Journal of General Psychology, 128*, 170–193. https://doi.org/10.1080/00221300109598906

Freeman, A., Felgoise, S. H., & Davis, D. (2008). *Clinical psychology: Integrating science and practice*. New York: Wiley.

Friedberg, R. D. (1996). Cognitive behavioral games and workbooks: Tips for school counselors. *Elementary School and Guidance Counseling, 31*, 11–20. https://www.jstor.org/stable/42869167

Friedberg, R. D., Gorman, A. A., Wilt, L. H., Buickians, A., & Murray, M. (2011). *Cognitive behavioral therapy for the busy child psychiatrist and other mental health professionals: Rubrics and rudiments.* New York: Routledge.

Friedberg, R. D., & McClure, J. M. (2018). *Clinical practice of cognitive therapy with children and adolescents: The nuts and bolts* (2nd ed.). New York: Guilford.

Friedberg, R. D., McClure, J. M., & Garcia, J. H. (2014). *Cognitive therapy techniques for children and adolescents: Tools for enhancing practice.* New York: Guilford.

Grave, J., & Blissett. J. (2004). Is cognitive behavior therapy developmentally appropriate for young children? A critical review of the evidence. *Clinical Psychology Review, 24,* 399–420. https://doi.org/10.1016/j.cpr.2004.03.002

Greenberg, R. L. (2000). The creative client in cognitive therapy. *Journal of Cognitive Psychotherapy, 14,* 163–174. https://doi.org/10.1891/0889-8391.14.2.163

James, I. A., Morse, R., & Howarth, A. (2010). The science and art of asking questions in cognitive therapy. *Behavioural and Cognitive Psychotherapy, 38,* 83–93. https://doi.org/10.1017/S135246580999049X

Kendall, P. C., Beidas, R. S., & Mauro, C. (2013). *Brief coping cat: The 8-session coping cat workbook.* Ardmore, PA: Workbook Publishing.

Kingery, J. N., Roblek, T. L., Suveg, C., Grover, R. L., Sherill, J. T., & Bergman, R. L. (2006). "They're not just little adults": Developmental considerations for implementing cognitive behavioral therapy with youth. *Journal of Cognitive Psychotherapy, 20,* 263–273. https://doi.org/10.1891/jcop.20.3.263

Kraemer, S. (2006). Something happens: Elements of therapeutic change. *Clinical Child Psychiatry and Psychology, 11,* 239–248. https://doi.org/10.1177/1359104506061415

Lageman, A. G. (1989). Socrates and psychotherapy. *Journal of Religion and Health, 28,* 219–223. https://doi.org/10.1007/BF00987753

Leahy, R. L. (1985). The cost of development: Clinical implications. In R. L. Leahy (Ed.), *The development of the self* (pp. 267–294). San Diego: Academic Press.

McGraw, A. P., & Warren, C. (2010). Benign violations: Making immoral behavior funny. *Psychological Science, 21,* 1141–1149. https://doi.org/10.1177/0956797610376073

March, J. S., & Mulle, K. (1998). *OCD in children and adolescents: A cognitive behavioral treatment manual.* New York: Guilford.

Martin, R. D. & Ford, T. (2018). *The psychology of humor: An integrative approach.* London: Elsevier Academic Press.

Mooney, K. A., & Padesky, C. A. (2000). Applying client creativity to recurrent problems: Constructing possibilities and tolerating doubt. *Journal of Cognitive Psychotherapy, 14,* 149–161. https://doi.org/10.1891/0889-8391.14.2.149

Padesky, C. A. (1988). *Intensive training course in cognitive therapy.* Newport Beach, CA.

Padesky, C. A. (1993, Sept.). *Socratic questioning: changing minds or guided discovery.* Keynote address at the meeting of the European Congress of Behavioral and Cognitive Psychotherapies, London, UK. Retrieved from https://www.padesky.com/clinical-corner/publications

Padesky, C. A. (2004). Behavioral experiments at the crossroads. In J. Bennett-Levy, G. Butler, M. Fennell, A. Hackman, M. Mueller, & D. Westbrook (Eds.), *Oxford guide to behavioral experiments in cognitive therapy* (pp. 433–438). Cambridge, UK: Oxford University Press.

Padesky, C. A. (2007, July). *The next frontier: building positive qualities with cognitive behavior therapy.* Invited address at the 5th World Congress of Behavioural and Cognitive Therapies, Barcelona, Spain.

Piacentini, J., & Bergman, R. L. (2001). Developmental issues in cognitive therapy with child-hood anxiety disorders. *Journal of Cognitive Psychotherapy, 60*, 1181–1194. https://doi.org/10.1891/0889-8391.15.3.165

Scarlet, J. (2017). *Superhero therapy: Mindfulness skills to help teens and young adults deal with anxiety depression & trauma*. Oakland, CA: New Harbinger Publications.

Schulberg, B. (Writer). (1954). *On the waterfront* [Film]. United States: Horizon Pictures and Columbia Pictures.

Shannon, J. (2015). *The anxiety survival guide for teens: CBT skills to overcome fear, worry and panic*. Oakland, CA: New Harbinger Publications.

Shannon, J. (2017). *A teen's guide to getting stuff done: Discover your procrastination types, stop putting things off, and reach your goals*. Oakland, CA: New Harbinger Publications.

Shannon, J. (2022). *The shyness and social anxiety workbook for teens: CBT and ACT skills to help you build social confidence*. Oakland, CA: New Harbinger Publications.

Shapiro, J. E., Friedberg, R. D., & Bardenstein, K. K. (2005). *Child and adolescent therapy: Science and art*. New York: Wiley.

Stallard, P. (2019). *Think good, feel good: A cognitive behavioural therapy workbook for children and young people*. Chichester, UK: Wiley.

Veith, R. (Writer). (2008). The new girl (Season 2, Episode 5) [TV series episode]. In Matthew Weiner (Executive Producer), *Mad men*. Weiner Bros. Productions; Lionsgate Productions; AMC Original Productions.

Weiner, D. J. (1994). *Rehearsals for growth*. New York: W. W. Norton.

Yerkes, R. M., & Dodson, J. D. (1908). The relation of strength of stimulus to rapidity of habit formation. *Journal of Comparative and Neurological Psychology, 18*, 459–482. https://doi.org/10.1002/cne.920180503

Zuckerman, M. (1979). Attribution of success and failure revisited or the motivational bias is alive and well in attribution theory. *Journal of Personality and Social Psychology, 47*, 245–287. https://doi.org/10.1111/j.1467-6494.1979.tb00202.x

10

Socratic Dialogue in Group Therapy

James L. Shenk

Celia: I got really depressed over the weekend. I was planning to go to the work party Friday night, but I really didn't feel like going. I just felt so tired and didn't want to see anyone. I don't know what to do. I don't think I'm getting any better.

John: (To Celia.) You told us last week that you were going to go to that work party. I mean, I think you're supposed to take action and push yourself out there if you want to make any real progress. (Turns to the other group members.) Isn't that right?

Celia appears more despondent after John's comment. The other members of the therapy group are quiet. Some members are looking at the floor, some at the therapist. As the group's therapist, you find yourself quickly contemplating your options. You can see that Celia is really feeling depressed. No one seems to be responding to Celia directly; no one is giving her any empathy. She may not feel safe in the group right now. You could validate her feelings, but maybe you should give other members the opportunity to respond first. Or maybe it would be best to continue the didactic portion you had planned for today. Shifting to that might ease the tension, and you are already are a little behind on this session's planned agenda. You could ask others about their feelings and automatic thoughts, but then, what about Celia's feelings? It would seem more genuine to just let others respond in a natural way, but no one is saying anything to her!

This vignette illustrates typical challenges and dilemmas therapists encounter in group therapy. A group therapist must discern whether to focus on Celia's needs in the moment, John's communication style, redirect to topics on that session's agenda, or focus on interpersonal cognitions, processes, and behaviors. Time-limited formats, common in cognitive behavioral therapy (CBT), compel therapists to maintain their focus during at least portions of each session on concepts and skill acquisition relevant to the session agenda. A group therapist must also attend to all participants at the same time, keeping them actively engaged while facilitating a sense of confidence that speaking up in group is valued and that responses will be generally supportive and constructive. Some therapists may assume that a natural, unfolding group interaction will lead to powerful learning and positive outcomes without much therapist involvement. Others may be inclined to respond directly to each group member, perhaps assuming that their advanced clinical training and experience will ensure the best outcomes. The differing personalities, clinical needs, and interpersonal dynamics of group therapy present many potential clinical traps for any therapist, or therapists, running a group.

Socratic Dialogue offers an elegant solution to the complex group therapy challenge of concurrently teaching relevant skills, involving members actively in learning processes, and responding to the emotional needs of participants. In the vignette above the therapist could employ Socratic Dialogue to:

1. Ask about Celia's or other members' automatic thoughts in response to John's somewhat critical comment and tone;
2. Facilitate empathic responses from John or other members;
3. Enquire regarding alternative perspectives on Celia's difficulty with her plans to attend the party; or
4. Ask members for strategies they have found helpful when feeling tired or discouraged about attending a social event.

Observe what happens when this group therapist begins to employ Socratic Dialogue:

Therapist: John, you're pointing out the value of pushing ourselves to do activities, as we discussed in the first two sessions. I appreciate you encouraging this (*summary; empathic listening*). Let's keep that goal in mind, but perhaps someone might first have a response to Celia about how she has been feeling, and how difficult it was for her to go to the party like she planned. Sometimes when we receive some understanding and support it helps us to feel more capable of taking action even when we feel depressed. (Attempting to facilitate *empathic listening* while also setting the stage for upcoming *informational questions*.)

Letisha: Well, I think I know how you feel, Celia. When I'm really depressed, the last thing I want to do is be with other people. I feel like I'd be no fun at a party, and that seeing others who are happy would just make me feel worse.

Celia: You got that right.

Therapist: Letisha, you seem to understand Celia's feelings, and the urge to retreat. Can you think of any reasons it might be important for Celia to reconnect with other people? And how can she begin to do that when feeling so sad?

Letisha: Sometimes just being with other people helps me feel less alone and sad.

Celia: It's true. I know I need to get out. I did feel pretty awful staying home all weekend.

Therapist: So Letisha, or someone else, when you are feeling tired and depressed, what can you do to give yourself encouragement to go out?

Letisha: I guess it could be what we talked about in the second session. Like, I could ask myself, or I guess I'd ask you Celia, what would you be able to do to help yourself feel better? Like maybe a small step, calling one friend to meet for coffee, or meet to watch a movie or something? (Celia remains quiet.)

Therapist: Do you think it would feel more doable to you, Celia, to take a small step?

Celia: Yes. I think I know who I can call, maybe tonight when I get home. Someone I've been putting off lately.

Therapist: Sounds good, Celia. Thanks for being open with us in group. To help you do that, today we will be talking about this very dilemma: what to do when we're feeling depressed and having negative, all-or-nothing thoughts such as, "I can't do anything when I feel this way." We're going to look at how to evaluate and test out those negative thoughts.

Group therapy provides an exciting and dynamic opportunity for therapists to bring guided discovery alive, drawing forth member participation by searching for experiential evidence, alternative perspectives, and empathy from the diverse backgrounds represented in a given group. Interpersonal responses and feedback among participants provide opportunities for learning and testing out ideas in ways that go beyond what is possible in individual therapy. Members learn from observing others and from active, sometimes lively participation in discussions and group exercises.

Clinical vignettes in this chapter illustrate how Socratic Dialogue provides a flexible vehicle for the group therapist to: (1) respond effectively to emerging interpersonal reactions even while staying structured and focused on a group agenda, (2) ensure that appropriate empathic responses and learning occur in moments of tension or vulnerability, (3) keep members actively involved rather than passively listening or observing, and (4) facilitate the application of cognitive techniques in a real, *in vivo*, social setting. As in the vignette described above, we also include illustrations of how to turn an empathic failure or conflict into a learning opportunity for the entire group.

An Introduction to Cognitive Behavioral Group Therapy

The structured and educational foci of CBT are very amenable to a group therapy format, and many research studies demonstrate the efficacy of group CBT for common psychological disorders (e.g., Brown et al, 2011; Söchting, 2014). A group application was described and advocated in the classic text on treatment of depression by Beck et al. (1979). A model for group CBT using the client workbook *Mind over Mood* (Greenberger & Padesky, 2016) has more recently been described (Padesky, 2020a).

Therapy provided in groups makes sense from a number of perspectives. The opportunity to receive social and emotional support from others who have a similar base of experience and understanding is appreciated by people experiencing psychological distress. Belonging to a group can reduce the sense of alienation and shame and help normalize personal struggles in a very powerful and therapeutic way. A group format makes therapeutic services more affordable and accessible, a notable benefit in times of rising health care costs, especially given the limited number of highly trained CBT therapists. In addition, group therapy can be offered via the Internet, making it much more accessible to people who have difficulty traveling to session. Finally, the complex, unpredictable interpersonal experiences of a group can actually approximate the challenging and often unpredictable events of daily life for our clients. Thus, the learning achieved in groups may more effectively generalize to real-life social situations and stressors, increasing resilience and higher levels of functioning in society.

Existential group therapists have a long history of focusing on learning opportunities that arise through natural interpersonal processes in groups. CBT therapists share a value on experiential learning and can gain an important understanding of group dynamics from reading DeLucia-Waack and colleagues (2013), Yalom & Leszcz (2008), and other authors who have devoted careers to the study of group therapy processes. There are, however, significant differences in conceptualization and levels of intervention in group CBT, particularly that CBT therapists provide more structure and guided discovery than is typically found in traditional process groups. Relying on natural interpersonal processes can result in conversations or sessions that do not facilitate learning relevant to problems or needs of the members. Socratic interventions can be informed by wisdom from the traditional group therapy literature and at the same time be thoughtfully guided by cognitive conceptualizations that lead to interventions that may improve the efficiency and efficacy of group therapies.

Socratic Dialogue in Group Therapy

Very little has been written or illustrated regarding how Socratic Dialogue can be implemented in a group therapy setting. Bieling et al. (2006) and Söchting (2014), in their comprehensive guides to CBT in groups, describe how the same strategies and teaching methods used in individual CBT are typically adapted for groups. They note that a CBT group therapist engages members in a process of *collaborative empiricism* and employs various processes of *guided discovery* along with other more specific techniques and strategies modified for groups. These texts provide some examples of Socratic Dialogue in group therapy. Padesky and Greenberger (Padesky, 2020a) also offer examples of Socratic Dialogue and other guided discovery exercises in group therapy.

Involving a diverse group of individuals in the process of collaborative empiricism is both a tremendous opportunity and a challenge. Therapists can employ all the principles detailed in Chapter 2 of this book in a *strategically guided group dialogue.* Informational questions, empathic listening, summaries, and synthesizing questions will likely elicit a wider range of responses and ideas, and potentially greater credibility for those ideas, than that which would be elicited in a single therapist–client dyad. Ideally, group dialogues increasingly involve members as active participants in the process of guided discovery.

Advantages of using Socratic Dialogue in group therapy

Group CBT provides a context in which Socratic Dialogue can be particularly dynamic and effective. Consider these seven potential advantages of Socratic Dialogue in group therapy:

1. **The important understanding that thoughts and beliefs are actually** *subjective* **interpretations and assumptions** can be quite easily observed and demonstrated by gathering the different viewpoints of participants regarding a particular incident or issue. The following vignette illustrates this process.

Therapist:	So Najeeb, what might go through your mind if she did reject you when you ask her out? Actually, let me ask each of you to imagine being turned down when you ask out a person you are really attracted to. What would go through your mind, most likely? (The therapist pauses, then turns to each, one at a time.)
Jose:	Hmm. Probably that, that I'm not attractive enough.
Najeeb:	That I must have approached her the wrong way. Maybe said something stupid.
Carl:	I'd just think that she's really stuck up, one of those cold women. I mean, she at least could be friendly and talk to me a little.
Therapist:	Isn't that interesting that each of you have a different viewpoint about this specific scenario. So, what does this difference in interpretation illustrate about our automatic thoughts in a particular situation? [*analytic question*]

2. A group offers a **more expansive pool of experiential evidence.** Each member's unique history of real-life experiences expand the data bank of potential evidence for understanding and evaluating a thought, belief, or clinical dilemma. The probability of accessing a relevant, *disconfirming* experience in response to a particular maladaptive thought or belief is increased substantially by the presence of multiple people. Further, there may be greater credibility when two or more members, based on their life experience, challenge an unhelpful cognition, or validate a helpful one. Consider the following Socratic questions posed by the therapist and imagine what might subsequently transpire in the group dialogue:

Michele:	I just know that people don't like to be confronted. I've never had a good experience trying that. I don't really want to talk to Jules about what he said to me or how I'm feeling.
Therapist:	(Speaking to the group.) Are there any exceptions to the rule that people don't like to be confronted and Michele's prediction that it won't work out well? (Pauses for group members to answer.) Has anyone experienced something positive when confronting someone who has hurt you? (Pauses for group responses.) From your experiences, does it matter how you go about that confrontation?

3. Group participants can help identify a **widened range and variety of** *alternative perspectives* **and creative** *solutions*. The differing personalities, careers, relationship constellations, and living situations present in

a group provide more opportunities to identify viable, alternative viewpoints or solutions that will be acceptable to a given group member. The expanded process of generating ideas is also likely to enhance awareness regarding the value of tenacity in finding solutions to problems.

Maria: It's just a dead end for me, trying to get into the paralegal program when I have a young child to care for. My mom coming to stay was my last hope, but now she says she can't come.

Therapist: How do the rest of you feel, when hearing about Maria's dilemma? (The therapist selects the word "feel" to facilitate empathic responses, anticipating that members will also suggest solutions.)

Jeremy: That's gotta be disappointing, when your Mom knows how important this is to you.

Cindi: But, isn't there something else you might try, to help out with the child care?

Maria: Believe me, I've thought of everything, and I'm just not willing to let a stranger take care of my child when I'm at school. I don't have any friends who could do it either.

Cindi: What about going to school online, is that an option?

Lou Anne: And what about really carefully interviewing babysitters, like ones who have been referred by friends? I had a babysitter for a while, and my kids loved her. She was great! The only problem was that I got a little jealous of how much my kids liked her.

Maria: Hmm. I don't know. Maybe going online, but I'd really have to think about the babysitter option. It seems scary, but maybe I should consider it.

4. Responses elicited from peers **may be experienced as more authentic, relevant, and unbiased than those coming from a therapist.** Sometimes feedback offered by a therapist is discounted because a client assumes the therapist is "just doing their job ... to make me feel better" rather than providing unbiased responses. Feedback elicited from peers who are experiencing similar emotions or challenges, such as economic hardship or low self-esteem, will likely be seen as relatively credible, not as representing some "agenda," and thus may more easily be assimilated by a client. Further, peer responses may actually be more realistic and relevant than those of the therapist, and thus may do more to assist a given client in their learning and recovery. Note how the therapist below is alert to involve other members.

Briana: It's so hard to get the courage to speak up to my boss when I feel like my job is on the line and there aren't a lot of other jobs out there. But I have to say something because I can't keep up with all the work she throws at me. It keeps piling up!

Therapist: (Observing other members nodding their heads affirmatively.) I noticed a few of you shaking your heads. What can you say about how hard it is to speak up like that?

In the Therapist's Mind

When therapists observe group members responding to a topic or to each other in nonverbal ways, this can be an indication of relevant, activated cognition and emotion, often a useful time for Socratic inquiry.

Jiang: Well it is hard, even if you planned a good speech and rehearsed many times. You just can't predict how the boss will respond. And it could be really bad to lose a job, to have to go out there again with the economy as it is. I was out of work for 10 months, and it was scary. If I were Briana, I would test the waters a little before saying anything too strong to her boss.

Therapist: (Facilitating Socratic Dialogue by rephrasing her words in a brief *summary* and then asking an *informational question*.) That's an interesting point, about testing the waters. What do you all think might be some effective ways to do that? Are there any minimal, low-risk ways Briana could begin being assertive with her boss?

5. Group therapy offers the potential for **immediate, meaningful confirmation and disconfirmation of thoughts and assumptions via social consensus and even nonverbal responses.** As mentioned earlier, group feedback can immediately strengthen or weaken an individual's beliefs. Socratically eliciting feedback or perspectives of other members comprises a form of *social data gathering*, a type of behavioral experiment that requires less delay and effort than homework assignments in individual therapy.

Being present when a client elicits group opinions or responses allows the therapist some degree of quality control in the conduct of this type of behavioral experiment. Group therapists and participants can directly observe and comment on actual interpersonal experiences in group, on feedback given, and on how an individual is interpreting that feedback. The immediacy of in-session behavioral experiments offers opportunities for contemporaneous learning from any critical reactions or other unexpected negative responses. *In vivo* observations of group interactions can also help detect and correct an individual's tendency for selective attention or misinterpretation of experiences. Consider the following example in which the therapist's observation of Sharon's tears is followed by an *informational* question that leads to a behavioral experiment:

Therapist: Sharon, I noticed that you got teary-eyed when Brian said he thinks your comment was very insightful. What went through your mind when he said that?

Sharon: I know he doesn't mean it. People are so disingenuous, always trying to manipulate you in some way or just trying to make you feel good when they don't mean it.

Therapist: (Stepping in immediately to prevent a possibly unproductive interaction between Sharon and Brian, and facilitating a behavioral experiment.) Would you be willing to check that impression out with others in the group? You can ask people to be really honest with you, because I can understand that feedback is not helpful if it is not authentic.

Sharon: I don't know. I guess so. So (to group), didn't that seem kind of phony when he said that I was insightful? Come on, be real with me you guys!

David: To tell you the truth, I think you are right, that Brian was just trying to play therapist. (To Brian.) I've noticed you seem to always say the "right thing" (gesturing the quote signs with his hands), like you're trying to win points or something.

Therapist: Sharon, how does it feel to have David validate your impression of Brian's remark?

Sharon: I'm surprised. I didn't expect anyone to be real.

Therapist: Do you think David is being honest and real?

Sharon: Yes.

Therapist: Maybe you should write this experience down in your positive core belief log where you are looking for evidence of people being honest and genuine.

Sharon: OK. (Gets out her notebook to write a brief summary of this exchange.)

Therapist: While Sharon is doing that, I wonder, Brian, how you are reacting to what David said?

In the Therapist's Mind

This therapist recognized the importance of constructively guiding the group discussion. He asks Sharon to notice and contemplate whether this new comment (by David) might be a form of authentic feedback, something she has not noticed in people even though it sometimes might be occurring. The therapist strategically brings attention to this experiential data which contradicts Sharon's core belief, people are disingenuous, and strengthens the alternative belief that some people are sometimes honest and genuine. The therapist conceptualizes that this belief might be relevant to her depression and he prompts her to make a written summary so this information is not lost.

At the same time, the therapist recognizes that Brian might be feeling attacked because David agreed his comment might be "phony." So the therapist shifts attention to Brian to begin to check out his reactions to David's judgment of his earlier comments.

---

6. **Group members may initiate or participate in Socratic Dialogue with different styles of communication or alternative word choices that are more meaningful and effective than what the therapist might offer.** Certain types of colloquial phrases or everyday life illustrations can capture and communicate ideas in ways that might be unfamiliar to a therapist. People in the group might come from particular subcultures (e.g., age, race, or neighborhood cohorts) or have shared rather unique situational or emotional experiences (e.g., sexual assault, or rejection by peers in high school). Experienced CBT therapists will elicit relevant group feedback and sometimes allow interactions to continue between members even if the history, words, and styles of communicating are not familiar or fully understood by the therapists. They do so by subtly initiating dialogue, then gracefully backing away when a constructive process of interaction is occurring in the group. Here is one example of this type of process:

Therapist: So, what do you think Abel is feeling and needing to hear right now, as he talks about his embarrassment with that woman in the store? (Inviting *empathic listening* responses from the group.)

Riana: I think that was really mean of her, to use the word "pathetic" like that. I think she was a bitch, a real bitch! Maybe she had some bad experience with a guy or something, but that's no excuse. I thought that what you said was really sweet, and brave, seriously!

Diane: Yeah, I wish a guy like you would come up to me and say something like that, I mean, I never had a man talk to me that way. I got a kinda nice feeling inside just listening to what you were saying to her!

These spontaneous responses from members may ring of authenticity in a powerful way for the client, and do not need to be "repackaged" by the therapist.

7. **Participants can gain an enhanced awareness of themselves and of cognitive change processes by observing and participating in the Socratic Dialogue with other members.** Listening to Socratic dialogues unfold with other participants can help group members learn and internalize the Socratic process in a unique way. Their own information processing is not as likely to be compromised by affective arousal, not as emotion driven as when they are confronting their own personal, "hot" issue. Observing other members' responses may lead to vicariously learning to question their own beliefs, formulate adaptive responses, and promote self-compassion. Group members also learn effective ways of relating to others, such as responding empathically, when they collaborate in group Socratic dialogues. They may even benefit by observing how certain responses actually block consideration of new or different perspectives. Participants potentially gain therapeutic understanding of their own and other's emotional responses, behaviors, or reluctance to take on challenges.

Strategic levels of Socratic Dialogue in group therapy

Therapists can use Socratic Dialogue in various formats and with varying levels of group participation. The advantages of involving all members in a Socratic Dialogue are espoused throughout this chapter. There are situations, however, when using Socratic Dialogue with only one individual in the group is more clinically appropriate. The therapist may even prompt group members to initiate Socratic Dialogue with peers. Such "co-therapist" participation is possible when group participants have truly learned the processes of collaborative empiricism and guided discovery.

Socratic Dialogue with one focal individual in group

At times it is prudent for the group therapist to engage in Socratic Dialogue briefly with only one individual. This may be useful to ensure that a sequence of unfolding questions and responses will illustrate a central, important concept for the group. Relevant examples include when a client with panic disorder insists that they do not have automatic thoughts during a panic attack like others in the group seem to have, or when a client with a "pure O" form of obsessive-compulsive disorder (OCD) reveals an intrusive thought about sex or violence. In these examples, in which group members may not have the clinical knowledge or training to respond in a direct, targeted, and constructive way, the therapist can use Socratic Dialogue with one client while simultaneously educating group members in an unobtrusive way that will likely facilitate more relevant and useful responses from them. Here are some informational questions a therapist might ask a client with a "pure O" form of OCD that might be unfamiliar to other group members:

- When you have that intrusive image of stabbing your daughter, I wonder what assumptions are you making about the image?
- What do you tend to do to manage your fear or otherwise to cope when the image occurs?
- I wonder what evidence you have about whether you would act on such an image?
- Do you have any history of acting out violently?
- Can you think of an alternative reason for why this image might reoccur so frequently?

Once the individual has reflected on and answered these questions, the therapist can turn to the group and ask them for additional ideas about the persistence of this violent image. The group's ideas can be written in a summary and then both the individual who had the original image and other group members can be asked analytical or synthesizing questions to construct an alternative view of these intrusive thoughts.

A Socratic Dialogue focused on a single individual might also be warranted when a member is revealing a very sensitive issue or is experiencing acute emotional distress. Group members have varying levels of emotional maturity, communication skills, and empathy. Sometimes they may make dismissive, disparaging, or distracting remarks at a sensitive moment. This risk would likely be higher in the first few sessions of a group when response propensities are unknown, in anger management groups, or in groups with members who have poorer social skills (e.g., currently experiencing psychosis) or when impulsivity or verbal aggressiveness are more likely to occur. The choice to limit Socratic Dialogue in this way may restrict group participation briefly but, in the bigger picture, it may prevent negative exchanges that would otherwise lead to broader inhibitions about participation. This cautious containment of the dialogue is best used sparingly. Often a skillful application of Socratic Dialogue will quickly allow for a transition back to the useful participation of all members, as will be illustrated later in this chapter.

A third scenario in which Socratic Dialogue might be focused on one group member for a limited time is when a participant has adequate internal resources but tends to rely excessively on the opinion or help of others. This may be true for those with dependent personality traits, OCD (reassurance seeking), agoraphobia, or low self-esteem. In these situations, therapist-driven Socratic Dialogues can guide the individual to access their own internal pool of knowledge, wisdom, and solutions rather than waiting to hear what others might offer.

Socratic Dialogue with the entire group about a common issue

Often the issues or problems addressed in group therapy are familiar to several or all members, particularly in homogenous groups. A Socratic Dialogue with the entire group can therefore be quite natural, asking questions, listening empathically, and making written summaries of responses from one, then another member, trying to ensure that all contribute and feel included in the discussion. For example:

Therapist: Some of you may have anxious thoughts about doing this exposure exercise. What are some ways that you might talk yourselves out of completing this homework assignment? Let's go around the room, and Sumiko, would you record each member's response on the board?

or

Therapist: What are some of those automatic thoughts that led you to stop taking your meds? For example, like Keneisha just mentioned (writing on a white board), when the depression seems to be lifting and you start feeling really energized?

Group members can also participate in providing a summary or synthesizing response after a group discussion:

Therapist: Who would like to summarize the main points of our discussion about...?

Involving others in Socratic Dialogue regarding an individual's clinical issue

Use of Socratic Dialogue keeps other group members attentive and actively engaged by bringing them into the discussion regarding an individual's thoughts, feelings, and responses. As discussed earlier, group observations offer diverse perspectives and ideas and can promote collaborative empiricism. The therapist can often guide participants to directly responding to automatic thoughts or assumptions of another member. For example: "Would one of you please identify a possible 'hot automatic thought' in what Raphael just said?" or "Marjan, when you heard David say he felt stupid after losing his keys at the office, you shook your head. Is there some alternative perspective you have about this? Any relevant evidence you can point out about his idea that he was 'stupid'?"

This chapter includes many examples of how other group members can be brought into a Socratic Dialogue when addressing an issue presented by one individual. Vignettes will illustrate how the group therapist can guide this process, actively directing and redirecting to facilitate empathic and constructive responses, while minimizing risk that a distressed individual feels embarrassed or criticized.

Involving other members as facilitators of Socratic Dialogue

After several weeks of modeling Socratic Dialogue in group, therapists can sometimes draw members into a leadership role of guiding a Socratic Dialogue. The therapist, for example, might prompt a member to ask informational or analytical questions to another participant or to the group as a whole. The therapist is thereby addressing group needs while also deepening the experiential learning of the person who is asked to take a facilitating role in the Socratic process. The therapist, of course, remains available to guide or redirect the process as needed. Consider these examples of involving group members as guides in Socratic Dialogue. Note how the therapist prompts reminders of what Socratic Dialogue might sound like:

- Would one of you take the role of helping Liam evaluate this assumption, that he would be a 'failure' if he does not pass his exam this time? Liam, I will ask you to do the same with another group member later. It can be helpful to practice these Socratic questions with each other. So, what can Liam ask himself to help focus on relevant evidence and alternative viewpoints? And direct those questions to Liam, please.
- Mike, could you be the one to ask each member about their homework, keeping in mind the Socratic questions we have discussed to maximize

learning from homework? You can refer to the review sheet I gave each of you last week.

- Elesha, knowing that you were finally able to talk more openly with your boss last week, would you help Cynthia develop a behavioral experiment about asserting herself with her new employer? And group members, help Elesha out with any questions or steps in the process that might be useful for Cynthia.

The practice of involving participants as "co-leaders" in Socratic Dialogue must be used judiciously to minimize risk that members feel condescended to by their peers or conclude that the therapist believes a "co-leader" is more intelligent than they are. The opportunity for members to experiment with using Socratic Dialogue, nonetheless, can potentially reinforce their depth of understanding and skill regarding questioning their own thoughts and behaviors. This experience can therefore increase their ability to apply these empirical processes in coping with their own life problems.

The therapist can also choose to incorporate group exercises that build cognitive therapy skills while guiding members to take on the Socratic role with each other. This might occur after 6–8 weeks of sessions. For example:

> Let's now break into dyads, one playing the role of "depressive thinking" and the other asking questions to guide their partner in evaluating their automatic thoughts. When you are the guide, remember the importance of including empathy. And include summaries that integrate the main points and conclusions. Remember, the one in the listener role is a guide to the other, mainly using questions rather than giving advice or suggestions. I wrote these guiding points on the board to help you remember.

Exercise for the reader: Strategic levels of Socratic Dialogue in group therapy

Consider the advantages and disadvantages of choosing Socratic Dialogue at one or another level of intervention with respect to the following example. Also, consider when in the sequence of group sessions the particular questions might be appropriate. Note that in the options presented below, only the therapist portion of the dialogue is included.

Susan: It just seems so real that I will lose control if I don't leave, or get away from the situation when I feel panic coming on. I get really shaky, and have those unreality feelings, and I feel like I'm losing it. It happened yesterday in the grocery store!

Option 1: Therapist speaks directly to Susan, modeling the process and allowing members to observe and consider emerging data.

Therapist: Susan, what have you learned so far about this fear of "losing control," about what really occurs when you are feeling panicky? (Susan responds.) What is the evidence that supports the counterpoint that you can choose to stay in a situation even if you feel panic surging to high levels? (Susan responds.) How would you summarize these different points you just made? (Susan responds.) How confident are you right now that you will lose control when you feel panicky?

Option 2: Therapist involves the entire group in Socratic Dialogue without directly addressing Susan.

Therapist: (To group.) What have you all learned so far about this fear of "losing control," about what is really happening in panic and what would actually occur if you stayed rather than fleeing when you start to feel panicky? (Various group members respond.) How could we summarize these different points? (Several group members make suggestions.) How confident do you each feel right now that you will lose control when you feel panicky?

Option 3: Therapist involves other members in a Socratic Dialogue in responding to Susan.

Therapist: (To group.) Who can offer a relevant question or response to Susan about how she thinks she will lose control when she feels panicky? (Several group members speak to Susan.) What have you all learned so far about this fear of "losing control"? What can you say to Susan based on your experience? (Group members respond.) Susan, how would you summarize these different points made by others in group?

Option 4: Therapist Socratically guides members to take lead roles in the Socratic process.

Therapist: (To group.) You know the types of questions that can help Susan evaluate her fearful thoughts. Who would be willing to take on that role of asking Susan questions to help her examine the evidence about her fear of panic, of losing control if she does not escape or leave?

Specific applications of Socratic Dialogue in group therapy

There are many opportunities to integrate Socratic Dialogue into group therapy, even in very focused, short-term models. Three common situations encountered in group CBT are discussed as illustrations of typical applications of Socratic Dialogue.

Early didactic, skill-building stages

Adopting Socratic Dialogue for the more didactic portions of group therapy, such as socializing members to the cognitive model or learning to identify and evaluate automatic thoughts, is fairly straightforward. Padesky's 4-Stage Socratic Dialogue Model (Padesky, 2020b), as articulated in Chapter 2, is applied with an added awareness to balance interactions across all group participants, actively drawing out the quieter ones as well as those who are more outspoken.

Consider the following examples of contrasts between a purely didactic (D) versus a Socratic (S) style of teaching in a group:

Example 1: Therapist (socializing the group to CBT in the first session)
  D. Some examples of behavioral changes that occur when people are depressed include …
  S. What are examples of behaviors that change in your daily life when your depression gets worse?
Example 2: Therapist (speaking to group)
  D: Several months after losing a long-term romantic relationship, a person who is more depressed is likely to have all-or-nothing thoughts such as … In contrast, they are more likely to recover if they recognize that their thinking may not be totally accurate and they look for exceptions or evidence of how things can get better over time, with thoughts such as …
  S: Imagine it is several months after losing a longterm romantic relationship and you are still feeling deeply depressed. What types of automatic thoughts could be maintaining your depression? And in contrast, what types of thoughts would support movement toward feeling better? I will record your responses on the board in two columns, "Depressive Thinking" and "Feeling Better Thinking."

Experiential exercises and homework assignments

Socratic Dialogue can facilitate access to here-and-now evidence regarding automatic thoughts during experiential exercises, such as behavioral experiments or role-plays conducted in group. Similarly, when developing homework assignments, Socratic Dialogue can enhance motivation, elicit a wider range of relevant ideas, and help group members anticipate potential obstacles or challenges. Note this therapist's use of the third and fourth stages of Socratic Dialogue (summaries and analytical or synthesizing questions) in the following discussion which occurred after listening to participants' responses to informational questions about a role-play exposure in a social anxiety group.

Therapist: So there does seem to be a common dilemma here. All of you are aware of certain symptoms of anxiety that might be noticed by others. When this happens, you have a strong fear of being judged, or rejected. (*Summary*) What does this suggest that people have to do to make progress, to overcome inhibition, when they have anxiety symptoms that people might see? (*Analytical question*)

Celia: Well, the thought records only help me a little, not so much for this kind of thing, so I guess we have to eventually do those exposures you talked about. That's supposed to make the anxiety come down, right?

Therapist: (Deliberately ignoring that question for now.) Good point, Celia. And those exposures would mean that others could see that you have some anxiety, right? So what can we do to prepare for this experience of people noticing? (*Analytical question*)

Celia: We have to go out and face situations on our hierarchies, like for homework?

Therapist: What might we do here in group as a preliminary step before going out there to do the assignments, to build some confidence for those next steps? (*Analytical question*)

Alejandro: I guess we could try this out here first, in group. But I don't really know if that will help, because when we just practice it's not real.

After some discussion, the therapist was able to engage Alejandro in a simulation of talking to a girl he is interested in.

Therapist: So Alejandro, do you think you experienced some real anxiety during that role-play? (*Informational question*)

Alejandro: Yeah, it surprised me, but I know I was sweating kinda like I do with other girls. It really got me going when you had Susan ask me why I was sweating so much.

Therapist: (Incorporating a spontaneous behavioral experiment in group.) Alejandro, would you be willing to ask others whether they noticed your sweating, and what thoughts went through their minds about you? (Alejandro is reluctant but willing. Susan and two others say that they noticed he was sweating a little.)

Therapist: So, some people, and it seems it was the ones closest to you in this room, did notice the sweating. Now, would you ask them to say what they thought of you, or what they would think if they saw you talking to them in public and sweating like that?

Alejandro: So (to Susan), what were you thinking, really, when you saw me sweating?

Susan: Honestly, Alejandro, you just looked shy, a little nervous, but to someone like me, that's not such a bad thing. Actually, what I noticed more was that you were looking at the ground when you were talking. A lot of women don't like the guy to be too full of himself, and would find you less threatening if they noticed you were a little shy. But the eye contact thing, I just think eye contact is much more important with women.

Therapist: (Recognizing the value of guiding the dialogue toward the empirical data most germane to his "hot" automatic thoughts.) Alejandro, did Susan seem sincere to you in her feedback? (Alejandro nods affirmatively.) How does this feedback relate to your original automatic thought about looking "disgusting" when you sweat? (*Synthesizing question*)

Alejandro: I don't know; maybe it's true that some people will just think I'm nervous. But I still don't like to look nervous.

In the Therapist's Mind

The therapist ignored Celia's early question about whether exposure would reduce anxiety. In the short run, exposure exercises are likely to increase anxiety and the point of exposure is not to lower anxiety but to test out beliefs about the consequences of anxiety. However, that discussion would have been off-topic at this point in this group. One of the challenges of group therapy is that various emotions, thoughts, and concerns will emerge for each person during group interactions. It is important for therapists to listen empathically to client comments and respond to those that benefit the group's progress. At the same time, therapists are cautioned not to direct the dialogue only to simple, "pleasant" responses that might feel validating. Thus, the therapist is quiet when Susan talks to Alejandro about eye contact. This is useful information for him to learn. If the therapist redirects away from negative comments or emotions too quickly the meta message could be that "only positive feelings can be expressed here (in group)." Thus, clients may refrain from expressing doubts or dysphoric emotions, and the therapist may remain in the dark about relevant thoughts or assumptions that block integration of new evidence and perspectives. Empathic listening, summaries, and relevant follow-up questions help preserve an authentic and open process of collaborative empiricism.

As the therapist continues the group discussion above, she recognizes the opportunity to respond empathically and also to clarify and enhance Alejandro's synthesis of new information:

Therapist: You know, Alejandro, it makes sense that you don't like feeling that way, that you really would want to appear calm and feel more at ease. I bet others of you (looking at the group) can relate to that feeling. (Some heads nod affirmingly. She then turns back to Alejandro.). Yet, is this difference significant, that perhaps you would be seen only as "nervous" rather than "disgusting"?

Alejandro: (Pausing.) Yes, I guess it is quite different, really. Maybe I need to work on the eye contact thing, at least.

Therapist: That sounds useful, Alejandro. Now can any of you think of a good follow-up learning assignment to do this week to test out your automatic thoughts and assumptions about appearing anxious?

Addressing interpersonal issues that emerge in group

Automatic thoughts related to presenting problems are often primed by interactions and interpersonal dynamics in a group setting. Bieling and colleagues (2006) note that responses in group are much more than "incidental," that they provide unique learning opportunities by focusing on a "significant relational component that is rarely addressed in traditional CBT protocols" (5). Participants in groups for depression or social anxiety, for example, will often experience a priming of schemas about inferiority, rejection, dependency, or social alienation triggered by group interactions or by self-comparisons with others in the group. Group CBT provides a unique opportunity to observe and respond Socratically *in the moment* when these social cognitions are "hot." Doing so allows therapists to illustrate concepts and apply CBT skills in a powerful way while also addressing group reactions in order to facilitate a cooperative, cohesive group experience.

In contrast with the more common practice in traditional process groups of letting interactions unfold "naturally," based on the assumption that some therapeutic benefit will spontaneously occur, the cognitive therapist is prepared to guide the discovery process, informed by a cognitive conceptualization and the overall cognitive therapy model. Clinical judgment is highly involved in decisions about when and how to intervene. Therapists function best when remaining true to collaborative empiricism, avoiding the urge to direct the content or conclusions toward some preconceived conclusions as illustrated in the following group interaction.

Manny: Uhh, Yoshi, or Yo-shoe, or whatever your name is, could you please stop interrupting me when I talk? You think that what you have to say is more important than what I say.

Yoshi: That's just not true! I just had something I wanted to say too.

Therapist: (Recognizes the risk of letting this dyadic exchange escalate and also sees opportunity to use this as an educational opportunity.) This is an opportunity to look at interpretations, or automatic thoughts, that can help make sense out of what each of you are feeling right now. Manny, what went through your mind when Yoshi interrupted you?

Manny: That he doesn't think what I have to say is important. He thinks he is better than me.

Therapist: I imagine that would not feel very good, *if* that is what he is implying by interrupting. Would you be willing to ask him about that, to ask if that was his motive or if perhaps there might be some other explanation for his talking over you a few minutes ago?

Manny: I can ask, but he'll probably just deny it or make up something, so what's the point?

Therapist: Well you will be the final judge of whether his responses seem credible to you. And, if Yoshi is willing, you can feel free to probe with other questions to help see if his explanation seems valid or not. Is that fair?

Manny: Yeah, maybe. I guess so. Well, why did you interrupt me like that? You did it at least three times this evening.

Yoshi: You know, Manny, I actually feel inferior to you in this group. I mean, you have a college degree, and I don't. And you seem to always come up with good things to say. So no, it has nothing to do with me feeling better than you. I'm kinda impulsive and say things without thinking sometimes. My boyfriend hates when I do that, and tells me I have ADHD. And I do it with others, if you haven't noticed.

Therapist: Manny, any response to what Yoshi just revealed?

Common Clinical Traps in Group CBT

CBT group therapists face a challenge that is typically more complex than interacting one to one with an individual therapy client. They must concurrently (1) consider differing individual needs, (2) maintain focus on the group objectives, and (3) address emerging conflicts and other interpersonal issues in group. Group therapists need to make many decisions in the moment, such as when to focus Socratic Dialogue toward an individual or toward the entire group and when to explore an interpersonal interaction or return to a didactic topic planned for the day. The interplay of differing needs and issues results in many potential clinical traps that could interfere with optimal group participation and learning. The rest of this chapter guides therapists in recognizing, avoiding, and responding more effectively to clinical traps in group therapy through judicious use of Socratic Dialogue.

Clinical traps in group therapy can derive from individual participants, from group member interactions, or from therapist factors. The list in Box 10.1, "Common Clinical Traps in Group Therapy," is not exhaustive, but

---

Box 10.1 Common Clinical Traps in Group Therapy

Participant-driven Traps
Trap 1
A group member strongly expresses emotional needs, exhibits intense re-activity, or otherwise dominates group therapy time in a way that interferes with the educational focus of the group or with the opportunity for others to participate in the therapy process.

Trap 2
There are large discrepancies among members in readiness or ability to engage in the therapy process: differing levels of motivation, homework adherence, participation, comprehension, or skill acquisition. This leads to the therapist offering imbalanced attention to group members.

Trap 3
Interactions among members become harsh or hostile, or result in conflicts that are potentially damaging and could lead to emotional withdrawal, clinical crises, or dropout. The therapist tries to control or cover over the conflict rather than using it as a learning opportunity.

Therapist-driven traps
Trap 4
The therapist dominates the group through didactic presentations rather than actively engaging the participants.

Trap 5
The therapist elicits group participation but then takes a laissez-faire approach in which they rely excessively or indiscriminately on participant interactions, providing too little guidance in the unfolding group dialogue.

provides a useful guide for discussion and illustration of how therapists can use Socratic Dialogue to transform potential traps into learning opportunities. Regardless of the origin of the clinical trap, a therapist's assumptions are likely to be important because these directly influence how we do or do not respond. Therefore, throughout this section, therapist assumptions about each trap are considered.

Trap 1

A group member strongly expresses strong emotional needs, exhibits intense reactivity, or otherwise dominates group therapy time in a way that interferes with the educational focus of the group or with the opportunity for others to participate in the therapy process.

The first trap occurs when someone in group repeatedly responds with very intense affect or a domineering style of interacting; others may feel threatened or intimidated, leading them to retreat emotionally and even physically from the group. Members sometimes also stop attending or engaging, due to boredom or feeling excluded, if the therapist allows an individual to talk on for an extended period of time. Some therapists fall into a trap of passivity, allowing these patterns to interfere with the agenda or with opportunities for other members. Other therapists confront the member in a way that is counterproductive. Socratic Dialogue allows the therapist to respond to Trap 1 by bringing others into the discussion, involving them in a truly collaborative process that provides learning and support for the focal individual while also keeping others engaged in a learning process that feels safe and constructive.

A cognitive conceptualization of the phenomenon of an unbalanced group, one in which a member or members dominate discussions, can guide the therapist to determine how best to respond. This conceptualization will ascertain relevant beliefs and cognitive processes of the dominant individual(s), the less active participants, and most importantly the therapist who ostensibly is guiding and managing the levels of participation.

An outspoken, highly expressive group member may be operating with a cognitive deficit of simply not noticing the presence or needs of others, particularly when their core beliefs are activated. Alternatively, a more expressive member who is biased by beliefs common with narcissistic or dependent personality traits may assume that their own needs supersede those of others. For example: "Others aren't suffering like I am. When I feel this bad I deserve ... " or "I am so overwhelmed ... I can't handle this ... I need help, now!" In other cases, dominant members may simply lack a good support system, concluding that "This is the only place where I can get help ... where people will understand me!"

Sometimes the cognitive biases or habits of a therapist lead to one member dominating and a lack of balanced participation across all members. Some therapists have a strong tendency to engage at length with the more "interesting" or expressive members in a group. They can operate with tunnel vision, responding to highly expressed affect or distress of one individual without adequately considering or valuing the needs of others. They may hold overgeneralized, unbalanced assumptions such as "I should always (directly) respond when others are in pain. I'm being insensitive if I don't."

These types of biased thinking in therapists can occur due to an extensive history of providing individual therapy and a lack of training or supervision regarding work with groups. The therapist may not have developed the ability to scan members with the goal of attending to relative levels of participation. Similarly, some therapists engage in 1:1 interactions excessively due to their own anxiety about leading a group or based on unexamined assumptions such as "I need to always manage strong emotions very carefully in group; otherwise things will get out of control ... Other members will not know what to say ... will say the wrong things." Some therapists are inclined to respond 1:1 based on a strong need to show how competent they are, or for the gratification of feeling emotionally engaged and valued at every moment in their work as a therapist. Finally, some passively allow a member to dominate due to excessive fears about the outcomes of confronting aggressive members.

This trap of allowing members to dominate a therapy group brings several clinical risks. Less active members may experience a reinforcement of core beliefs such as "I'm not important." Other members may conclude that the therapy group, or CBT in general, will not be of personal value to them. Further, if a therapist engages in extensive, in-depth interactions with one member, that client could end up disclosing more than they feel ready to expose to their peers. If that happens, they could feel vulnerable and anxious about how others will perceive them, and may even choose not to return to group. Conversely, others in group might worry: "What if the therapist draws out my hidden issue … my incest experience/unfaithfulness/feeling of being worthless?" In all these various ways, this trap can lead to resentment, anxiety, or loss of interest, possibly leading to dropout from group but most certainly resulting in diminished benefits for some members in the group.

Socratic Dialogue allows the therapist to involve others even when specific members tend to dominate. The therapist can expand the focus by asking others to disclose whether they have had similar feelings or experiences, can involve others in providing information, feedback, or empathy, or request that others synthesize concepts or provide summaries. At times an individual's needs might go beyond that which could be provided in a time-limited therapy group. Even in this situation the therapist can involve others by way of informational questions regarding solutions or resources in the community, concurrently strengthening their sense of worth and value as "helpers."

Notice in the group dialogue below how Socratic Dialogue provides an effective way to address the trap of a dominant member by inviting and guiding the participation of others. In this vignette, Suzanne is feeling overwhelmed with grief about being left by her boyfriend. She has been tearfully expressing her pain and despair in the depression therapy group for more than 10 minutes and other members are starting to look uncomfortable. Others have made empathic comments, but Suzanne continues on tearfully. The therapist is aware that the group comments are not expressed to Suzanne with much warmth, and that she does not appear to be listening.

Suzanne: It feels like a pain so deep that I don't know how to get through it. I don't see how I can go on alone, after being with him for 8 years. I'm getting older, and I feel I gave up everything for him. (Tears flowing.) (Group members appear sullen and remain quiet.)

Therapist: Suzanne, I can certainly see and imagine that this is a tremendous loss for you, a very painful time right now. Would it be OK with you, Suzanne, to hear some responses from other members right now? (This word choice emphasizes collaboration and also increases the likelihood that Suzanne will pay attention to the responses of others.)

Suzanne: I don't know if anything will help, really.

As the discussion continues, the therapist guides group members toward empathic listening, delaying for a moment any movement toward coping strategies. A focus on Stage 2 of Socratic Dialogue, empathic listening, is very important when a client is highly vulnerable. It encourages group members to respond to emotional reactions while also increasing the distressed individual's receptivity to other forms of feedback. Notice how the therapist's careful word choice below reduces the likelihood of a comment that might feel unbelievable or invalidating to the client, such as "I know what you are feeling. I went through the same thing."

Therapist: I know that none of us can completely understand what Suzanne is going through. Yet some of you may have lost someone you really cared about deeply and perhaps can sense some way of offering understanding or support. Is that true for anyone here?

Ryan: I know I felt like my life was coming to an end when my wife left me. She had been my high school sweetheart, the only woman I had ever loved.

Ryan's response is not really directed empathically toward Suzanne and therefore the therapist guides the process back toward her, speaking first to Ryan and then turning his head toward Suzanne.

Therapist: So Ryan, from your experience, what words of understanding and support would you be able to say to Suzanne at this time?

Ryan: I just know, with time, you will be OK, even though it doesn't feel like it at all right now. After a while you might reconnect to people that you used to spend time with, before that relationship. I started getting back together with some of my old buddies, and even started jogging again for the first time in years. I mean, it was a couple months before I wanted to do anything, but I gradually started getting out there, and I found out that I still could have a life.

Therapist: (Elects to continue involving others rather than returning the focus back on Suzanne quite yet.) Thanks, Ryan. Did anyone else have some feelings or thoughts when you heard what Suzanne is going through?

After eliciting responses from a few other members, the therapist recognizes an opportunity to focus back onto the agenda. He chooses to provide a summary rather than asking a participant to do so, thereby assuring a gentle segue back to the group agenda.

Therapist: Suzanne, I hope you sense some caring from the group, that others have at least some understanding that this loss is really painful and will take time. How do you feel about the feedback, in particular about getting out again with friends, and about pursuing some of your own interests and hobbies?

Suzanne: I know I can try to get back into my swimming. I'm pretty sure that will help. But I just don't have close friends to talk to now because I was so exclusive with John. (Tears again well up in her eyes.)

Therapist: (Realizing she will need additional social support outside of group; directs an *informational question* to all members.) Does anyone know of a support group or resources in our community that might be helpful to Suzanne?

Juwan: My sister went through a divorce and found a good support group at the Woman's Health Center, near downtown. I'm sure it's open to anyone going through a separation.

Therapist: Could you perhaps write down the name, and even the phone number for Suzanne if you have it? Thank you so much, Juwan. (Pause.) This week we are continuing to look at our automatic thoughts. We've heard a number of Suzanne's automatic thoughts about her breakup. What types of automatic thoughts did the rest of you notice this week?

Trap 2

There are large discrepancies among members in readiness or ability to engage in the therapy process: differing levels of motivation, homework adherence, participation, comprehension, or skill acquisition. This leads to the therapist offering imbalanced attention to group members.

It is not uncommon for group members to have different levels of engagement, motivation, comprehension, or pace of skill development. Socratic Dialogue with a group can create meaningful bridges that reach across differences to enhance participation and learning. Decisions about how to employ Socratic Dialogue is best made when informed by a conceptualization of client differences and also of the therapist's own response tendencies.

Members may appear less motivated or active due to automatic thoughts, assumptions, and core beliefs such as:

- I don't have anything interesting/intelligent enough to say … If I speak out I will sound stupid.
- Everyone else is smarter/further along/better than I am. I won't do that assignment as well as the others and the therapist will make a spectacle of me in front of the group. Or, in contrast,
- This exercise is not going to help me. I already know this stuff. I know more than the others so why should I have to do this assignment?

Socratic enquiry provides an educational, collaborative way to identify and address these types of obstacles and to promote participation and motivation. For example, if a client in a group for psychosis is not participating in a discussion about a psychiatrist leaving the clinic, and that client clearly had been very attached to this doctor, the therapist might ask, "Aaron, I noticed that you remained quiet during our discussion about Dr. Chavez leaving, yet I know you were quite attached to him. What was going through your mind when I asked each of you to express your feelings about his leaving?" If low self-esteem is central to Aaron's case conceptualization and this inhibits him from expressing his own reactions, his therapist might take this into account and ask the question this way, "Aaron, you formed a good relationship with Dr. Chavez. How do you think his leaving will affect patients here?"

Therapists' assumptions, interpretations, and biases regarding differences among group members will influence their responses and vulnerability to this second clinical trap. Consider how the following thoughts would discourage a therapist from using Socratic Dialogue with the entire group:

- Raul is just asking too many questions, slowing the group down. It's best to ignore him.
- Briana is the only one really doing assignments, the only one really working hard in group. She deserves my attention the most.
- David feels inferior to the others. I need to build him up.
- Saed is always giving the best answers. He's going to make others feel bad. I've got to cut him off when he talks.

Therapist assumptions that lead to these types of interpretations and direct a therapist into the trap of offering imbalanced attention to group members, include:

- If I just wait longer, then quiet clients will eventually decide on their own to participate.
- Some people learn best by just observing.
- If I say something about lack of participation, then she or he will feel embarrassed/bad/irritated and they might drop out.
- People should bring their own motivation to therapy. It's their responsibility to make an effort if they want to get something out of the group.
- Dominate members sometimes need to be humbled a bit in order for them to back down and give others a chance to participate.

Keep in Mind

Group therapists need to self-assess and conceptualize their own cognitive vulnerabilities that can undermine their role in group, examining their own assumptions about people, motivations, group process, and their role as therapist. One effective method to do so is to record sessions, or invite an experienced group therapist to sit in on sessions. Then examine data that does and does not support the idea, "I am using Socratic Dialogue to involve members in a balanced and effective way." At those moments when the statement is not supported, the recording or consultant feedback can help you identify and address relevant automatic thoughts and underlying beliefs that are interfering.

One simple strategy to address differences in participation, motivation, or competency is to direct Socratic Dialogue toward the less active or advanced members in an effort to equalize their involvement or enhance their rate of learning. Notice how the therapist in the dialogue below involves a shy member, Juliana, in the advanced stages of summarizing information and providing a synthesis of the group dialogue. Here we continue the vignette about Suzanne, who lost her boyfriend of 8 years.

Therapist: Juliana, I noticed that you were listening attentively to what Suzanne said and how others were responding. What do you think are the most important points for Suzanne as she goes through this process of recovery from her loss?

Juliana: I guess that you just have to get on with things and get busy with life again.

Therapist: Juliana, your point is so important for Suzanne and all of us, to find a way to get moving forward, even when, or especially when, going through real losses and difficulties.

Even though Juliana's response was not particularly comprehensive or elegant, the therapist supports her comments in the hope this will strengthen her confidence to participate in group.

Simplistic efforts to balance attention and dialogue to ensure equal participation of all can leave more skilled members insufficiently challenged, even feeling neglected or bored. This potential trap can be addressed by asking members to respond to the obstacles or learning deficits of other group members, and to do so in ways that minimize risk of being seen as preferential or condescending, as illustrated in the following example:

Simona: I just don't seem to have automatic thoughts before purging. I just find myself in the bathroom, doing it, not really thinking about it.

Therapist: It is difficult to identify automatic thoughts when you've done something many times, like a habit. (*Empathic listening*) Who in the group can describe a way to access thoughts in a situation like this, when you've binged and felt the urge to purge? (*Informational question*)

Shirleen: I know what Simona means about not really even thinking about it, but that incomplete sentence technique we talked about helped me. Like when I asked myself, "If I didn't do it, if I didn't purge, then I would worry that 'x' would happen." For me it was, I would worry that I would look like a fat pig again.

Therapist: (To reduce the risk that Simona feels singled out, and to ensure that others are involved, the therapist opens the dialogue to the entire group.) Shirleen, would you just write that incomplete sentence on the white board here, and let's go around the group and see if it helps identify more relevant trigger thoughts, or the "permission giving thoughts" we talked about. Simona, could you start by imagining that time on Friday? Imagine yourself finishing the box of Krispy Crème doughnuts you talked about . . .

The therapist in the next vignette engages the participation of Sierra, who is learning to approach her OCD more effectively, to help Amir, who the therapist realizes has not been doing the exposure and response prevention (ERP) learning assignments between group sessions.

Therapist: Amir, what has been holding you back from ERP assignments? What goes through your mind when we talk about them, or when you are home and thinking about doing them?

Amir: I'm afraid of what could happen, but I know everyone in group says they are too. I think it mainly is that I can't get motivated enough, you know, to be willing to feel that anxious.

Therapist: Sierra, you have been on a roll with your ERP, doing more than was even assigned. What helps you to be motivated, specifically, what helps you start the exposures?

In a social anxiety therapy group, another therapist addressed several discrepancies:

Therapist: Can anyone ask those questions that help identify automatic thoughts? Maybe help Daren in this process a bit?

Faris: (To Daren.) So, what does go through your mind, I mean what is the worst you think would happen if you talk to someone you're attracted to?

Daren: My face turns red so easily; I think it is right now. I just feel like I look nervous.

Therapist: (Seeks to ensure an *empathic*, supportive response for Daren.) That helps makes sense out of your anxiety feeling, but I noticed, Faris, that you were shaking your head. Do you have a comment, or follow up question would help clarify Daren's thoughts and assumptions?

Faris: Yeah, like Rolando was saying, what's the worst—if you do look nervous?

Daren: I guess I feel like I'm weak, and pathetic, when I get nervous like that. I hate it!

Therapist: I think you are getting to the relevant thoughts, Daren. That's good. So Thomas (turns to another member), did hearing Faris's questions, or Daren's automatic thoughts, help in identifying any of your thoughts and hesitations about approaching an attractive guy?

Thomas: Yeah. I feel like I'll sound, and look, like a ridiculous person who isn't intelligent. Afterwards I feel really bad, like I ruined a good opportunity.

Therapist: These questions and automatic thoughts are worth writing down. (Looking at Viktor, who has limited English skills and who missed the prior session on identify automatic thoughts. The therapist sees Victor is taking notes but not participating.) Viktor, did this discussion help clarify how to identify automatic thoughts?

Viktor: I think so, yes.

Therapist: What do you see that is common among these thoughts about meeting someone and getting anxious? (*Synthesizing question*)

Viktor: I think everyone feels like the other person is going to judge you or criticize you. And I think this is true for me too.

As shown in these brief illustrations, the flow of the group can be maintained even when there are significant differences between members. Therapists are encouraged to balance enquiries among individuals, involve more skilled members in helping others, and elicit summaries or clarifications from members who are not otherwise speaking up. These flexible applications of Socratic Dialogue keep members of all skill and motivation levels involved. It supports the entire group's learning when members are allowed to take roles that utilize their growing knowledge and skills. The therapist can orchestrate this process judiciously to ensure that all participants feel stimulated, valued, and respected.

Trap 3

Interactions between members become harsh, hostile, or result in conflicts that are potentially damaging and could lead to emotional withdrawal, clinical crises, or dropout. The therapist tries to control or cover over the conflict rather than using it as a learning opportunity.

Aggressive comments or conflicts between group therapy members are challenging for any therapist and can lead to clinical trap 3. Intense interpersonal reactions, or even those that are subtle and blunted, can divert attention away from the group learning and can be counterproductive. At the same time, hostility and conflict can provide excellent opportunities for inquiring about "hot" automatic thoughts and to illustrate CBT concepts and skills *in vivo*. These types of group interactions are most likely to become constructive learning opportunities if the therapist addresses conflict using Socratic Dialogue rather than falling into the trap of trying to control or cover over the situation.

Some therapists respond reflexively to criticism or conflict in a group by trying to defend a perceived "victim," quickly diverting attention to another topic or confronting the perceived "perpetrator." Relevant therapist thoughts and assumptions contributing to these reactions include:

- That client is vulnerable … needs my help … can't defend themself.
- I cannot allow cruel, insensitive behavior in the group. I must confront anyone who tries to put down another member.

Conflict can elicit anxiety in group members as well as the therapist. A therapist who lacks experience employing Socratic Dialogue in a group may default toward excessive attempts to control "for the sake of the group" based on beliefs such as:

- Conflict is … bad, dangerous, and not therapeutic.
- Things are getting out of control. I must get this under control now!
- I don't know what to do. I'd better just return to the agenda topic.

An experienced, self-aware therapist can use Socratic Dialogue to constructively guide the group through emerging conflicts, facilitating helpful learning as illustrated below.

Carl: You make me sick with your petty complaining about everything. You have no idea what it's like to suffer. I did two terms of duty in Iraq, and we would have laughed to hear a man whine and cry like you do, about nothing.

Darren: Well f**k you! You think you have your act together, but you are just useless when it comes to dealing with people! You just hide behind the military thing, and never even talk about yourself, about your own issues. You can't even keep a job, so why don't you deal with your own stuff rather than jumping on others?

Carl: Well I can run circles around guys like you. And you think working behind a desk and wearing a tie makes you a hot shot?

Therapist: Darren, and Carl, it sounds like you each have very legitimate feelings activated here. I'd like to ask you both to work with me a bit, to bring this discussion back in line with our goals in group. You know how we were talking about "hot thoughts" and how powerful they can be in triggering strong emotions? (Both members are glaring at each other.) Work with me here, both of you for a minute. Now Carl, when was the moment, or what was the thing Darren said that triggered you to became angry?

Carl: He was whining; he was saying how difficult it is when you have to find a replacement for his secretary. And then …

Recognizing the importance of guiding the discussion toward the topic of the day, "Finding Evidence Regarding Automatic Thoughts," the therapist chooses to interrupt Carl:

Therapist: So, when he talked about the secretary, something was triggered in you. What went through your mind at that moment?

Carl: It's just … What a trivial thing, to have to take over the secretary's tasks, to maybe stay a little late at work for a few days, and to put out a help wanted ad. It's bullshit!

Therapist: Carl, it seems like something more got triggered here. What else was going through your mind, other thoughts, or images, or memories that might help make sense out of how intensely you reacted? I imagine you have some good reasons for your feelings about this. (*Empathic listening*)

Carl: (Pauses, as if unsure of whether to go on.)

Therapist: It might be really helpful if you are willing to talk about this.

Carl: Well if you … if you want to talk about having to replace someone. (Carl appears to be trembling a bit.) If one of the guys in your battalion gets blown away, and he happens to be the guy who has had your back for the past 3 months in combat. Talk to me about what is hard to do and I can tell you more shit than you want to hear!

In the Therapist's Mind

This comment suggests Darren's comments may have triggered a post-traumatic stress disorder (PTSD) reaction in Carl. Processing PTSD material goes beyond the objectives for this depression group. Therefore, the therapist decides to keep the focus on interpersonal thoughts and begin by modeling empathic listening.

Therapist: Carl, what an incredible loss. More than us civilians could even comprehend. (Turning to Darren.) Darren, does that help make sense out of Carl's reactions, knowing what got triggered in his mind?

Darren: Well I don't like being attacked like that in group, but yeah, I get it. It does make a lot more sense. Hey Carl, I, I really am sorry about what happened with your friend out there. Really. I guess my problem is kind of trivial compared to that.

Sometimes empathic listening can be phrased in ways that also reinforce other key CBT principles. Here, the therapist draws attention to the idea that Carl's strong emotional reactions were related to thoughts and memories experienced within Carl, rather than being due simply to what Darren said about his office manager.

Subtle interpersonal reactions are even more common in therapy groups than these strongly expressed ones. When these are noted, therapists have the choice of exploring the reactions or electing to remain focused on the agenda or current topic of discussion. They may, for example, continue the topic in progress or the planning of post-session learning assignments rather than inquiring about the feelings between group members. Neglecting to address signs of interpersonal tension, however, can result in missed opportunities for important learning, and can result in escalation of conflict or withdrawal. Socratic Dialogue, fortunately, often provides a method for addressing interpersonal responses while also linking these to the topic of the day in a group. The following example from a therapy group for people with bipolar disorder illustrates this well.

Therapist: Sirena, I noticed that you were really active in our discussion about evaluating automatic thoughts, then you suddenly stopped participating and seemed distracted. Was there something that just occurred in group, or something significant that went through your mind a few minutes ago? (*Informational question*)

Sirena: Not really, I'm just a little tired.

Therapist: I realize this is an evening group, and a work day. (*Empathic listening*) I did notice, though, that your reaction seemed to occur just after Sandy said she thought you were mind reading a lot. What did you feel just then? What went through your mind when she said that she thought you were mind reading a lot? (*Informational questions*)

Sirena: I think she is rather arrogant, judging me and telling me that my thoughts are wrong, thinking she is better than me.

Therapist: Maybe we can explore this with Sandy in a moment, but I appreciate you are willing to say what went through your mind just then. Were there any other thoughts or images, anything else that went through your mind when you heard her say that?

Sirena: Well it didn't exactly make me feel good about myself.

Therapist: What did it mean to you, hearing that comment? (*Informational question*)

Sirena: It seems that I just can't do anything right. That people don't like me, just as I said earlier in group.

There is no single best intervention at any point in a therapy session. The following section illustrates three of the many alternative directions that the therapist might take at this moment in the dialogue above. Compare these possible responses to the one you devised. The potential risks and benefits of each response are noted.

Option A: The therapist focuses on the priority of having all members involved.

Therapist: Are there others in the group who feel that way at times, that you are being judged or that you can't do anything right?

PROS/CONS: This question will invite the participation of others and might lead to productive discussion, especially if the therapist fosters a Socratic Dialogue about member responses. However, this question alone might be considered *pseudo Socratic* in that it is ambiguous, not guiding the discussion toward learning a relevant concept or skill, and not necessarily leading to empathy for Sirena. It is just as likely to move the topic onto another group member's story rather than following up with Sirena's thoughts and feelings, and it may distract away from a valuable learning opportunity.

Option B: The therapist focuses on two priorities: responding to Sirena's feelings and reaction, and involving others in the agenda topic of evaluating automatic thoughts.

Therapist: It's understandable you could feel hurt or frustrated when it seems that someone is judging you. Would you be willing to hear how other people viewed, or interpreted, Sandy's comment?

PROS/CONS: This dialogue gets others involved actively and collaboratively, and is focused on alternative thinking and interpretations. It can help demonstrate the subjectivity of cognition and possibly generate an alternative perspective that would seem credible to Sirena. There is some risk, however, that this way of involving others could leave Sirena on the sidelines too long, engendering a sense that she is not as capable as others in being objective or evaluating her own thinking. It could reinforce a negative self-schema of being inadequate. Further, it does not directly involve the most relevant source of data in evaluating her initial automatic thoughts, Sandy. And it might even alienate Sandy by not giving her the chance early on to clarify her intention and feelings about Sirena.

Option C: The therapist directs dialogue onto the agenda topic of evaluating automatic thoughts but keeps the focus primarily on the responses of the two members involved in the relevant interaction.

Therapist: So Sirena, would you be willing to do a brief behavioral experiment right here in group? Would you be willing to test out your automatic thoughts by asking Sandy her intention in making that comment about mind reading? Just ask her in whatever way you think could give you an honest, believable response.

PROS/CONS: This therapist response could facilitate the most direct way for Sirena to gather relevant evidence for evaluating her automatic thoughts. This also provides opportunity for group members to observe a very focused process of identifying and evaluating relevant automatic thoughts, similar to the internal thought testing process that they are learning to use in everyday life. Further, members can observe how a conflict between two people can be addressed through objective inquiry rather than reactivity. On the other hand, this approach could carry a risk of further escalation between the two members by keeping them engaged with each other rather than diffusing the focus by involving others. Further, it could leave other members on the sidelines for an extended period.

Any of the three options above could be fruitful as long as the therapist is alert to redirecting the discussion if and when problems and opportunities emerge in the unfolding group process. For example, Option C could be quite effective if the therapist continued on to involve other members in providing observations, summaries, or synthesis of relevant concepts.

> **Trap 4**
>
> The therapist dominates the group through didactic presentations rather than actively engaging the participants.

Important opportunities for active learning are curtailed when the therapist relies extensively on a didactic approach in group therapy. Periods of didactic education are clearly prudent in time limited groups, particularly in the early stages of concept and skill acquisition. The experiential involvement of all members, however, enhances relevant learning, offering opportunities to integrate new ideas when emotions and core beliefs are activated by the dynamic social context of a group.

The didactic Trap 4 is perhaps a greater risk for beginning group therapists or for those who have perfectionistic assumptions regarding the need to convey a "full picture" (i.e., greater detail or breadth of information) to the group. Too much time devoted to didactic presentation interferes with opportunities for active, experiential learning. Relevant therapist assumptions include:

- There is so much for them to learn, so I better keep moving through teaching all the important material.
- This group won't be effective if I leave things out.

This didactic trap can also be triggered, and not questioned, for group therapists who were or currently are classroom instructors, because of the stimulus similarity between the two settings.

Consider what would have been lost in the therapy vignettes earlier in this chapter if the therapist had attempted to teach by simply conveying information about CBT and using hypothetical examples, rather than taking a Socratic approach. For example, in the vignette concerning anger between Carl, who fought in Iraq, and Darren who wore a tie and worked in an office, the excessively didactic therapist could have responded as follows:

Therapist: These strong emotions Carl and Darren are expressing are no doubt triggered by automatic thoughts just as I have been describing to you today. With anger we usually have judgmental thoughts about others, whereas with depression the thoughts are more likely to be about ourselves. Let's review the list of cognitive distortions ...

Clearly many opportunities for three-dimensional learning are lost with such a narrow focus on conveying didactic information. While some formal teaching is quite useful in CBT groups, relying too much on a didactic style often leads to group passivity, boredom, and missed or weakened learning opportunities.

Trap 5

The therapist elicits group participation but then takes a laissez-faire approach in which they rely excessively or indiscriminately on participant interactions, providing too little guidance in the unfolding group dialogue.

A lack of guidance by the therapist can be equally damaging to group learning. When a therapist relies indiscriminately on group interaction, a group can begin to drift aimlessly, potentially moving in directions that are not helpful, that result in counterproductive conflict or confusion, or that diverge away from the goals and needs of the group members. While a less directive role by a therapist may allow for relevant process issues to materialize spontaneously, it will limit opportunities for learning treatment principles and skills. Low levels of therapist guidance would not work well in time-limited groups for mood-related disorders such as depression, panic, or social anxiety.

It is advisable to identify and conceptualize one's own thoughts and assumptions about how much structure and direction to provide in group whenever you notice you frequently deviate from your agenda, fall behind on the timeline for the group, face interpersonal conflicts, or experience time periods with little productive group participation. These can be signs you are falling into the clinical trap of inadequate group guidance. Relevant therapist beliefs and assumptions can include:

- If I interrupt the discussion, group member(s) will feel hurt, offended, not understood.
- If I just allow the discussion to go further, someone will provide good empathy, ideas, or solutions. It's best to give it more time.
- The best learning always comes in spontaneous interactions, because each individual and the group as a whole are fully capable of helping each other in recovery.
- I'm not sure what would be right to say or do here. It's best to not say anything if I'm unsure.

Note that the assumptions above, and those identified earlier in the chapter, are not necessarily incorrect or invalid. The traps responsive to them will emerge when these therapist beliefs are rigid, unbalanced, or excessive in the given group therapy context. Again, therapists are encouraged to conceptualize and address their own assumptions. Discussions with a consultant or colleague can often help when your individual efforts do not lead to improved group interactions or outcomes.

Socratic Dialogue allows group therapists to vary their level of involvement as needed to ensure productive use of therapy time so that members are actively engaged in meaningful learning. As illustrated throughout this chapter, Socratic Dialogue helps the group therapist guide group interactions and exchange of ideas and also facilitates and enhances spontaneous learning experiences.

When is Socratic Dialogue not appropriate in group therapy?

Socratic Dialogue can become second nature for therapists, even within the complex dynamics of group therapy. There are a few situations, however, when other therapy methods would be more prudent. As indicated in the preceding Traps section, a more directive approach is sometimes superior when intense emotions or conflicts arise, such as when a member experiences a PTSD flashback, or when a participant is acutely depressed and at risk of suicide. Using Socratic Dialogue with a highly agitated group member, or trying to involve other group members in this type of situation, could result in further escalation or excess levels of stress and anxiety for group members.

In situations of high agitation or volatility, therapists can briefly respond empathically to the relevant member or members, and then explicitly explain that they believe it best to return to the topic planned for the session. At this point, a brief didactic module can effectively diffuse the situation and segue back into a more constructive group interaction. When a highly agitated member does not calm down, the therapist can offer to talk to them privately after the session, or even ask them to leave the group if necessary and within the boundaries of clinical safety. For example, inpatient groups sometimes include patients who are highly aggressive toward others or self-harming and they might need to leave the group for a time and receive staff supervision.

In a situation when one member is experiencing a panic attack, or a flashback from a traumatic event, involving group members carries higher risks of unhelpful or counterproductive responses. Clear guidance from the therapist can help ensure a constructive outcome for the individual, teach a sequence of therapeutic skills, and also illustrate that intense emotion can be managed effectively. This observation can strengthen the confidence of other group participants regarding exposure work.

A directive interaction with a suicidal patient in group would often be more prudent than a Socratic one. Therapists can thus ensure that an initial suicide risk assessment is completed in group, even if they plan to continue the assessment after the session. Other members would rarely be involved in Socratic Dialogue with a highly suicidal member. Most group therapy members are not trained to deal with suicide risk and they would likely have anxiety about what to say or not say given the inherent gravity of the situation. Group members may not respond helpfully and could feel anxious or guilty about what they said after the group session, especially if the suicidal person did not respond well to their comments or made a suicide attempt following the group meeting.

Key Ideas Regarding Socratic Dialogue in Group Therapy

- Group therapy provides a dynamic opportunity to maximize the benefits of Socratic Dialogue, using experiential evidence and alternative perspectives from members with diverse backgrounds.

- Having multiple participants invariably provides a wider range of alternative responses and solutions for beliefs or problem situations.

- Group therapists function best when they respect the educational value of natural, unfolding social interactions yet recognize the opportunities to incorporate Socratic guidance to ensure optimal learning.

- Group members may accept the empathy, feedback, summaries, and conclusions of other members more than those coming from the therapist. Feedback of peers can be perceived as, and actually may be, more credible and relevant to their own particular needs and life situation, and may be communicated in more meaningful ways.

- Group interactions provide opportunities for priming and testing relevant interpersonal cognitions in real time while emotions are "hot."

- Socratic Dialogue can be employed at different levels within the group: sometimes it is prudent to focus on only one member at a given moment, but typically it is most effective when actively involving all group members, eventually guiding their involvement even as collaborators in Socratic Dialogue as they become more experienced with the method.

- The group therapist can employ Socratic Dialogue to effectively address clinical traps triggered by individual needs, characteristics of the group members, interactions among members, or the therapist's own propensities and vulnerabilities in a group setting.

- The ability to recognize, understand, and address clinical traps is best guided by a cognitive conceptualization of relevant beliefs and behaviors. Therapists function best when they self-assess and conceptualize their own patterns, along with a conceptualization of individual and group responses to them.

Summary

Socratic Dialogue offers many unique opportunities to enhance client learning in group therapy. Its use can be quite valuable in avoiding or addressing the clinical traps described in this chapter. Maintaining a Socratic stance in groups can be challenging and requires a broad attentiveness to multiple members with differing needs and competencies, as well as strategic responses to interactions among members. The awareness, understanding, confidence, and skill of the therapist in working with groups and employing Socratic Dialogue in this setting will likely determine how well group therapy challenges are met and transformed into opportunities for learning. Less experienced therapists will benefit from reading or observing relevant training resources (e.g., Chapter 2 of this book; Padesky, 2020a; Padesky's video demonstration (Padesky, 1996) of Socratic Dialogue) and seeking consultation from experienced group therapists.

Engaging in Socratic Dialogue with a group can be stimulating and rewarding for the therapist. It is personally meaningful to participate in a communal experience where members collaborate in a common endeavor of learning and self-growth. Even though group therapy involves some added complexities, the same confidence and ease developed with Socratic Dialogue in individual therapy can be achieved in group therapy when therapists are willing to experiment and receive feedback. It can be quite gratifying to witness how participants begin to assist one another by using the very principles and skills that the therapist has endeavored to teach, including the ability to initiate Socratic Dialogue with their peers in group.

Reader Learning Activities

Now that you've learned about the use of Socratic Dialogue in group therapy,

- Try to increase your use of Socratic Dialogue in your therapy groups.
- It is often helpful to begin by using Socratic Dialogue to debrief learning activities group members tried or practiced between therapy sessions.
- Consider rating your use of Socratic Dialogue using the Socratic Dialogue Rating Scale and Manual (Padesky, 2020b), available from https://www.padesky.com/clinical-corner/clinical-tools/.
- Record a group therapy session and listen to it to see whether you use Socratic Dialogues with individuals, dyads, or the entire group.
- If you fall into the traps described in this chapter, review those sections to see how you might respond to those situations more effectively.
- For any traps you experience frequently, identify your own underlying assumptions and behavioral tendencies that might contribute. If you feel stuck, seek consultation or supervision from an experienced CBT group therapist.

References

Beck, A. T., Rush, J. A., Shaw, B. F., & Emery, G. (1979). *Cognitive therapy of depression.* New York: Guilford Press.

Bieling, P. J., McCabe, R. E., & Antony, M. M. (2006). *Cognitive-behavioral therapy in groups.* New York: Guilford Press.

Brown, J. S. L., Sellwood, K., Beecham, J., Slade, M., Andiappan, M., Landau, S., Johnson, T., & Smith, R. (2011). Outcome, costs and patient engagement for group and individual CBT for depression: a naturalistic clinical study. *Behavioural and cognitive psychotherapy, 39*(3). 355–358. https://doi.org/10.1017/S135246581000072X

DeLucia-Waack, J. L., Kalodner, C. R., & Riva, M. T. (Eds.) (2013). *Handbook of group counseling and psychotherapy.* Thousand Oaks, CA: Sage.

Greenberger, D., & Padesky, C. (2016). *Mind over mood: Change how you feel by changing the way you think* (2nd ed.). New York: Guilford Press.

Padesky, C. A. (Guest Expert). (1996). *Guided discovery using Socratic Dialogue.* [Educational video]. Retrieved from https://www.padesky.com/clinical-corner/publications-video/

Padesky, C. A. (2020a). *Clinician's guide to CBT using mind over mood (2nd ed.).* New York: Guilford Press.

Padesky, C. A. (2020b). *Socratic Dialogue rating scale and manual*. Retrieved from: https://www.padesky.com/clinical-corner/clinical-tools/

Söchting, I. (2014). *Cognitive behavioral group therapy: Challenges and opportunities.* Chichester, UK: Wiley.

Yalom, I. D., & Leszcz, M. (2008). *The theory and practice of group psychotherapy* (5th ed.). New York: Basic Books.

11

Supervision and Therapist Beliefs

Helen Kennerley and Christine A. Padesky

> We would never dream of turning untrained therapists loose on needy patients, so why would we turn untrained supervisors loose on untrained therapists who help those needy patients?
> —C. E. Watkins, Jr. (Ed.) *Handbook of psychotherapy supervision*
> (1997, p. 606)

Following Watkins' astute statement in 1997, we have seen a rise in the attention given to CBT supervision. It is now seen as crucial in developing and maintaining adequate standards of CBT (Beidas et al., 2012; Liness et al., 2019; Rakovshik et al., 2016). In the past decade, in particular, we have moved beyond accepting that supervision is simply a matter of a more experienced practitioner talking with a less experienced one, or a session of therapy-by-proxy. Supervision is recognized as a complex interaction of relationships and tasks. Guided discovery methods have a firm place in contributing to successful outcomes.

The way that we use guided discovery methods in supervision is very similar to the way that we use them to generate and test hypotheses in in our clinical practice, so nothing fundamentally is new for the experienced practitioner. As you observe Harold's supervision of Stella below, see if you can recognize his methods and motives based on what you have already learned from the other chapters.

Stella mentioned that her client Kae had said that she sometimes wished that she wasn't here. Harold immediately entertained the hypothesis that Kae was suicidal so he asked direct questions to ascertain risk. Stella's responses indicated that Kae was probably not at risk but that Stella had been rather vague in her assessment of risk. More direct questioning revealed that Stella actually knew risk assessment procedures, but that she had not used them with this patient. Socratic Dialogue revealed why:

Harold: (Hypothesizes that Stella does not take risk assessment seriously enough.) Why do you think I am asking you about her wish not to be here?

Stella: Because you think that she might be suicidal.

Harold: Yes. Now that we've discussed it here, what do you think was the right course of action?

Stella: To ask her, of course. I realize that. Even though she's probably not at risk, I should have gone through the risk assessment just the same.

Harold: I wonder why you didn't.

Stella: I don't know—it's as if I just wanted to get past it as quickly as possible. I'm not sure that I know why I felt like that but it seemed the right thing to do at the time.

Harold: (Now hypothesizes that Stella was afraid of asking direct questions.) What do you think might have happened if you had asked Kae what she meant when she wished that she wasn't here?

Stella: Well, I suppose I thought that if she hadn't already considered killing herself my questions might put the idea into her head.

Harold: And that would mean?

Stella: That I could have made her suicidal—and that would have been awful.

If Harold had simply reminded Stella that suicide assessment should always be done, he might not have uncovered Stella's belief that asking direct questions about suicide can increase a client's risk. By using Socratic Dialogue to check out his own assumptions, Harold was able to discover what had prevented Stella from carrying what she knew to be good practice. He then used guided discovery methods to encourage Stella to review her prediction that discussing suicide would make a person more suicidal. He and Stella agreed she would do some Internet research and carry out a survey of colleagues to test the validity of her prediction.

Once Stella had collected data from her fellow therapists she shared her findings with Harold. Out of 10 therapists who responded, none had found that talking about suicide resulted in a suicide attempt and 90% confidently rated that it was unlikely that talking would put the idea into someone's head. Harold then simply posed the most basic Socratic question, "What do you make of that?", which prompted Stella to look at her findings and conclude for herself that it is safe to make enquiries about suicide risk. Harold then asked her how she might use this information to inform her sessions going forward. Stella said that she would now always carry out a proper risk assessment if she felt that a client might be considering suicide.

The Many Tasks of Supervision

Even though guided discovery methods work similarly, the tasks facing a therapy supervisor are not precisely the same as those facing a therapist, and we need to adapt our methods accordingly. Although the specific definitions of supervision tasks are still debated, there is general agreement that the welfare of the client is central (Bernard & Goodyear, 1998) and that there are three discrete supervisory functions (Milne 2007):

- **Educative/formative**: the supervisor facilitates the supervisee's acquisition of relevant information and skills;
- **Supportive/restorative**: the supervisor provides a forum for exploring difficulties, keeping the supervisee on track, and facilitating supervisee self-care; and
- **Managerial/normative**: the supervisor ensures that standards of practice are maintained.

Sessions will, and should, shift in focus to reflect need. A supervisory meeting might focus on task one moment and swiftly shift to process as the necessity arises. One session might emphasize a supervisee's developmental requirements and the next address client risk management or case management in response to client service demands. Early supervision sessions might offer didactic modeling while later sessions require a supervisee to take more initiative. This thoughtful flexibility is also required in using guided discovery and other methods to achieve the goals of good supervision.

Again, there is a general consensus rather than an empirical foundation indicating the core skills of supervision (Roth & Pilling, 2008), but they are usually cited as:

- Contracting (including agenda setting),
- Goal setting,
- Structuring,
- Giving and eliciting feedback,
- Evaluating performance, and
- Developing and working with the therapeutic alliance.

We will see how these important skills can be developed as we go through the chapter exploring where and when to use guided discovery most effectively.

Even more than in therapy, our role as a supervisor demands skilled "juggling." As already noted, supervisors must consider the appropriate focus of a

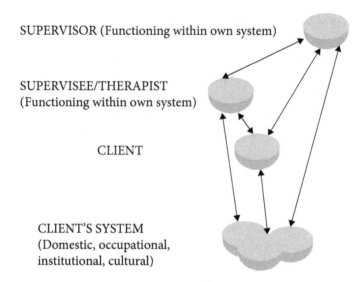

SUPERVISOR (Functioning within own system)

SUPERVISEE/THERAPIST
(Functioning within own system)

CLIENT

CLIENT'S SYSTEM
(Domestic, occupational,
institutional, cultural)

Figure 11.1 The "system framework" of CBT supervision.

session and be responsive to need, while concurrently attending to the proper execution of core skills and the education of the supervisee. But there is even more to juggle: a supervisor should be self-reflective *and* also attuned to the perspectives of the supervisee, *while* considering client needs and perspectives *and* the needs of those who have significant relationships with the client *and* the characteristics of those relationships. To challenge us further we must be able to appreciate that clients, supervisees, and supervisors are all embedded within dynamic systems (home, work, institution, culture) along with children and partners with whom they have a reciprocal role. The "bigger picture" becomes even more complicated when interpreters are involved or when we supervise in groups.

So, although the overt relationships are between supervisor and supervisee and between therapist and client, you can see that there is much more to consider (see Figure 11.1). All this needs to be held in mind during a supervision session as we attend to the array of supervisory tasks laid out earlier. At times, supervision can feel as though we are juggling with batons, balls, and fire!

Common Traps in Supervision

What we have said so far about education, scope of supervision, and the complexity of those involved begins to point us toward the traps we can fall into,

---

Box 11.1 Common Traps in Supervision

Trap 1
Education trap: Taking the expert position and instructing supervisees too much of the time: failing to get the balance right and thus failing to enhance learning.

Trap 2
Neglecting therapist and supervisor assumptions.

Trap 3
Losing sight of the bigger picture. Not thinking beyond the therapist and client.

Trap 4
Neglecting the supervisory relationship. Failing to be sensitive to, respectful of, and consistently mindful of the need to maintain the working alliance between supervisor and supervisee.

---

summarized in Box 11.1, "Common Traps in Supervision." Each of these traps will be addressed in turn in this chapter.

Supervisees often prefer supervisors who spend time offering didactic instruction because this takes the pressure and scrutiny off them. However, supervisee learning is usually enhanced when supervisees present their own thinking and reasoning processes. Clinical presentations and discussions help both the supervisee and supervisor identify and address knowledge and practice gaps.

Trap 1

Education trap. Taking the expert position and instructing supervisees too much of the time: failing to get the balance right and thus failing to enhance learning.

Supervision to enhance learning—getting the balance right

One fundamental supervisory challenge is deciding how much time in each meeting to spend in the "expert" didactic teaching role and how much time to spend guiding supervisees to think and process information for themselves. Are you getting the balance right in your own supervision? How would you know? There are two simple steps that you can take to find out if you fall into this trap. The first is eliciting feedback from your supervisee (one of the core skills in supervision). The second is to record your supervisory sessions and periodically review these to enhance your own awareness and learning. We recommend you take the first step every supervision session and that you schedule reminders to periodically take the second step.

Asking for and giving feedback

At various points during and certainly at the end of a supervision session we need to ask our supervisee(s) about their experience. This readily lends itself to the straightforward question: "What was most helpful and what was least helpful about the supervision session today?" Perhaps a more experienced and confident supervisee can give a full response and combine constructive criticism with favorable feedback in response to this question, signaling an openness to both types of feedback. However, many supervisees struggle to structure their response and to feel comfortable giving what they consider negative feedback to a supervisor who often has evaluative power over them.

Thus, it can be very helpful to preface a feedback enquiry with a rationale:

> As a supervisor I want to make sure that I'm meeting your needs and I want to become an even better supervisor over time. Therefore, every time we meet I am going to ask you for your views and feedback on supervision. Essentially, I need to know what you find helpful about supervision—so that we can build on that— and I need to know how you think supervision might be made even more useful or helpful. Perhaps you can bear this in mind during our meetings so that you can give me honest feedback. I truly welcome it, negative feedback as well as positive.

Asking what has gone well and what might make the session even more productive will encourage even the reticent supervisee to offer constructive criticism. By doing this, you increase the likelihood that you will gain relevant information. Also, your enquiry becomes more Socratic in that it poses an invitation for your supervisee to review and consider deeply enough to help you discover a novel perspective. When asking for feedback, also remember to give your supervisee enough time to reflect and respond. Otherwise, they might find it hard to generate useful feedback.

Similarly, feedback that you as supervisor will give your supervisee can and should be discussed at the outset as you formulate your contract for working together (another core skill of supervision). See how Tomas (below) sets up the expectation for supervisory feedback in his first session of supervision with a new therapist, Alice.

In the Supervisor's Mind

Tomas realized Alice probably had little idea of the range of ways in which he could give her feedback. He planned to use Socratic enquiry to help her refine her ideas about the best approach for her, but he realized that he might have to "seed" the discussion with some examples just so that she had relevant knowledge about feedback in supervision.

Tomas: Part of my role as a supervisor is to give you feedback. I want to encourage you to recognize and build on your strengths and to appreciate where you might develop and improve your therapeutic skills.
Different people have different preferences for receiving feedback—
some of my supervisees say things like "Give me the bad news first—
don't dress it up!" I hope that my feedback never sounds like "bad
news" but I know what they mean. Others ask that I start with what
went well in their work and then move on to areas for development.
I want you to be in the right frame of mind to hear feedback, so perhaps you could begin thinking about what works best for you . . .

... I hope to listen to a recording of at least one full therapy session
each term. Some supervisees like me to do this on my own and then
give them feedback. Some prefer to have written feedback before we
next meet so that they can mull it over, others don't. I am also happy
to review a recording "live" alongside you, commenting as we go.

Once Tomas laid out these options, he gave Alice a written summary of these general expectations and guidelines for her review. He could then more confidently ask questions such as:

"So, how do you think you'd like to receive feedback?"
"Is there anything else that would make it more memorable?"
"How might we judge if we are getting the right balance for you?"

Although Tomas asks Alice how she would like to receive feedback, keep in mind that every session's feedback to supervisees should include a description of what they did well. It is important to highlight therapist skills, good intentions, and moments in which they managed challenges in competent ways. Positive feedback is encouraging and also reinforces good behaviors, attitudes, and reasoning processes that serve the supervisee and their clients well. We recommend you also require supervisees to identify what they did well in any of their session recordings they review. This helps mitigate against the human tendency to focus more on errors and flaws than on strengths and what is done well.

Recording and reviewing supervision sessions

A second step that you can take to judge if you are creating the best milieu for learning is listening to or watching recordings of your supervision sessions. You can then ask yourself guided discovery questions about what you observe and set up behavioral experiments to try out alternative approaches. As noted in the previous paragraph, it is crucial you also note what you did well in the supervision session. You can do this yourself and/or you can ask a peer or your own supervisor-of-supervision for an appraisal.

Tomas had his own supervisor-of-supervision and would take recordings of his sessions along for feedback on specific stuck points and overall evaluation. However, these meetings were not as frequent as he would have liked and sometimes he found himself facing a supervisory problem alone. He then made time for *self-supervision*. He turned his supervisory skills on himself. While listening to recordings, he paused to ask himself, "How did I feel at that point?" "What was going through my mind?" "How could I check that out next time I meet Alice?" "What else do I need to know—what am I missing?" "Where will I get that information?"

Just as Tomas is doing for himself, listening to one's own or supervisees recordings is a good opportunity to help avoid the second supervision trap.

Trap 2

Neglecting therapist and supervisor assumptions.

Tomas noted some particular recurrent behaviors such as running overtime on his sessions with Alice. Even when he tried to change these behaviors, it was difficult for him to do so. He had learned in his CBT training that behavioral habits that were hard to change were often maintained by underlying assumptions (see Chapter 6 and also Padesky, 2020). He worked to identify relevant underlying assumptions such as "If I end on time and we have not fully addressed Alice's questions, then the next session with that client will go wrong," and tested these out with behavioral experiments.

Engage supervisees in structuring session learning

A pragmatic step that you can take to increase the likelihood that you will address your supervisees' learning needs is to ask them to prepare a specific supervision question prior to coming to your meeting. Good supervision questions are specific, realistic, and backed up by enough information that allows them to be addressed.

Tomas met his regular supervisee Alice and asked her what her supervision question was for this meeting. She replied, "It's Wim. Where did I go wrong?" This was clearly a pressing question on her part but not very specific so Tomas enquired further to elicit a more precise supervision question.

Supervisor: I remember your patient, Wim. In fact I've got my notes here with your initial formulation of his depression. But could you update me—set the scene for me? Remind me just what you were doing in the session that concerns you.

Alice: It's session 4. Although he was very closed and defensive at the beginning of therapy, I thought that we were now working well. He was getting active, cutting down on his drinking; he was honest in telling me about suicidal thoughts. I felt that we had a good alliance. The review of his homework went OK, and then I began to explore things a bit more with him—trying to get more detail for our formulation. Then it just fell apart—he looked cross, he wasn't open anymore and he asked to leave early. I'm not sure what was going on.

Supervisor: So your supervision question would be . . . ?

Alice: I'm still not really sure.

Supervisor: Let's imagine that it's the end of our session and your supervision issue has been addressed—what will you know then that you don't know now?

Alice: I will know what I might have done to trigger withdrawal in a client who had been cooperative for the early part of the session and in sessions before that.

Supervisor: So your question would be: "What might I have done to trigger withdrawal in this usually cooperative client?"

By using questions and prompts, Tomas helped Alice to shape her very general request into a specific supervision question—this meant that they were more likely to address her learning needs (and, at the same time, probably better serve the client's needs).

Padesky (1995) provides a structured worksheet for supervisees to complete prior to the supervision meeting that helps them prepare a useful supervision question and spend time thinking it through for themselves in advance. In this way it offers a Socratic framework, prompting supervisees to explore the knowledge they have and, where possible, generate their own ideas. Her worksheet form also includes a variety of tips and recommendations for its best use. The worksheet begins asking the supervisee to write a specific supervision question and then asks successively for the case conceptualization, a description of an evidence based treatment plan, a self-assessment of their knowledge and skills to carry out the treatment plan, and various types of hypotheses about roadblocks that could be limiting treatment progress. She recommends this form be filled out starting with the supervision question at the top and then moving through the subsequent steps until the supervisee no longer knows what to say. As a beginning therapist, Alice might write her question and the beginning of a conceptualization but not know what to write for a treatment plan, so she would stop filling out the worksheet there.

This structured worksheet has three built-in advantages for supervision:

1. When supervisees need to think about a specific question prior to supervision, it focuses their thinking beyond the usual, "What should I do next?" or "What did I do wrong?" Often, in filling out the form, the supervisee figures out an answer to their initial question (by reviewing the conceptualization, for example) and develops a more refined question to ask.

2. Supervision can be helpfully focused on improving the supervisee's understanding of each step on the form. The supervisor can generally identify knowledge/skills gaps by reviewing what is written on the worksheet and also by seeing where the supervisee stopped writing because they "drew a blank." This is often a good focus for that supervision session.

3. The supervisor can review what has been written on the form to identify gaps in the supervisee's knowledge and skills. One can quickly assess whether the conceptualization and treatment plan seem adequate or are missing key elements. Subsequent discussions of the same client can simply add new information to the worksheet, with new questions highlighted.

Employ active learning methods in supervision

Another strategy for enhancing supervisee learning is to employ active learning methods, using Socratic Dialogue to extract learning from them. Active learning methods in therapy include written summaries, imagery, behavioral experiments, and role-plays (Padesky, 2019). The same is true of supervision. By using a variety of these action methods in supervision, learning can be made more memorable than it is when you simply discuss case issues week after week. Table 11.1 shows a sample of supervision options that can be used to increase supervisee skills and learning, drawing on the ideas discussed in Chapter 1.

Imagine the different learning experience working with a supervisor who only uses case discussion and didactic teaching (column 1) in supervision compared to one who uses all the methods in this chart. A skilled supervisor will not only vary methods and the foci in supervision but also select the methods and foci best suited to meeting the supervisee's current learning needs. Thus, a novice therapist might benefit initially from case discussion and didactic learning. Then this information can come to life when the supervisor does a role-play demonstrating the methods discussed, followed by a role-play with the supervisee in the therapist role.

No therapist can be expected to consistently identify what they don't know or what they might be doing inadequately in therapy. Live observation or the review of session recordings is the best ways to assess supervisee skills and knowledge gaps. As therapists become more knowledgeable, they can sometimes review their own recordings and pinpoint sections of a session that will benefit from supervisory review.

Didactic explanations can appear clear and simple and yet practice of these same ideas in role-plays often reveals subtle aspects of a method that are difficult to carry out or that were not fully understood. Imagery exercises can be fruitfully employed to help a therapist recall their own thoughts and feelings in a past session, to imagine an intervention from the point of view of their client, or to envision carrying out therapy steps in a future session to assess how this might unfold.

Behavioral experiments can be used in a supervisory session to try out a variety of approaches or to test out supervisor or supervisee underlying assumptions. Similarly, supervisee assumptions or the utility of particular therapy approaches can be evaluated through behavioral experiments with clients. The supervisor can model good practices in use of behavioral experiments by asking the supervisee to make predictions in advance about the outcomes of these experiments based on current and alternative beliefs.

Table 11.1 Supervision Options to Enhance Learning.

Focus	Methods paired with Socratic Dialogue to extract learning					
	Case discussion/ didactic	Live or recorded observation	Role-play	Imagery exercise	Behavioral experiment	Written summary
Case conceptualization						
Specific therapy skills						
Client–therapist relationship						
Treatment plan						
Therapist reactions						
Supervisory relationship/ processes						

The 4-Stage Model of Socratic Dialogue (see Chapter 2) will support learning no matter what methods from the grid in Table 11.1 are chosen in supervision. Recall from Chapter 2 that Socratic Dialogue is used in therapy at the beginning of therapy sessions to debrief between session learning and at the end of therapy sessions to make a written summary of take-home learning and plans for how those ideas can be used in the coming week. Socratic Dialogue can frame supervision sessions in the same way. Feedback on the utility of actions taken since the last supervision session can be gathered using Socratic Dialogue and yield a written summary of learning for the supervisee to carry forward. Each supervision session can end with a written summary of what was learned and a plan for how to carry these ideas forward with clients. Using Socratic Dialogue processes in these ways provides a bridge between supervision sessions and also models these processes for supervisees who will be trying to use these same practices in their therapy sessions.

Reflective practice

Throughout this book we have described how guided discovery methods can be skillfully used to enhance learning. A related approach widely promoted in CBT supervision is reflective practice. This is a two-fold task as it requires a supervisor to:

- self-reflect on supervision and
- encourage self-reflection by the supervisee.

Reflective practice goes beyond simply looking back on experiences and reviewing actions; it is the capacity to reflect on an action to engage in the process of *continuous* learning. The psychologist John Dewy first promoted this concept in the 1930s (Dewy, 1960). Then, as now, it very much embodied asking oneself questions and the approach has taken a firm position in the practice of CBT supervision. There have been many elaborations of Dewy's concept, most notably Lewin (1946), Kolb (1984), Gibbs (1988), and Bennett-Levy (2006). But it is not always possible to hold in mind complicated frameworks when we are active in supervision, and that is why we would remind you of Borton's (1970) simple, and therefore memorable, heuristic comprising three questions: What? So What? Now What?

Even the most stressed supervisor or supervisee can generally keep Figure 11.2 in mind!

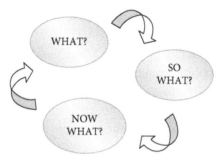

Figure 11.2 Borton's reflective framework.

Schön (1984) furthered Dewey's concept by making an important distinction that is very relevant to supervision, namely that reflection offers a dual opportunity:

- **Reflection-*on*-action**: conscious retrospective appraisal through self-review, discussion, keeping a reflective journal.
- **Reflection-*in*-action**: the conscious or unconscious ability to "think on one's feet," as we carry out tasks and approach problems.

Keep in Mind

Learning is a process of active enquiry and this is facilitated by a supervisor who prompts reflective practice. This means asking:

What?	Pause and then review what the supervisee tells you.
So what?	What does this mean? What does this tell us? What are we learning?
Now what?	What will we do with this new perspective or understanding?

The value of these three questions is illustrated in the following supervision example. Alice's supervisor Tomas listened to an excerpt of her therapy recording. She had isolated this part of the session because she felt that it represented what she called "the poor practice that alienated Wim" and she hoped for constructive feedback from Tomas. As they listened to the recording she indicated the moment that she thought that she had stopped being collaborative. Thomas used a Socratic prompt to help her reflect *on* her actions:

Alice:	(Pauses the recording.) There—that's where he detaches and begins to sound cross.
Supervisor:	At that point you ask about his children. What was behind your decision to do that?
Alice:	I was trying to develop the formulation. When we first met he was less communicative so the formulation was rather "minimalist." Now he was opening up so I was keen to take the opportunity to include everything that was relevant.
Supervisor:	That's a good motive. What then prompted you to pinpoint this as your example of "poor practice"?
Alice:	That's where things started to go wrong. Wim suddenly seemed wrong-footed and that's when I felt that we lost our collaboration.
Supervisor:	Do you have any thoughts about the reasons for that?
Alice:	I'm not sure—it seemed so out of the blue. (Pauses to reflect.) I wonder if I touched a nerve, maybe?
Supervisor:	Why do you say that?
Alice:	Well I realize that he has only just been allowed to see his children again unsupervised. Now I'm wondering if he thought that I was questioning his fitness as a parent. I was kind of excited to think that we were talking more and that I could start to get a more detailed conceptualization of his difficulties. I think I forgot to consider his situation and feelings.
Supervisor:	OK, this leaves me with two trains of thought—one is to ask you how you might check out your hunch and the second is to ask you what you have learned from this and what you might do differently as a result.
Alice:	Checking it out is easy—I'll suggest that we give some time to reflect on this when we next meet. I think that he'll welcome me being open about it. The second question is harder for me to answer. I think that I've learned not to jump in too quickly, to maybe stand back and summarize, pause, give myself time to consider the pros and cons of my questions.
Supervisor:	That sounds excellent—but how will you make sure that you do that?
Alice:	I don't know—you see, I kind of know all this already and yet in that session, I just leapt in.
Supervisor:	Do you recall just what was going through your mind at the time?
Alice:	No—even when I listen to the recording I'm not sure. I listen to it, thinking: "Don't do that Alice!" and I did it and I don't know why I did it.

Tomas was pleased that Alice was so open to exploration. In order to help her get in touch with the feelings and thoughts that had driven her to question Wim about his children at that moment, Tomas offered to role play the scenario. In this way he hoped to help her "relive" the situation so that his questions might be more fruitful. At regular points, when Tomas hoped that they might catch a "hot cognition," he paused their role-play and asked a Socratic question in order to prompt Alice to participate in reflection *in* action:

Supervisor: (Comes out of role.) Right now—what's going through your mind?
Alice: He mentioned his children—this is good—I have to have a sys-
                     temic formulation. This is my chance.

They resumed the role-play and Tomas re-enacted the client's detachment from therapy and his discomfort, while Alice continued to ask questions about the relationship with the children. Again Tomas interrupted:

Supervisor: (Comes out of role.) More questions—what's the benefit of these
                     enquiries right now?
Alice: He's disengaging and I might lose my chance. I have to hang
                     in there.
Supervisor: And how are you feeling?
Alice: I'm anxious—feels like I'm losing him and I need to hold on.
Supervisor: No wonder there is such urgency in your questions. Can you tell
                     me more?
Alice: No—that's it really. I feel driven to keep questioning him because
                     I fear losing his cooperation. That one backfired, didn't it?

At this point they ended the role-play and were able to *reflect on action* again. Tomas helped Alice formulate an understanding of her fears that led to her unproductive questioning and then asked her what she would now do differently given her new perspective. She volunteered a more moderate and considered approach to her assessment questions and they devised some alternative assumptions to help her in such situations. They then role-played Alice holding back, seeing the bigger picture, keeping calm. Finally, they co-created a plan for Alice to monitor her tendencies to give priority to procedural tasks over the therapy relationship. Thus, within the supervision session she had been able to reflect in action, reflect on her actions, and engage in a process of continuous learning at an intellectual and a behavioral level. Tomas was able to both model and promote a reflective practice that was more than a cursory review and which reflected good guided discovery processes.

This need not be the end of the reflective process. Tomas will carry out his own reflection on his supervision. When he reviewed his supervision notes and thought back on his experience, he recalled that in the role-play he was tempted to take on an aggressive personae. He asked himself, "Now, what was that about?" He quickly recognized his own Achilles heel—he had a tendency to get cross when therapists put procedures before process as Alice had done. He felt so strongly about this that, in the past, he had tended to promptly "tutor" his supervisees about this. Within the role-play—perhaps because he was in role-play—he had controlled his feelings and this had resulted in a productive session with Alice in which she had also come to appreciate for herself that she had lost the therapeutic alliance because of her dedication to procedure. This reminded him that it was often the best decision to not jump in and "correct" a novice therapist—better to let them make their own discoveries if possible. He mentally added this to his "data log" of experiences that reinforced a more guided discovery approach to formative and restorative supervision. Like many of us, Tomas often used *self-supervision*. Just like in other-supervision, self-supervision is more productive if it is structured and incorporates guided discovery methods.

The reflective process would also continue when Alice and Tomas next met because their agenda would contain a review of her subsequent therapy session with Wim. Teaching supervisees to critically review each session and consider their reactions and actions is one of the most valuable lessons of supervision. When therapists record and review sessions, keep their own thought records, and try out behavioral experiments to test out their own assumptions, they develop a better understanding of their own strengths and vulnerabilities. Learning to keep a close eye on the content and processes of each therapy session helps therapists to stay on track by formulating difficulties within each session and predicting problem issues and stuck points.

Using thought records and reviewing behavioral experiments are excellent guided discovery methods for self-supervision. Many roadblocks in therapy and supervision can be solved through this type of reflective practice. When roadblocks are not resolved in self-supervision or significant issues arise, these can be taken to supervision or supervision of supervision. And as described earlier, "good" supervision begins with a "good" supervision question. Therapists familiar with reflective practice will be well-versed in the skills necessary to think about what they want to learn from supervision.

This process is illustrated by the therapist Jonas who set aside time to review recordings of his meetings with his client Philip. He was concerned about his therapy with Philip because he they seemed to be making little progress and Jonas felt heavy hearted when they met. His supervision questions for himself were "How can I understand my feelings of 'stuckness'?" and "What might I do differently to get 'unstuck'?" When he listened to the therapy session, Jonas tried to attend to the content, the therapeutic relationship, and his own thoughts and feelings. He did notice some "ruptures" in the session when he was aware that his own feelings of frustration and hopelessness were coming through, but he still felt at a loss as to what to do with this insight. So, he decided to take this to his next supervision session.

With his supervisor's help, Jonas identified a key unhelpful thought:

> I can't possibly ask him to tell me more about his experience of being abused by the priest—he will view that as further abuse by a man in a trusted position.

Jonas quickly realized that he was jumping to conclusions and becoming caught up in a cycle of avoidance which prevented him and Philip from developing a shared formulation and which would hinder them in testing and restructuring Philip's beliefs about his abuse.

As they looked at the cycle of avoidance, his supervisor asked Jonas questions:

- How can you modify this cycle—what can you change?
- Have you been in similar circumstances? What helped then?
- How will you set this up with Philip? What do you need to share?
- What needs to be in place for change to occur?

Jonas decided that there were two main tasks ahead of him. First, to clarify with Philip just how Philip felt about Jonas exploring his history in more detail, he asked a simple question:

> I would like to know a little more about the abuse you experienced at school—how would you feel about that?

Jonas discovered his prejudices about Philip were unfounded. Phillip was open to talking more.

His second task was to share the unhelpful interpersonal cycle that he had identified. He did this by stating that he wanted to put on their session agenda an item to look at ways of improving Philip's progress. Philip was happy to include this item and then together they reviewed the cycle and ways of breaking it. This collaborative practice gave both men a sense of hope.

Trap 3

Losing sight of the bigger picture. Not thinking beyond the therapist and client.

Seeing the bigger picture

Standing back and reviewing the full implications and impact of our supervision sessions allows us to appreciate when factors beyond the supervisor–supervisee–client triad play a role. This means posing questions that will stretch your supervisee's perspective:

- … And when this person leaves a therapy session and goes back to their job, what is the impact of their workplace and domineering boss?
- Are their children at risk?
- How might you help achieve these goals within a service that is under-resourced?
- Who else might help or hinder your client's recovery?

You also need to make sure that you are aware of the "bigger picture" that is pertinent to you and ask yourself relevant questions such as:

- I have problems in my family relationships at present; am I imposing some of my personal fears in this supervision session?
- I'm feeling very protective towards the client and irritable with my supervisee—what's that about?
- What else do I know about the client that can bolster my hypotheses?
- Can I really support this therapist in the time available to us?
- I feel unhappy about the expectations of my supervisee's boss. How can I best explore/express this?

You can see how keeping the bigger picture in mind will so often relate to beliefs—our own, our supervisee's, and others "outside the room."

Keep in Mind

Use Socratic enquiry to maximize your appreciation of the wider and deeper systems in which each person is embedded. This means:

- Look beyond the "room." Regularly ask yourself and your supervisee, "What else?" and "Who else?"
- Attend to thoughts and feelings: Your own and those of the people on whom the supervision impacts.

On occasion additional factors add to the complexity of the bigger picture. For example, when therapy or supervision is carried out through an interpreter there are additional factors to consider as illustrated in the following two examples.

Rachel, a German therapist, was working for a year in Bangladesh helping develop a CBT training course. In addition to teaching therapists in a tutorial setting, she was contracted to offer them live supervision of their clinical work. In order to do this she needed to use an interpreter. It was the most rewarding and also the most difficult supervisory practice of her career. In one session, she supervised Raja's live therapy with Shanti, a man with anxieties, with an interpreter giving Rachel a concurrent translation of the session.

Jenna worked in a service for the deaf and she herself was deaf; thus, her supervision (with a hearing supervisor) took place with two interpreters present. They translated into sign language what the supervisor said and then articulated what Jenna signed. The practical issues of needing a larger room and more time for supervision were relatively easily overcome, but the supervisor was uncomfortable with an ever-changing team of interpreters.

In these two scenarios, the supervisors initially neglected to understand the impact of these sessions on the interpreters and this blind spot limited the usefulness of supervision. Rachel had presumed that her male interpreter would be able to translate precisely what Shanti said—but it turned out that there were certain issues that the translator was embarrassed to disclose to a female. Jenna simply welcomed the two interpreters into her office without discovering that neither had been briefed that they might hear accounts of trauma and one of the interpreters was clearly overwhelmed by the recounting of a clinical session.

These problems could so easily have been averted by proper contracting before the sessions began. Knowing what to put in such a contract is underpinned by thoughtful and thorough Socratic enquiry as illustrated by Rachel's experience:

In the Supervisor's Mind

Although Rachel had not carried out this sort of live supervision before, the charity that she worked for had committed her to this. With hindsight she wished that she had discussed this with her boss because she now felt out of her depth. However, she did know that she had the opportunity to discuss this with Raja and the interpreter who were both more experienced with use of interpreters than she was. Rachel realized that she could use Socratic enquiry with both of them to get a better understanding of the setup (by asking direct information-gathering questions) and that she could discover top tips for how to overcome problems. A written summary of what they discussed could form a rough outline of a contractual agreement between the three of them.

In the ideal situation, Rachel would have developed a contract with the therapist (her supervisee) and the interpreter before they even met the first patient. This had not happened because the organization that Rachel worked for imposed a standard contract and there was an assumption that "one-size-fits-all." Very soon, she realized that arrangements needed to be more bespoke. She set up an additional meeting so that she, Raja, and the interpreter could refine their agreed way of working.

Rachel: You have both done this before; can you tell me how we best set up the therapy/supervision session? Do you have any suggestions for making it as useful as possible for both the client and the therapist? (Turning directly to the interpreter.) And is there anything that you have found makes your job easier? Maybe we could start with Raja. You have done this before, I haven't, so could you tell me some of the obstacles that you have encountered when using an interpreter in a clinical session with live supervision?

Raja: It's certainly not without problems. The main one for me is that it does interfere with the flow of therapy because it is distracting for both me and my client.

Rachel: I'm writing this down—let's "brainstorm" and then return to the list to consider solutions. Can you think of more obstacles?

Raja: The gender mix can make a difference, I find that a male might be more reserved with a female interpreter and also with a female supervisor—especially a Western, educated woman. I am sorry to say that this can make things difficult, but you need to understand that it can.

                      . . .

Rachel: (Later turning to the translator.) And what difficulties have you discovered during your time translating in these clinical sessions?

Translator: The pressure to translate quickly can pose problems. Sometimes I substitute the best word I can because I don't have time to reflect on the nuances of the patient's speech.

Rachel: Mm, that could be quite significant. Are there other issues around the precision of the translation?

Translator: Well, sometimes I sense that the patient is reluctant to say exactly what's troubling them and so they use euphemisms for their condition or their behavior—then it really is hard to work out what they mean, then translate and keep up with the session! You do know that I am a general translator and not specialized in therapy work? So sometimes, when I realize what the patient is trying to say, I feel embarrassed about sharing it. Sometimes I am shocked by what I hear and feel very upset.

If they had actually had this meeting before they saw the first patient together the session could have been much more productive because they would have anticipated problems and been able to take proactive steps in dealing with them. As it was, they could now spend time clarifying the obstacles and problem-solving the difficulties so that they could make the most of a challenging setup in the future.

You can see that the Socratic enquiry itself in this scenario is not particularly sophisticated or unique, but it is aimed at the right people at the right time for it to make difference to the outcome of the supervision session. This is so frequently the case—"good" use of Socratic Dialogue is not simply about what you say or even how you say it but also when you say it.

The supervisory relationship

Considering the complexities of the "bigger picture" necessarily involves being sensitive to aspects of the supervisory relationship. As well as taking into account all the issues that we have already indicated, you need to be aware of, develop, and maintain a supervisory alliance that facilitates good supervision. This relationship needs to be so much more than a comfortable supportive discussion. It should be a forum where your supervisee feels safe in sharing concerns (without it becoming therapy). It is a medium for enabling your supervisee's therapeutic knowledge, skills, and reflective abilities and not therapy-by-proxy for the client.

Trap 4

Neglecting the supervisory relationship. Failing to be sensitive to, respectful of, and consistently mindful of the need to maintain the working alliance between supervisor and supervisee.

The supervisory relationship needs to be honest, authentic, and enabling. This can be achieved through investing time in developing a written supervision contract, being open about potential difficulties, negotiating how to give and receive feedback, and setting clear and agreed-upon supervision goals and boundaries. All these aspects will contribute to developing a safe, productive working alliance. However, this can prove to be quite a juggling act and even more so when we provide group supervision. In Chapter 10 of this book, Shenk described the ways in which guided discovery methods are best used in group settings. We recommend that chapter as a companion to this one when you are offering group supervision.

Keep in Mind

- The supervisory relationship is for supervision of therapeutic practice. It is not therapy-by-proxy or therapy for your supervisee.
- The supervisory relationship provides a milieu for growth and development: Therefore, co-design it to stretch and challenge your supervisee.
- Ruptures in the alliance/relationship need to be addressed swiftly and sensitively.

Christiana was an experienced supervisor for a university-led training course. She routinely took on a small group of supervisees. This semester she had three supervisees including Ruby, who offered support to trauma victims via a charitable organization. Within the supervision session Christiana recognized a repeated pattern of internal escalating tension when she addressed Ruby's question. She was unhappy to observe herself adopting a very didactic, authoritative approach with Ruby. After the session she listened to a recording of the supervision meeting and realized:

"I'm getting anxious. The longer I work with Ruby, the more anxious I feel."

She took this issue to her Supervisor-of-Supervision, Noa. Her question for him was: "How can I stay calm and attend to Ruby's supervision needs in a more Socratic fashion?"

Noa needed to put this supervision question into context so he asked a series of questions to clarify the problem. He asked information-gathering questions to help him appreciate the scope of the problem. He learned that Ruby's charitable organization operated on very little money and yet took on large numbers of clients who had been recently traumatized. As a result, all the therapists were under pressure to see people quickly and for little pay and with sparse supervision. He also needed to understand the dynamic between Christina and Ruby and between group members in general, so he asked Christiana about the interaction between her and Ruby—how Christina felt, what she did, and how Ruby responded.

In the Supervisor-of-Supervision's Mind

After gathering this contextual information, Noa thought that a role-play of their supervisory interaction could bring alive the dynamics of Christiana and Ruby's relationship. At the same time, he hypothesized that Christiana's reactions had something to do with her own assumptions and not just her supervisory relationship with Ruby. Therefore, he also thought he might suggest that Christina role-play being one of the other group members when the supervision focus was on Ruby. He hoped this shift in perspectives would help her identify some helpful insights into what was going on. He held these options in mind and intended to be open to whatever discovery occurred and prompt Christiana to use her own knowledge and skills as much as possible.

Noa: (Sharing a capsule summary.) So Ruby is in a pressured position: she tends to bring several supervision issues at once and although she has developed clear supervision questions, there is often too much to deal with in your session.

Christiana: That's right and I feel very stressed about it. I expect that is why I need your help learning how to stay calm.

Noa: Let's stay with how you feel and what you are thinking at the time. Can you tell me more about that?

Christiana: I'm a bit all over the place, I get so tense … there I'm feeling it now and I can't think straight!

Noa: Why don't we try to pinpoint a specific moment—preferably a recent one—and then role-play it? We can take our time and unpack what's behind the confusing tension.

They then role-played with Noa regularly pausing, coming out of "Ruby" role and prompting Christiana to reflect on her thoughts, images, and emotions.

Noa: Just then—what was happening for you?

Christiana: It's the thought that there is too much to cover in a session—I get anxious that I can't address Ruby's questions.

Noa: Anything else?

Christiana: Angry with her for putting me in this position month after month.

Noa: Anything else?

Christiana: Cross with myself for feeling like this and then even crosser with myself because I start to lecture her on how to treat trauma victims. I'm trying to fix her clients at a distance and I'm not thinking of her development as a therapist. And I ignore the rest of the group.

Noa: Go on …

Christiana: And when I think about the rest of the group I feel really ashamed that I'm neglecting them and I dread asking them for feedback on the supervision in case they tell me how bad a supervisor I am.

Noa: Goodness—such a lot going on for you. Is there anything else going through your mind?

Christiana: I don't think so—I think that's quite enough!

Noa: So how would you summarize what you've picked up from the role-play and debrief?

Christiana:	It's no wonder that I'm overwhelmed because Ruby brings big, often disturbing issues and she is stressed and stretched so it's no wonder that she drops it all at my door. I can also see why I get cross with her and then with myself—even thought I don't think this is justified. I need to sort that out.
Noa:	That's a neat mini-formulation. How do you feel now that you've devised that?
Christiana:	I feel calmer—just getting to the position where I can say, "It's no wonder that …" helps me appreciate my position and be more empathic towards Ruby. I think that I feel compassion for her rather than frustration and I think that will make it less likely that I ignore her developmental needs.
Noa:	Sounds good—but what will you actually do to make sure that things change?
Christiana:	I'll write down my mini-formulation and I'll look at that before the session. I think that I'm going to ask the group if I can record the meeting so that I can do my own debrief afterwards—monitor how I am with Ruby.
Noa:	Sounds good—but I wonder if you have more thoughts about taking things forward. I'm really interested in what you said about "need to sort that out" in terms of feeling cross with Ruby and yourself. What thoughts did you have when you just said that?
Christiana:	Doing this exercise has made me realize that I need to revisit my contract with Ruby and I need to ask my boss to look at the contract that we have with this charity. I suspect that we are promising more than we can deliver and I worry about the ethics of this. She may need individual supervision rather than group.

Christiana felt confident about approaching her boss and also revisiting Ruby's contract so this was not something that she and Noa needed to focus on. He did, however, pick up on Christiana's concern that she was neglecting the other group members.

Noa:	You said that you felt "ashamed" about "neglecting" other group members. Is that something that we also need to look at?
Christiana:	I think that it is. I haven't brought that as a supervision question because I really only thought about it today.
Noa:	We are about halfway through our session. You had another item about preparing yourself for your re-accreditation. Do you think

	that we should aim to address both issues, or prioritize one over the other this session?
Christiana:	I think that the accreditation question could be tackled elsewhere—it is quite a concrete, practical question and I've a couple of colleagues going through the same process—I could talk with them. I'd rather use supervision time to look at my relationship with the group members. The question that I'd like to address is: What is going through their minds and how do they feel when I focus on Ruby?
Noa:	I don't know that we can mind-read what's going on for your group members—but we can certainly develop some hypotheses and think of ways of testing them. And we could also focus on what's going through your mind and how you feel and react.
Christiana:	That would work—looking at my part in this. Yes—could we start there?
Noa:	Certainly—let's set the scene. Can you recall a recent incident when you were aware that you felt that you were neglecting the other group members and talk me through it?

As Christina recounted a recent supervision session with her group, Noa asked her to pause and reflect on her feelings, thoughts, and actions and the reactions of various group members. By doing this, she developed a formulation of the supervision issue, which she drew out on Noa's whiteboard. She saw that, as she became stressed and very didactically focused on Ruby, Christiana was aware of others in the room being neglected yet she avoided eye contact lest they interrupt her. She became even more didactic in an attempt to finish Ruby's supervision so that she could give time to the others. At the end of the session she did not give group members time to offer authentic feedback and so Christiana never really learned how they felt about the session. Given this cycle, she would enter the next session with the same concerns and she would follow the same pattern.

In the Supervisor-of-Supervision's Mind

Noa knows that Christiana is an experienced therapist who knows how to use a formulation to test hypotheses and devise interventions. He decides he needs to do very little other than prompt her. This will improve her confidence that she can handle issues regarding the supervisory relationship.

Noa:	Look at your formulation. What is it telling you?
Christiana:	That I should give my supervisees time for feedback so that I can begin to understand how they feel and what they need?
Noa:	Okay—why don't you write that down and we can come back to it? Now what else is it telling you?
Christiana:	That I avoid eye contact and don't encourage collaborative supervision and this means that I probably lose their interest and I certainly don't tune into their reactions and needs . . . (Christiana compiles a list of conclusions and hypotheses.)
Noa:	Now look at your list—let's take the first hunch, that it would be a good idea to gather meaningful feedback at the end of the session. How will you ensure that you do that?

Using only minimal prompts, Noa was able to elicit from Christiana a formulation, hypotheses, and ways of testing them. When he asked her to look back on their work he asked what she had learned from supervision in terms of ways forward, the supervisory alliance, and herself. She reported that she was relieved to now have practical "plans" to improve her sessions but more than that, she had learned how to stand back and appreciate the supervisory interactions better and that her own thoughts, feelings, and behaviors played a part in this. She also realized that had she set aside the time, she might have been able to self-supervise on this issue. Noa then asked, "And knowing this, what will you do differently in the future?" Once again, this is an excellent analytic Socratic question in so many situations.

Managing a supervisory rupture

We have already described supervisory discomfort in Christiana—she felt uncomfortable because she perceived she was imbalanced in her attention to group needs. She was able to analyze what was happening and take steps to address her contributing behaviors. This was likely to remediate the situation.

There are instances, however, when the "rupture" in the supervisory alliance requires more active involvement of the supervisee. In 1990, Safran and Segal developed an approach for dealing with interpersonal ruptures within therapy sessions and their guidelines lend themselves well to managing interpersonal issues within supervision as well. It is particularly applicable to this chapter as their approach, like Socratic Dialogue, includes processes of hypothesizing, exploring, and eliciting issues and resolutions from the other person.

In brief, Safran and Segal recommend that we use ourselves as sources of information by reflecting on our sessions and looking out for interactions that jeopardize the working relationship. When we suspect that there is a rupture in our alliance we:

- **Observe** the hypothesized interpersonal pattern and collect enough data to assure us that it is not an aberrant issue: we should avoid jumping to conclusions too soon;
- **Formulate** the problem interaction between the involved individuals and make sure that if the rupture reflects our own issues, we take this elsewhere;
- **Own the "dilemma"** that we have in the session—state what *we* are struggling with;
- **Share** the dilemma: "I have difficulty …"; "I am concerned that I … "; "There is something that I need help in understanding…"; and
- **Problem solve** collaboratively.

The following supervision example illustrates this process. Conrad struggled supervising Bill because he initially thought that Bill was over-compliant within their supervision meetings, and rather discursive. He reflected on this and recognized that he quickly became disinterested in what Bill was telling him and then detached and found his attention wandering. Conrad realized his reactions might at least partially explain the limited development in Bill's therapy skills.

Conrad was not quite sure what to do about this so he took it to his supervisor-of-supervision who helped him "unpack" his own part in this problem's interaction. Conrad was able to develop some hypotheses about Bill's inner world.

Supervisor-of-Supervision (SoS): Can you set the scene for me? Take me to a moment in supervision when you are aware that you are detaching.

Conrad: Bill has only recently completed his CBT training although he has a long history of being a counsellor and he is older than I am. He is polite and almost, well, obsequious—I'm sorry to sound judgmental but that's how it feels—and his presentations will be rather textbook "blah blah" and he only ever presents patients that are doing well. I don't trust him—I think that he is not being honest about his practice and that could be dangerous. Again I'm sorry to sound so damning of him but as I think about it I realize how much he gets under my skin. I think that he's taking me for a ride.

SoS: It's good that you realized that he got under your skin—that's an excellent clue that something needs attending to. Does knowing that he has this effect help you move forward?

Conrad: Not really, no. If anything I just feel a bit more hopeless about my skills as a supervisor. Really—I should be able to rise above this!

SoS: Could we stay with that for a moment? You think that you should be able to rise above this supervisory rupture and you feel hopeless about your skills as a supervisor.

Conrad: I have been supervising for two years now. My workplace takes the "See one, do one, supervise one" approach and to be honest I've always felt untrained and therefore inadequate. When I see that I'm not supervising Bill well then it confirms that I'm a bit of a charlatan.

SoS: That's an interesting and relevant insight—it's come to mind as we've reflected on the session; does it come to mind in the session?

Conrad: I think that it does, and I think that I get annoyed with my organization and with Bill and then I feel bad about having those feelings and then I mentally and emotionally "check out." And now I feel annoyed with myself for not seeing this earlier and for being so petty.

SoS: It sounds as though Bill's use of supervision concerns you for ethical reasons, and because he is possibly not open, and that the dilemma you face with him reminds you that your organization has not given you the training and support that you need to deal with supervisory ruptures. In turn, this leaves you feeling annoyed with them and subsequently annoyed with yourself for not resolving the situation. Quite a heavy load—I'm thinking that it might be no wonder that you "check out."

Conrad: I suppose . . . (Silence.)

SoS: Does that summary give you any ideas about how to move forward?

Conrad: Well it reminds me that there are three players: my organization, Bill, and me. I could bring up the issue of lack of training at our departmental meeting. I'm sure others feel the same way. That should be easy enough. I need to tackle Bill—not sure how to confront him—and I need to sort out my own reactions. I need to be able to get some perspective in the session that allows me to stand back rather than "check out." I don't know who to focus on: me or Bill.

SoS: Or a third option might be to look at your interaction with Bill . . .

> ### In the Supervisor-of-Supervision's Mind
>
> Conrad's supervisor was pleased that Conrad was now viewing a "bigger picture" of the interaction with Bill and the influence of his own organization. There were several ways forward for the supervision. She considered continuing to explore the bigger picture and perhaps looking more closely at Bill's organizational and personal background, or at Conrad's personal situation, or hypothesizing about Bill's motivations and working out ways of testing these hypotheses. Conrad had already said that he was not a confident supervisor so she thought it best she not "play the expert" and make this decision because that would only reinforce his views that he was not fully competent. Instead, she decided to ask Conrad to make the decision about the way forward. He chose to try to formulate the interaction between himself and Bill.

SoS: Given what you have observed in yourself and given what you know about Bill, how would you now conceptualize the rupture between the two of you?

Conrad: When I'm not on the spot with Bill I can appreciate that he is still quite a novice CBT therapist. If I were to speculate I would say that he's not very confident but is perhaps embarrassed about bringing his difficulties to supervision. He copes by being a supervisor-pleaser (and avoids revealing his struggles and mistakes) which leaves me thinking that he is insincere. I get annoyed, I lose interest and detach. When I realize what I'm doing, I feel guilty and suddenly take charge of the supervision session and become didactic. He then closes down. This isn't helping him develop his confidence and skills and so we get caught in an unproductive cycle.

SoS: That sounds like a succinct formulation. How might you break the cycle?

Conrad: Well the least I can do is take charge of my own behavior. I'm going to keep a copy of the "rupture formulation" in my notes to help me stay empathic towards Bill and I am going to try to be open and curious as I know I can be with other supervisees.

SoS: Sounds good—but I'm going to play devil's advocate and ask what might sabotage your best intentions?

Conrad: Bill continuing to defend himself in the same old way. I don't feel comfortable confronting him with what I think is going on for him.

SoS: So ... ??

Conrad: I could ask him, couldn't I? I don't have to "confront"; I could simply offer him the opportunity to give me some real feedback on how we could improve our sessions.

SoS: Absolutely—but again I'm going to play devil's advocate and ask what might sabotage your best intentions?

Conrad: If he is so insecure and defensive that he continues to say all is well, that the supervision is great, and that he has no clinical difficulties?

SoS: Yes, based on your description, that might happen. So it might be good to have another option—one that would not risk putting him on the spot. An option that would allow him to be more open and not lose face.

In the Supervisor-of-Supervision's Mind

Conrad's supervisor thought it was now a good time to introduce the option of presenting the supervisor's dilemma (adapted from Safran and Segal, 1990) rather than a confrontation. Since Conrad indicated he has no familiarity with this strategy, she used a didactic approach, giving Conrad a verbal overview and also directing him to reading material. Together they shaped an authentic statement about Conrad's difficult position.

SoS: So, the idea is that you genuinely own the supervision dilemma that you face. No tricks, no veiled message of blame, just an honest statement of your difficulty as a supervisor. What might you say?

Conrad: I could start my saying that when he present things as being fine, I feel ... ?

SoS: Can I just pause there—how might he interpret "when you do x, I feel ..."?

Conrad: Yeah—I see. He could take that personally and get defensive.

SoS: Quite. So, in order to avoid that risk, could you phrase things so that your statement simply reflects your difficulties, your dilemma?

Conrad: This is harder than I thought.

The two of them then worked together on developing a statement that would be an honest appraisal of Conrad's position. They role-played and refined it until Conrad felt that it was acceptable and that he was confident that he could share it with Bill.

Conrad: Here goes—"Bill, there is an item that I'd like to put on our agenda. I am concerned about my supervisory practice and the quality of supervision that you get from me. You see, sometimes I 'lose the plot' in our sessions. Things seem to be going so smoothly, I find myself not being able to pin-point real 'issues' and then I find myself not focusing properly. Losing focus is bad enough—but I'm also worried that I'm missing important issues and this isn't good for you or your clients. I wondered if we could explore this, get your take on it. Would that be ok with you? Then perhaps we could see if we could work together to improve things."

SoS: And that feels true?

Conrad: Yes. Yes it does.

SoS: And you feel confident in saying it?

Conrad: Yes—because it is true and it's non-blaming. Actually I feel quite calm—more than that I feel quite excited to explore this with Bill. It will be good to work *with* him for once!

In the Supervisor-of-Supervision's Mind

Conrad had shown lots of good supervisory skill in sharing and formulating this problem and in developing a way forward that took into account the "bigger picture" and which was encouraging and empathic towards Bill. His supervisor-of-supervision did not want this to go unappreciated. One option would be to summarize all that Conrad had achieved; another way was to elicit this from Conrad.

SoS: You had concerns about your ability as a supervisor. Having done this work—what would you say you have learned about yourself in that role?

Conrad: I've still got a lot to learn! But I also feel that you helped me appreciate how much I already know—you nudged me to do the work. I think that I lost my way with Bill because of my own feelings of guilt and anger and if I can learn to catch that and formulate the relationship in the way that we did today I can probably self-supervise when I encounter ruptures and I can probably work through many of the issues I face.

Additional problems in supervision

There are many more types of problems you will encounter in supervision. We hope this chapter inspires you to use guided discovery methods to understand and work through the various roadblocks you encounter. For example, when a supervisee fails to carry out agreed-upon tasks you can use Socratic Dialogue to discover why. When members in a supervision group appear to act in concert to pull you into a didactic role, you can identify this process and use guided discovery methods such as role-play and behavioral experiments to give the group experiences using other options. Next, you can use Socratic Dialogue to prompt group members' reflection on the benefits of these more active learning methods compared to a didactic presentation.

When Other Methods Might Be More Appropriate

While this chapter illustrates the use of guided discovery methods in supervision, there is also a place for more didactic approaches when these are a better match for achieving supervision goals. For example, supervisors are encouraged to assign preparatory reading to supervisees on topics pertinent to their supervision learning goals. Watching demonstration videos or modeling particular therapy approaches during supervision can be efficient ways of kickstarting skills development. And when a supervisee has knowledge gaps that can more easily be addressed didactically than by using Socratic Dialogue it is certainly appropriate to use more didactic methods in supervision. Of course, if the majority of the time you assess didactic methods will be more efficient, you may have fallen into the first trap listed in this chapter: taking the expert position too much of the time and failing to get the balance right to enhance learning.

Therapists need to develop skills for self-development that they can practice throughout their careers. Therefore, it is a good idea to sometimes direct supervisees to use Internet searches to find evidence-based information regarding particular client issues or treatment protocols rather than providing this information didactically in supervision. The supervisee can be asked to provide a summary in the next supervision session of what they learned and how they determined whether an Internet source was authoritative. This is an important skill to develop because therapists will encounter many novel clinical dilemmas throughout their careers and need to have strategies for self-development.

At times, supervisees may show evidence they are wanting personal therapy from the supervisor. One sign of this is when they ask to dive deeper and deeper into their own thoughts and emotional reactions that arise when doing therapy or when they keep raising personal issues during supervision. Of course, Socratic Dialogue could take a supervisor down a route of exploring these deeper issues. However, in supervision, this is only appropriate if the focus of this discussion is on the impact of these reactions on therapy with their client. If it seems their interest (or need) is more personally focused, it is appropriate to explore the benefits of the supervisee seeking their own therapy for the issues of concern.

Summary

Supervisors can rely on guided discovery methods to enhance supervisee learning, understand and resolve common traps, and manage the supervisory relationship as well as ruptures that occur. Although there are many competing tasks to attend to in supervision, there are a number of ways supervisors can enlist the collaboration of supervisees to maximize the learning potential of these meetings. It is good supervisory practice to set up supervision agreements in advance, structure sessions, exchange regular feedback with supervisees, and provide guidance on the types of preparation you expect them to make prior to a supervision session. A worksheet was described that can help supervisees prepare specific supervision questions in advance and organize relevant information so they can get the help needed to answer it (Padesky, 1995).

Common supervision traps were highlighted along with guided discovery methods to help navigate them. In particular, supervisors can guard against being overly didactic by employing action methods in supervision rather than relying solely on case discussions and mini-lectures. Regular use of Socratic Dialogue guides supervisees to access and broaden their own knowledge base and reflective abilities. When doing this work, supervisors are advised to pay attention to therapist and supervisor assumptions, the bigger world and social context outside of therapy and supervision, and the supervisory relationship.

Although concern for the client is central to all clinical work, supervision is meant to build supervisees skills and reflective abilities. Therefore, the supervisor's job is not one of therapy-by-proxy or acting as an evaluator critic when the supervisee makes clinical errors. Instead, being a supervisor requires flexibility, attunement to both supervisee and client needs, and a keen interest in fostering learning, competence, and growth. Guided discovery methods paired with reflective supervisory practice are essential tools to help supervisors juggle the many requirements of competent supervision. Finally, as illustrated in a number of the clinical examples, supervisors can regularly benefit from self-supervision and/or consults with a supervisor-of-supervision.

Reader Learning Activities

- Do you recognize that you fall into any of the traps in the chapter? Draw out a conceptualization of your personal patterns and look for ways of breaking free of them using ideas from this chapter that you think will be helpful.

- Do you have a written supervision agreement that you individualize to guide your supervision? If not, write out some ideas and begin to create one.

- Do you regularly ask for feedback in every supervision session? How do you set the stage so supervisees are willing and able to give you honest and constructive feedback? Based on what you learned in this chapter, what can you do to improve this?

- Do you regularly give feedback to your supervisees about what they do well and where their strengths lie as well as giving them feedback on areas of practice that they need to improve? If not, why not? How can you ensure that you offer balanced feedback to all your supervisees? Write down ideas with a plan to implement them.

- Print out Table 11.1. Over the next month, check the boxes that apply for each supervision session. Analyze which activities you do regularly and which ones you tend to neglect.

- Based on what you learn in the previous step, make a plan to experiment using some of the other action supervision methods and foci that you have been neglecting. Get feedback from your supervisees. Do these approaches foster additional or different types of learning?

- Record a supervisory session in which you practice using Socratic enquiry in at least one juncture when you typically might begin didactic teaching. Listen to the recording and reflect on how you did, what you might have done better, and how you can carry your learning forward into future sessions.

- Schedule a self-supervision or supervision-of-supervision session at least once a month. For each of the next few upcoming sessions, focus on a relevant section of this chapter and see what ideas prove helpful as you reflect on what you did well and what you can improve.

References

Beidas, R. S., Edmunds, J. M., Marcus, S. C., & Kendall, P. C. (2012). Training and consultation to promote implementation of an empirically supported treatment: A randomized trial. *Psychiatric Services, 63*(7), 660–665. https://doi.org/10.1176/appi.ps.201100401

Bennett-Levy, J. (2006). Therapist skills: A cognitive model of their acquisition and refinement. *Behavioural and Cognitive Psychotherapy, 34*(1), 57–78. https://doi.org/10.1017/S1352465805002420

Bernard, J. M., & Goodyear, R. K. (1998). *Fundamentals of clinical supervision.* Boston: Allyn & Bacon.

Borton, T. (1970). *Reach, Touch and Teach.* New York: McGraw-Hill.

Dewy, J. (1960). *How we think: A restatement of the relation of reflective thinking to the educative process.* Lexington, MA: Heath. (Original work published 1933)

Gibbs, G. (1988). *Learning by doing: A guide to teaching and learning methods.* London: Further Education Unit.

Kolb, D.A. (1984). *Experiential learning.* Englewood Cliffs, NJ: Prentice-Hall.

Lewin, K. (*1946).* Action research and minority problems. *Journal of Social Issues, 2,* 34–46. https://doi.org/10.1111/j.1540-4560.1946.tb02295.x

Liness, S., Beale, S., Lee, S., Byrne, S., Hirsch, C. R., & Clark, D. M. (2019). The sustained effects of CBT training on therapist competence and patient outcomes. *Cognitive Therapy and Research, 43,* 631–641. https://doi.org/10.1007/s10608-018-9987-5

Milne, D. L. (2007). An empirical definition of clinical supervision. *British Journal of Clinical Psychology, 46,* 437–447. https://doi.org/10.1348/014466507X197415

Padesky, C. A. (1995). Supervision worksheet. Retrieved from https://www.padesky.com/clinical-corner/clinical-tools/

Padesky, C. A. (2019, July 18). Action, dialogue & discovery: Reflections on Socratic questioning 25 years later. Invited address presented at the Ninth World Congress of Behavioural and Cognitive Therapies, Berlin, Germany. Retrieved from https://www.padesky.com/clinical-corner/publications/

Padesky, C. A. (2020). *The clinician's guide to CBT using Mind Over Mood* (2nd ed.). New York: Guilford Press.

Rakovshik, S. G., McManus, F., Vazquez-Montes, M., Muse, K., & Ougrin, D. (2016). Is supervision necessary? Examining the effects of internet-based CBT training with and without supervision. *Journal of Consulting and Clinical Psychology, 84*(3), 191–199. https://doi.org/10.1037/ccp0000079

Roth, A. D., & Pilling, S. (2008). A competence framework for the supervision of psychological therapies. Retrieved from https://www.ucl.ac.uk/pals/research/clinical-educational-and-health-psychology/research-groups/competence-frameworks

Safran, J., & Segal, Z. (1990). *Interpersonal processes in CT.* New York: Basic Books.

Schön, D. A. (1984). *The reflective practitioner: How professionals think in action.* New York: Basic Books.

12
Dialogues for Discovery: What Next?

Christine A. Padesky

Chance favors only the prepared mind.

—Louis Pasteur

We began this book by inviting you to consider the many ways in which discovery can be transformational. We hope you experienced many new discoveries in the process of reading and that, in turn, these discoveries have begun to transform your therapy practice to make it even more effective and engaging for your clients.

All our chapter authors modeled collaboration and curiosity in therapist–client dialogues, both hallmarks of our approach. At the same time, each chapter author demonstrated their own "therapy voice" and taught us that there are many ways to personalize Socratic Dialogue to fit with therapist personality and specific client needs. You are encouraged to develop your own therapist voice as you practice Socratic Dialogue and other guided discovery methods in the years ahead.

This text offers a rare opportunity to see expert therapists' minds in action and to appreciate the subtleties and complexities of good practice. Although we, the editors, were experienced in the use of Socratic Dialogue, hearing the perspectives of other authors propelled us on our own journey of discovery. Collectively, the chapter authors illustrated a versatility, adaptability, and creativity that enabled us to go beyond our current thinking. They also gave us a better appreciation of the therapeutic scope of good Socratic Dialogue as well as its limitations within certain contexts.

You also had an opportunity to see what I call the "3 speeds of therapy" in action (see Chapter 2 and Box 12.1). Our expert authors, all steeped in theoretical awareness and clinical wisdom, reminded us that really good Socratic Dialogue is underpinned by a sound grounding in clinical knowledge (a part of the first speed: fastest) and, without this, our practice can suffer from

---

Box 12.1 3 Speeds of Therapy

1. Fastest speed: thoughts racing through the therapist's mind.
2. Slower speed: what we actually say aloud to the client.
3. Slowest speed: what we ask clients to do between sessions.

---

limited hypotheses to explore in our Socratic Dialogues. The authors used their clinical knowledge to also guide their choices of what is appropriate to discuss with clients and at what time (second speed: slower) in order to create the right foundation for fruitful discoveries. Over and over again we saw the sophisticated thought processes of these experienced therapists making key decisions about what to say, what not to say, when to say it, using client language, and gauging optimum timing. Engagement in a session can be lost if therapists make too many false moves during this speed. Finally, we saw speed awareness in action as client and therapist evolved between-session assignments to encourage ongoing guided discovery in order to achieve progress toward therapy goals (third speed: slowest).

Discoveries Found

This book encourages a deeper understanding of discovery processes in psychotherapy. Here we briefly consider the sudden gains in psychotherapy research and then we recap many of the ideas you learned throughout this book.

Research findings: Sudden gains in psychotherapy

If, as Pasteur asserts in the quote at the beginning of this chapter, "Chance favors only the prepared mind," it is interesting to speculate whether guided discovery methods, including use of Socratic Dialogue, function as one of the driving forces for sudden gains in psychotherapy (Tang & DeRubeis, 1999). Sudden gains refer to the times in the course of therapy in which significant symptom improvement is measured between sessions. Sudden gains are associated with more positive therapy outcomes as well as maintenance of improvement. Originally observed in depression treatment, sudden gains have since been reported for many additional diagnoses in over 100 published studies (Shalom & Aderka, 2020).

Regular use of Socratic Dialogue prepares both therapists and clients for the possibility of new and unexpected discoveries. With this preparation, when a significant discovery or relevant new idea occurs, therapists and clients are more likely to acknowledge it and make good use of it which could lead to sudden gains. This may be especially true when the 4-Stage Model of Socratic Dialogue detailed in Chapter 2 is being used. Significant new ideas are written down in a summary and the client is asked analytical and synthesizing questions to consider how to best apply those ideas in their life: "How can this idea help you going forward?" and "What could you do differently this week now that you know this?"

Research cited in Chapter 1 is consistent with this sudden gains hypothesis. Recall that therapist use of Socratic questioning predicts session-to-session symptom change in cognitive therapy for depression (Braun et al., 2015). Other research suggests that the relationship between Socratic questioning and symptom change is mediated by cognitive change (Vittorio et al., 2022). As demonstrated in all the chapters throughout this text, cognitive change is fostered when Socratic Dialogue is paired with behavioral experiments, imagery, role-plays, and other guided discovery methods.

4-Stage Model of Socratic Dialogue: Recap

For some, the 4-Stage Model of Socratic Dialogue I developed (Padesky, 1993; 2019; 2020a) and detailed in Chapter 2 was a new discovery. Your use of this approach going forward has the potential to transform the psychotherapy you offer. Keep this text nearby and refer to it as needed to troubleshoot any difficulties that arise. To track your progress, use the Socratic Dialogue Rating Scale (Padesky, 2020a) to measure your current skill, identify gaps, and follow your improvements over time.

4-Stage Model of Socratic Dialogue

1. Informational questions.
2. Empathic listening.
3. Summary of information gathered.
4. Analytical or synthesizing questions.

For those therapists already familiar with my four-stage approach, I hope the elaborations of it described throughout this book deepen and enrich your understanding and use of it. Use of the Socratic Dialogue Rating Scale to measure your fidelity to this model can bring into focus any areas that need improvement on your part.

Many of these chapters detail applications of 4-Stage Model of Socratic Dialogue that are novel to some readers.

1. **Mental imagery:** Many therapists avoid identification and exploration of mental imagery in therapy because they are uncertain what to do with it. Chapter 5 described a variety of applications of Socratic Dialogue with mental imagery. Some of these interventions involved dialogue alone to explore and evaluate imagery. Other interventions (e.g., use of a continuum, work with kinesthetic and hallucinatory imagery) embedded Socratic Dialogue into written exercises, role-plays, and behavioral experiments.
2. **Depression and anxiety disorders:** While many CBT therapists are familiar with use of Socratic Dialogue in therapy for depression (Chapter 3) and anxiety disorders (Chapter 4), non-CBT therapists may be less familiar with the role this method can play in therapy for these issues.
3. **Group therapy, children and adolescents, supervision:** Even therapists with extensive experience using Socratic Dialogue in therapy for depression and anxiety are often less familiar with how to apply it in group therapy (Chapter 10), with children and adolescents (Chapter 9), and within supervision (Chapter 11). Chapters on these topics illustrate the robust nature of Socratic Dialogue and its adaptive flexibility to various clinical populations and formats.
4. **Inflexible beliefs, impulsive and compulsive behaviors, serious adversity:** Therapists at all levels of experience who use Socratic Dialogue often struggle in its applications with inflexible beliefs (Chapter 6), impulsive and compulsive behaviors (Chapter 7) and clients experiencing serious adversities (Chapter 8). Those chapters lay out specific processes and methods for addressing the common traps encountered either when therapy intentionally addresses those issues or when those issues interfere with therapy progress.

Discoveries Still to Come

Research

It is unfortunate that Socratic Dialogue was neglected by empirical research until recently. We could be much further along in our understanding of its role in psychotherapy outcomes and processes for change. It is our hope that this text spurs future research on the impact of Socratic Dialogue in psychotherapy. Further, we encourage researchers to measure and evaluate skillful use of all four of its stages (informational questions, empathic listening, written summaries, and analytical/synthesizing questions) rather than simply measuring the number of questions used. Preliminary research suggests that quality as well as quantity of Socratic questions is important (Kazantzis et al., 2016). Therefore a more careful investigation of different elements of these procedures is warranted.

We are gratified that researchers have begun to pay attention to these therapy processes and look forward to their new discoveries. In Chapter 1, we suggested a number of research questions regarding Socratic Dialogue that could be fruitful to explore. Now that you have read this book, we propose additional questions that merit study:

Fertile Areas for Research on Socratic Dialogue

- Are there times or circumstances in therapy in which use of Socratic Dialogue shows clear advantages over other therapy approaches?
- Does the 4-Stage Model of Socratic Dialogue featured in this text make it easier for therapists to learn effective Socratic Dialogue processes?
- Does use of this model of Socratic Dialogue increase the likelihood of sudden gains in therapy?
- When is Socratic Dialogue a sufficient intervention in its own right and when is it best utilized as a means for debriefing behavioral experiments, role-play learning, imaginal exercises, and other types of interventions?
- Are there certain types of people or issues that respond better to use of guided discovery and others that respond better to other therapy approaches?
- Does adding an imagery component to guided discovery increase its impact?
- Are there benefits to ensuring that clients have learned the skill of Socratic self-enquiry?
- Does the use of Socratic Dialogue enhance learning for supervisees?

These and hundreds of other questions await your studies and answers. To help you investigate them we offer a clear (a) 4-Stage Model of Socratic Dialogue, (b) reference a measure of its effective use (Padesky, 2020a), and (c) provide numerous clinical and supervisory illustrations of how to pair it with other therapy methods in order to guide client and therapist discoveries.

Individual therapists

Some therapists, especially those who find the ideas in this book new and compelling, could be inclined to regret discoveries lost to former clients who might have benefited from greater use of these Socratic processes. Others who think they are clumsily using methods described in these chapters might worry that their clients are not making as many discoveries as they could. For these readers we offer encouragement. The editors of this text have engaged in these processes for more than half a century in combined years and we still learned many new ideas from chapter authors and also from our own renewed thinking about the many topics discussed here. Potential discoveries are still there to be found. And we believe therapists who follow the guidance offered in these pages can learn how to help their clients make those discoveries more quickly.

Keep in mind that not all discoveries are equal. Therapists are advised to carefully consider what discoveries are likely to be most meaningful for your clients and what guided discovery methods offer the clearest path to help uncover them. We believe evidence-based models for understanding human strengths and distress provide good roadmaps for identifying lynchpin themes to explore with clients. For example, we know that people who struggle with anxiety (Chapter 4) are likely to benefit from learning to investigate their overestimations of danger as well as their underestimations of their own internal coping abilities and external help resources. We know that people with impulsive behaviors benefit from identifying the personal meanings of these behaviors, recognizing the signs of their fluctuating motivations to change, and consideration of safer, substitute behaviors (Chapter 6). Thus, we aren't looking for just any discoveries; we are searching for the most relevant and helpful discoveries for a particular individual. Each of this book's editors has written other texts describing evidence-based models for a variety of clinical issues as well as detailed guidance on how to implement them using guided discovery (Kennerley, 2021; Padesky, 2020b).

We encourage you to consider your own optimal speeds for putting what you have learned into practice. Reading this book is most likely the fastest speed of your learning. In the section "Developing your 'dialogues for dis-covery' skills," we provide some reflective practice exercises for you to do at a slower speed to help you plan ways to incorporate the ideas you found most meaningful into your clinical practice. You can anticipate that the slowest speed will be your deliberate clinical practice of Socratic Dialogue and other guided discovery methods. Plan to practice these methods and review your progress over many months to give yourself the best chance of developing your own expertise in their application.

Developing your "dialogues for discovery" skills

Each chapter of this book ended with a series of "Reader Learning Activities." If you chose to do some of these activities after reading a chapter, it is highly likely you made new discoveries about yourself as a therapist, how to practice more effective psychotherapy, and ways to manage the traps addressed in that chapter. If you did not do any of these learning activities, we highly recom-mend you make a plan to do so in the near future for whichever chapters have most relevance for your current clinical work. Just as clients who complete learning assignments have better psychotherapy outcomes (Kazantzis et al., 2016), therapists who put new learning into practice and reflect on its im-pact are more likely to develop improvement in their psychotherapy practice (Davis et al., 2015).

Bennett-Levy (2006) distinguished three systems of learning in therapist skill development to account for the differential rate of development of var-ious skills: declarative, procedural, and reflective. The first system, *declarative knowledge*, can be thought of as "book knowledge." After reading this book, you have acquired declarative knowledge about guided discovery, the four stages of Socratic Dialogue, and many other topics. Because of this declarative knowledge you can describe what you learned to other therapists.

The second system in Bennett-Levy's model is *procedural knowledge*, which means development of the skills to apply what you have learned with clients. Reading alone will not build procedural knowledge. The Reader Learning Activities after each chapter are designed to provide initial structured practice and application of the ideas taught. It is often helpful to practice one area of learning with multiple clients rather than trying to expand your procedural knowledge across many skills with a wide variety of clients. For example, ther-apists new to ideas addressed in this book might focus on using the 4-Stage Model of Socratic Dialogue on a regular basis with a certain type of client (focusing on Chapter 2 and the most relevant other chapter for that type of client). Or they might begin by using Socratic Dialogue to debrief between session client learning activities (aka homework) as described in Chapters 1 and 2. Practice of this one clinical application with a number of clients can speed your development of your procedural skill in the use of Socratic Dialogue. And if you lack confidence about applying Socratic Dialogue at all, remember that rehearsing in imagination can lay the foundation for real-life practice, as can role-play with a colleague or supervisor.

It can take considerable practice to develop flexible and skillful application of the ideas taught in this book. This is one of the reasons we emphasized common traps in each chapter that can interfere with carrying out the strategies taught (for a summary, see the "Traps Guide" in the Appendix on pp. 505–507). Hopefully, many of the difficulties you encounter in developing your procedural skills will be addressed in chapter discussions for how to manage these traps. If we have done our job well, this book will save you time in learning to overcome them.

The other practice that will help you become proficient more quickly is to employ Bennett-Levy's third system of learning, *reflective practice*. Reflective practice is considered essential to therapist skill development because it requires therapists to reflect on and build their declarative knowledge and procedural skills once these have begun to develop. "The reflective system is typically called into action when a problem arises in clinical practice (e.g. mismatch between expectations and outcome). Following reflection on the problem, the reflective system may be used to refine declarative knowledge and procedural skills" (Bennett-Levy et al., 2009, 573). For more experienced therapists, these reflections can lead to more refined "when this happens, do this" rules (Bennett-Levy, 2006). Solutions proposed for traps addressed throughout this book are the result of each chapter authors' reflective practice in their areas of expertise. In addition, many of the principles that chapter authors have gleaned from their own reflective practice are captured in the "Keep in Mind" boxes that pepper each chapter.

Reflective practice does not, and should not, simply arise from difficulties in practice. Therapists are encouraged to regularly do deliberate reflective practice. Bennett-Levy and Padesky (2014) found that therapists who attended a 2-day workshop were more likely to practice new skills and think about workshop learning on a regular basis in relation to their therapy if they filled out "reflection worksheets" in the weeks following the workshop. These worksheets were personalized in that the initial ones (completed during the workshop and one week later) asked therapists to identify the main things they had learned from the workshop that were pertinent to their own clinical practice and how they planned to practice those skills during the upcoming month. Subsequent worksheets (4 and 8 weeks post-workshop) asked therapists to reflect on what workshop learning they had practiced or implemented, barriers to doing so, and changes they might make to more fully implement their learning. Those therapists who completed these reflection sheets reported a greater awareness and practice of skills learned than a control group who were not given reflection worksheets or instructions to reflect on their learning post-workshop.

In a similar way, we recommend you begin a reflective practice right now. The section "Reflective Practice Worksheets" introduces three Reflective Practice Worksheets to help you focus more directly on how you can carry your personal learning forward to continue your *Dialogues for Discovery* progress. These worksheets are printed in the Appendix. Fillable PDF versions can be accessed by searching for this book's title on the Oxford Academic platform at academic.oup.com.

Reflective Practice Worksheets

Reflective Practice Worksheet 1 is the first worksheet we recommend you complete (see Appendix, p. 502). It will take about 15 minutes. Do it now if you can. Otherwise, schedule a time to do it soon so the ideas in this book are still fresh in your mind. It asks you to list the key ideas you learned in this book that could benefit your therapy practice and reflect on how greater proficiency in these ideas could help you, your clients, and your supervisees. Then you are asked to choose one area of learning to practice over the upcoming month. It asks you to set a goal and we recommend this goal be specific and achievable. For example, rather than "Get better using Socratic Dialogue" your goal could be: "use all four stages of Socratic Dialogue with at least three clients per week" or "Be sure to make a written summary with at least three clients and ask them the analytical and synthesizing questions listed in Chapter 2." We recommend scheduling a weekly review of your plan. Recording one or more of your sessions during the upcoming month will allow you to reflect on your actual performance rather than your retrospective recall.

Reflective Practice Worksheet 2 on page 503 should be filled out one month from now. Set aside a 30- to 60-minute reflection session to review your progress. A series of questions on this second worksheet asks you to consider what you have done well, what improvements you can make, and to make a plan for the coming month to continue progress and overcome any roadblocks.

Reflective Practice Worksheet 3 on page 504 can be filled out a month after you complete the second worksheet and every month thereafter until you achieve all your learning goals. Set aside 20–60 minutes each month to review your progress and reflect what else you can do to consolidate and expand your skills using Socratic Dialogue and other forms of guided discovery. This worksheet also prompts you to consider whether there are other resources you could use to support your progress such as consultation, supervision, video or audio demonstrations, peer role-plays, and review of chapters or articles. Schedule when to use these and other resources.

Tips for successful reflective practice
Socratic Dialogue with oneself can guide your reflective practice. Notice that the first question or two on each Reflective Practice Worksheet (in the Appendix) are broad informational questions (Stage 1, Socratic Dialogue). As you frame your responses to these questions, try to listen to your responses with empathy instead of self-criticism or judgment (Stage 2, Socratic Dialogue). Perfectionism kills a learning spirit. Therefore, it is really important to recognize personal progress or persistent attempts as steps in the right direction. Make a list to summarize what you have done better this month (Stage 3, Socratic Dialogue). This could include a particular portion of a session with one client, recognizing traps when you fall into them, or remembering to use certain methods more often. Subsequent questions on the Reflective Practice Worksheets are analytical or synthesizing questions (Stage 4, Socratic Dialogue). Refer to your written summary to answer these. In thinking about your answers, you might recall additional things you did well or struggled with during the month. Add these recollections to your written summary.

Add action steps
To make sure your reflection is not simply an intellectual exercise, add in some action steps:

1. Use imaginal rehearsal—to plan how you would like to implement a skill you are working on with one or more clients or supervisees in the coming weeks.
2. Role-play the skill—with a trusted colleague or supervisor. Practice can help build your confidence.
3. Select some sessions to record—to help you recall pivotal moments when you practiced new skills.
4. Be empathic with yourself and use positive self-encouragement when you review your sessions or listen to/watch recordings of them.

5. Focus first on identifying 3–4 things you are doing well in a portion of a session—attentional focus on positives can help counter the common human tendency to emphasize flaws over improvement in one's performance.
6. Identify any difficulties or errors you detect.
7. Make a constructive action plan for how to ameliorate these issues in future sessions.
8. Practice your action plan in imagery or via role-play—to increase the likelihood you will remember it and attempt to implement it going forward.

Future of Dialogues for Discovery in Psychotherapy

The future of "Dialogues for Discovery" in psychotherapy is in your hands. Throughout this book, we presented our case for the benefits of incorporating more guided discovery into therapy and supervisory practice and conducting more research on the impact of Socratic Dialogue. We hope you are inspired to try out these ideas and conduct your own research, whether single case studies or larger research designs.

CLINICIANS/SUPERVISORS: If you are primarily a clinician or if you are also a supervisor, we hope you use the Reflective Practice Worksheets in the months ahead to improve your skills in implementing these processes. Be curious, collaborative, and keep your mind open to new discoveries. Employ guided discovery with yourself as well as your clients.

STUDENTS/RESEARCHERS: If you are a student or researcher, consider all the fertile areas for research still waiting your exploration. Most of the important questions regarding guided discovery in general and the 4-Stage Model of Socratic Dialogue illustrated in this text are still unanswered. You can be a pioneer in this field.

Summary

If you read this entire book or even a number of its chapters, you have now completed quite a journey. In Chapter 1 we described the origins and history of use of Socratic questioning and the evolution of Socratic Dialogues and the 4-Stage Model of Socratic Dialogue in psychotherapy. We addressed the questions: "What" "Why" and "When" do we use Socratic Dialogue and other guided discovery methods in psychotherapy. Subsequent chapters answered a series of "How" questions. How are these methods used and adapted for particular issues or clinical populations? How can Socratic Dialogue help us navigate common traps that block therapy progress? Finally, by completing Reader Learning Activities, you practiced implementing what you learned in order to build and broaden your procedural learning skills.

This chapter encouraged you to personalize the answers to the questions: "What," "Why," "When," and "How." You were asked to reflect on what you have learned and throughout this chapter, you were encouraged to ask yourself:

- What methods discussed in this book do I want to incorporate into my clinical or supervisory practice and/or use as a springboard for new research?
- Why do I think these avenues of practical application will be helpful? Why will this research make a difference?
- When do I plan to try these approaches? With what clients or issues?
- How will I carry out my plan? What methods will I use? How will I guide my own discovery as I do so?

As illustrated throughout this book, we advocate active learning methods that require doing and not just "reading, thinking, or talking about something." Active learning methods can lead to deeper understanding, be more memorable, and make greater contributions to expertise in the long run. Our hope is that you actively practice and investigate the methods taught and illustrated here. It is through this active engagement that you make personal discoveries. By doing so, you participate in moving forward the collective edge of our understanding of the roles that "Dialogues for Discovery" and action-based guided discovery play in the effective practice of psychotherapy.

References

Bennett-Levy, J. (2006). Therapist skills: A cognitive model of their acquisition and refinement. *Behavioural and Cognitive Psychotherapy*, 34(1), 57–78. https://doi.org/10.1017/S1352465805002420

Bennett-Levy, J., McManus, F., Westling, B. E., & Fennell, M. (2009). Acquiring and refining CBT skills and competencies: Which training methods are perceived to be most effective? *Behavioural and Cognitive Psychotherapy*, 37, 571–583. https://doi.org/10.1017/S1352465809990270

Bennett-Levy & Padesky, C. (2014). Use it or lose it: Post-workshop reflection enhances learning and utilization of CBT skills. *Cognitive and Behavioral Practice*, 21(1), 12–19. https://dx.doi.org/10.1016/j.cbpra.2013.05.001

Braun, J. D., Strunk, D. R., Sasso, K. E., & Cooper, A. A. (2015). Therapist use of Socratic questioning predicts session-to-session symptom change in cognitive therapy for depression. *Behaviour Research and Therapy, 70*(7), 32–37. https://doi.org/10.1016/j.brat.2015.05.004

Davis, M. L., Thwaites, R., Freeston, M. H., & Bennett-Levy, J. (2015). A measurable impact of a self-practice/self-reflection programme on the therapeutic skills of experienced cognitive-behavioural therapists. *Clinical Psychology & Psychotherapy, 22*(2), 176–184. https://doi.org/10.1002/cpp.1884

Kazantzis, N., Whittington, C., Zelencich, L., Kyrios, M., Norton, P. J., & Hofmann, S. G. (2016). Quantity and quality of homework compliance: A meta-analysis of relations with outcome in cognitive behavior therapy. *Behaviour Therapy, 47*(5), 755–772. https://doi.org/10.1016/j.beth.2016.05.002

Kennerley, H. (2021). *The ABC of CBT*. London: Sage Publications.

Padesky, C. A. (1993, September 24). *Socratic questioning: Changing minds or guiding discovery?* Invited address delivered at the European Congress of Behavioural and Cognitive Therapies, London. Retrieved from https://www.padesky.com/clinical-corner/publications/

Padesky, C. A. (2019, July 18). *Action, dialogue & discovery: Reflections on Socratic Questioning 25 years later*. Invited address presented at the Ninth World Congress of Behavioural and Cognitive Therapies, Berlin, Germany. Retrieved from https://www.padesky.com/clinical-corner/publications/

Padesky, C. A. (2020a). *Socratic Dialogue Rating Scale and Manual*. https://www.padesky.com/clinical-corner/clinical-tools/

Padesky, C. A. (2020b). *The Clinician's Guide to CBT Using Mind Over Mood* (2nd ed.). New York: Guilford Press.

Shalom, J. G., & Aderka, I. M. (2020). A meta-analysis of sudden gains in psychotherapy: Outcome and moderators, *Clinical Psychology Review, 76*, 101827. https://doi.org/10.1016/j.cpr.2020.101827

Tang, T. Z., & DeRubeis, R. J. (1999). Sudden gains and critical sessions in cognitive-behavioral therapy for depression, *Journal of Consulting and Clinical Psychology, 67*(6), 894–904. https://doi.org/10.1037/0022-006X.67.6.894

Vittorio, L. N., Murphy, S. T., Braun, J. D., & Strunk, D. R. (2022). Using Socratic questioning to promote cognitive change and achieve depressive symptom reduction: Evidence of cognitive change as a mediator. *Behaviour Research and Therapy, 150*, 104035. https://doi.org/10.1016/j.brat.2022.104035

APPENDICES

REFLECTIVE PRACTICE WORKSHEET 1
Use after reading *Dialogues for Discovery*
(Padesky & Kennerley, 2023)
Estimated time: 15 minutes

1. List the key ideas from this book that you think could benefit your therapy practice.

2. How would greater proficiency in these areas help: You? Your clients? Your supervisees?

3. Make a plan to practice one of these over the upcoming month.
   My goal is to (make it specific and achievable):

   What will you do differently?

   More often?

   Less often?

4. Set a reminder in your schedule to review this plan on a weekly basis.

5. Consider recording one or more therapy and / or supervision sessions so that you can reflect on your actual performance and you are not limited to retrospective recall.

Adapted with permission from Bennett-Levy, J., & Padesky, C. (2014). Use it or lose it: Post-workshop reflection enhances learning and utilization of CBT skills, *Cognitive and Behavioral Practice, 21*(1), 12-19.

REFLECTIVE PRACTICE WORKSHEET 2
Use one month after Reflective Practice Worksheet 1
Estimated time: 30-60 minutes

Review recordings; look over your notes and the written plan you filled out last month on Reflective Practice Worksheet 1. Then ask yourself the following questions and write some notes in response to each for your future review.

1. What learning or skills from *Dialogues for Discovery* (Padesky & Kennerley, 2023) have I practiced or implemented this month to make progress toward my goals?

2. What has gone well? What have I done well?

3. What improvements can I make? What do I need to do to accomplish this?

4. What practices that I planned have I been unable to implement?

5. What has stopped me from doing this? What are the roadblocks?

6. Is there a way I could practice this in the next month? If so, how?

Adapted with permission from Bennett-Levy, J., & Padesky, C. (2014). Use it or lose it: Post-workshop reflection enhances learning and utilization of CBT skills, *Cognitive and Behavioral Practice, 21*(1), 12-19.

REFLECTIVE PRACTICE WORKSHEET 3
Use monthly until goals achieved
Estimated time: 20-60 minutes

Schedule a time for reflection each month until you achieve your goals. In each reflection session, review your notes from your previous reflections.

1. What learning or skills from *Dialogues for Discovery* (Padesky & Kennerley, 2023) have I practiced or implemented this month to make progress toward my goals?

2. What am I doing more of or less of?

3. How can I improve my skills in these areas in the next month?

4. What other changes do I want to make? If I've accomplished my current goal, I'll set a new one.

5. What do I need to do to achieve these changes / new goals?

6. Is there a way I could practice this in the next month? If so, how?

7. What learning from the book have I been unable to practice or implement? What has stopped me from doing this?

8. Are their additional resources I could use to promote my progress? If so, schedule it (consultation, supervision, video or audio demonstrations, peer role-plays, review of chapters/articles).

Adapted with permission from Bennett-Levy, J., & Padesky, C. (2014). Use it or lose it: Post-workshop reflection enhances learning and utilization of CBT skills, *Cognitive and Behavioral Practice, 21*(1), 12-19.

Traps Guide

Index

For the benefit of digital users, indexed terms that span two pages (e.g., 52–53) may, on occasion, appear on only one of those pages.

Tables, figures, and boxes are indicated by an italic *t*, *f*, and *b* following the page/paragraph number.